# food

# juice

# health

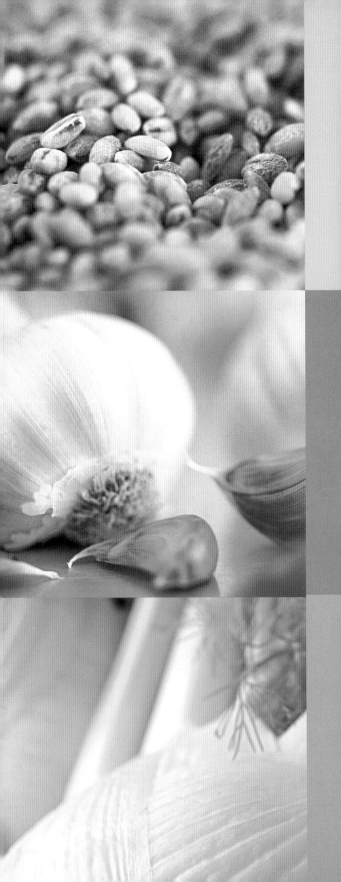
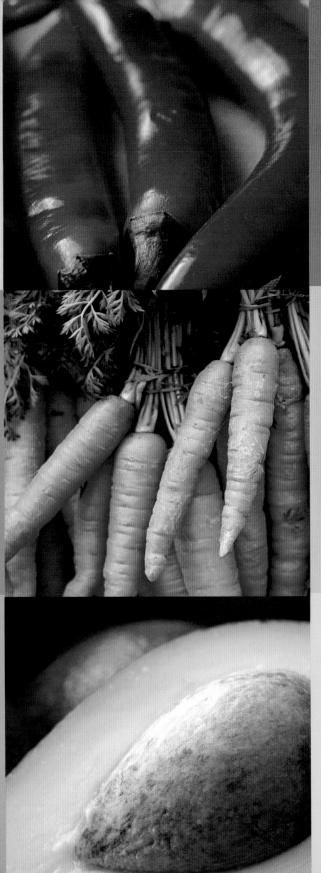

# food

# juice

# health

## michael van straten

MITCHELL BEAZLEY

**Super Food, Super Juice, Super Health**
by Michael van Straten

The recipes in this book are taken from
the following Michael van Straten titles:
*Super Hot Drinks*, *Super Cool Drinks*, *Super Juice*, *Super
Duper Juice*, *Super Soups*, *Super Duper Soups*, *Super Herbs*,
*Super Salads* and *Organic Super Foods*.

First published in Great Britain in 2009
by Mitchell Beazley, an imprint of
Octopus Publishing Group Ltd,
2–4 Heron Quays, London E14 4JP
An Hachette Livre UK Company
www.hachettelivre.co.uk

ISBN: 978 1 84533 486 4

A CIP record for this book is available from the
British Library.

Set in Kievit

Colour reproduction by Fine Arts in Hong Kong
Printed and bound by Toppan Printing Company Ltd
in China

**Dedication**
This book is the result of many years of fascinating
conversations with my wonderful patients and includes
recipes from Italians, Greeks, Chinese, French, Spanish,
Brazilians, Egyptians, English and many others. But all
the recipes have one thing in common; these are family
foods handed down from generation to generation.
Our great grannies did not need charts, tables and
nutritionists to tell them how to feed their children.
They simply cooked with love and tradition; I thank
them all for sharing their knowledge.

Of course, I also have to thank my wife Sally – with her
imaginative Irish creativity – for hours of trying, testing
and tasting.

Now that we live on the River Loir in France, we have a
whole new army of traditional cooks on our doorstep,
and their influence has added a certain *je ne sais quoi*
to the later recipes.

**Commissioning Editor** Rebecca Spry
**Art Director** Tim Foster
**Senior Editor** Leanne Bryan
**Copy Editor** Jo Richardson
**Proofreader** sandseditorial.co.uk
**Indexer** Helen Snaith
**Executive Art Editors** Pene Parker and
  Yasia Williams-Leedham
**Designer** Jon Morgan
**Photography** Peter Cassidy, Nicki Dowey,
  Francesca Yorke, Simon Walton
**Production Manager** Peter Hunt

# contents

# introduction

'Superfoods' is the new buzz word, but what does it mean? Can fruits and vegetables slow down ageing, lower blood pressure or even prevent some forms of cancer? As a complementary health practitioner; broadcaster, author and journalist concerned with natural health, food and healing; and having been an organic gardener since meeting Rachel Carson, author of *Silent Spring*, way back in the 1960s; I have become totally convinced that there are superfoods with the power to enhance and extend life.

With my colleague Barbara Griggs, I coined the term 'superfoods' back in 1990. Personally, I don't grow much in my organic garden that I can't eat, because fresh produce has the most nutrients and the best flavour. If it's organic, you get even more nutrients and avoid environmental- and health-damaging chemicals.

A superfood must have substantial levels of one or more essential vitamins and minerals, and/or be a rich source of the unique 'phytochemicals' – powerful natural substances that protect the body's cells from damage. Surprisingly, the two don't always go together.

Celery, for example, is pretty useless nutritionally: 95 per cent water and only 7 energy-giving calories in 100g (3½oz) – you burn more chewing it. But it has been valued as a medicinal vegetable since ancient Rome. The phytochemicals it contains provide flavour and calming properties. As a natural diuretic, it gets rid of surplus fluid, so it's perfect for women with monthly bouts of puffy hands, feet or breasts.

Superfoods affect whole populations and explain why southern European men have a 50 per cent lower risk of prostate cancer than the British – Spaniards, for example, eat more than twice as much fruit and vegetables as the average Brit. Their superfood diet also means fewer strokes, and less heart disease, bowel cancer and other ills.

As a practising naturopath for more than 40 years, I base most of my advice on the links between food and health. However, I'm not a member of the 'food police', and I certainly don't believe that one bar of chocolate, a cup of coffee, a jam doughnut or a dollop of cream on your strawberries will put your health at risk for the next 20 years.

I am deeply concerned about the many people I see – mostly women – who have become so obsessed with food that they worry about every forkful that goes into their mouth. Of course, it's great to eat organic food if you can, and it's important to consume less animal fat, salt and sugar, and more fruit, vegetables and wholegrain cereals, but healthy eating should never become a quest for the Holy Grail. The world has suddenly become inhabited by hordes of people convinced, only on the basis of extremely bogus and questionable tests, that they're allergic to dairy products, wheat, coffee, tea and a hundred other staple foods.

These poor obsessives come to your house for dinner with a brown paper bag containing a handful of sprouted mung beans, three grated carrots and a sprinkle of sesame seeds. They've suddenly become macrobiotic believers, vegans, fruitarians or, God preserve us, breatharians, who believe they can survive on fresh air.

For optimum energy, resistance to disease, protection of the heart, slower ageing and an extension of the vital faculties – such as reproduction, hearing, sight, memory, reasoning and the ability to revel in the joy of living – we all benefit from superfoods.

If you think superfoods are all the exotic, expensive things that ordinary people can't afford, you couldn't be more wrong. Here are 10 everyday foods and the reasons why they're super. You'll find them all spread around the recipes in the rest of the book.

**apples** Pectin and vitamin C reduce cholesterol; pectin protects against pollution by eliminating heavy metals; malic and tartaric acids relieve indigestion and break down fats; traditional with cheese, duck and goose; two a day help arthritis, rheumatism and gout; grated apple stops diarrhoea.

**avocados** Potassium relieves fatigue, depression and poor digestion; vitamins A, B, C and E make it an anti-cancer food; healthy monounsaturated oil; stimulates production of collagen; good for circulation, skin and fertility. Ignore all rumours that this nutritional powerhouse is fattening.

**bananas** Perfect fast food with potassium, zinc, iron, folic acid, calcium, vitamin B6 and fibre. Good for digestion and menstrual difficulties; essential for athletes; perfect food for old and young. With apples, rice and dry toast, it makes up the BRAT diet, the ideal treatment for sickness and diarrhoea.

**cabbage** Iron, chlorophyll, vitamin C, sulphur compounds and healing mucilaginous substances. Powerfully anti-cancer; vital for anaemia, stomach inflammation and ulcers; protective against stress, infection and heart disease. Best eaten slightly steamed.

**carrots** Super-rich in betacarotene – one supplies enough for a day; anti-cancer, especially of the bowel; puréed for infant diarrhoea; juiced for liver problems; also contains vitamins C and E, which ease circulatory disease, chest infections and skin and eye problems. Eat lightly cooked carrots two or three times a week.

**garlic** The king of healing plants. Modern science proves it reduces cholesterol, lowers blood pressure, stops blood from clotting and improves the circulation. It's antibacterial, antifungal, antiviral, anti-cancer and good for relieving chest infections and stomach bugs, too. Eat at least a clove each day.

**oats** Protein, polyunsaturated fats, B vitamins, calcium, potassium, magnesium, silicon and vitamin E. They're easily digested and soothing to the digestive tract. Oats help depression and reduce cholesterol – a daily bowl can lower levels by 20 per cent. They also help regulate sugar metabolism, so they're good for diabetics. They are the best and cheapest of all breakfast cereals.

**oily fish** The only source of all the essential fatty acids. These are vital during pregnancy and breastfeeding for the proper development of the brain in babies and infants. In children and adults, oily fish maintain brain function and can help in the treatment of dyslexia and attention deficit hyperactivity disorder (ADHD). They're also the most important source of vitamin D, essential for strong bones and many hormone functions. Great for the relief of arthritis.

**onions** They protect the circulatory system and are a powerful antibiotic. Good for chest, stomach and urinary infections, and their diuretic activity helps with arthritis, rheumatism and gout. A recent study in Newcastle gave a traditional fry-up breakfast to volunteers, but half of them got fried onions, too; the onion eaters' blood was much less likely to clot than the others; research in the USA shows that half a raw onion a day raises the amount of good fats in the blood by 30 per cent.

**potatoes** Even when boiled or baked, this wonderful vegetable is a source of fibre, B vitamins, minerals and enough vitamin C to keep scurvy at bay. They are best baked in their skins, which is where lots of nutrients, especially potassium and fibre, are. At less than a calorie per gram, cheap and very filling, potatoes are good news for slimmers; all the bad things you read about them are wrong, unless you only want to eat chips.

# 10 facts about superfoods

1 Two apples a day can reduce cholesterol by 10 per cent.

2 Eating 400g (14oz) of fruits, vegetables and salads daily halves your risk of heart and circulatory disease.

3 Eating one portion of any of the cabbage family daily significantly reduces the risk of lung, colon and breast cancer.

4 Two portions a week of spinach, sorrel or beetroot tops reduces the risk of adult macular degeneration (AMD) by 50 per cent.

5 The equivalent of six ripe tomatoes daily – whole fruit, purée, sauce, soup, ketchup, sun-dried or juice – halves the risk of prostate cancer in men and helps prevent blood clots and high blood pressure.

6 One clove of garlic daily reduces cholesterol and makes the blood less sticky, preventing blood clots.

7 Southern Europeans get 10 per cent of their energy from the protective fruit and veg superfoods. This is more than twice the percentage of energy that UK residents get from the same produce (4½ per cent)

8 The Mediterranean diet, with its high level of superfoods, means less disease and longer life expectancy – for example, Greeks have the lowest incidence of bowel cancer in the whole of Europe.

9 Vitamin pills are not a substitute for superfoods. All the studies using pills to replicate the benefits of the Mediterranean diet for heart disease have failed.

10 Superfoods explain 'the French Paradox' – cheese, pâté, sausage, wine and cigarettes but massive intakes of superfoods means 60 per cent less risk of premature death from heart disease than the UK.

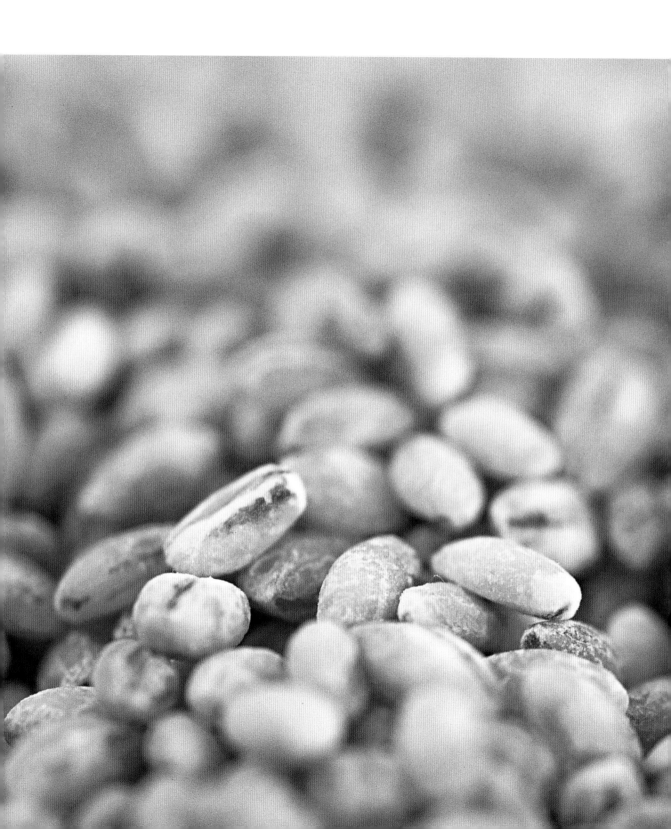

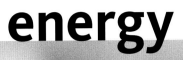

# energy

**E**verybody feels lethargic at times. Too many late nights, a gruelling day at the office, family problems, travel frazzle or just the need for a break... all of these can wear us down. Yet victims of chronic fatigue often have no idea why they feel listless, never have any surplus energy, even wake up tired. If that sounds familiar, then here are some of the answers.

Exhaustion is often the result of a combination of psychological and physical causes. Common psychological causes are stress, anxiety, depression, dissatisfaction, relationship problems, anger, frustration and boredom. Physically, specific illnesses can cause chronic fatigue. Anaemia is a common and often unrecognized cause, particularly among menstruating women and vegetarians who stop eating meat and don't substitute it with other good sources of iron. Thyroid problems, hormone problems and heart disease are yet more common causes of a constant lack of energy, as is poor posture, which is often the result of badly designed seating. Other causes are chronic pain, such as backache, arthritis, rheumatism, tension, headaches and migraines. Viral infections and their after-effects, surgery and all major illnesses often result in fatigue. Post-viral fatigue syndrome, ME (myalgic encephalomyelitis), is now recognized as a genuine physical problem.

Allergy, or sensitivity, to foods and environmental pollutants is another major cause of fatigue. According to Dr Stephen Davies, chairman of the British Society of Nutritional Medicine, 'waking tired' is one of the classic symptoms of food or chemical sensitivity. If you suspect this could apply to you, see a consultant in allergy medicine, as well as trying out the recipes in this chapter.

People who suffer from tiredness often lack the energy for exercise, without which the body's absorption of iron and other vital minerals is poor. They become trapped in a vicious circle of dwindling energy, which leads to less exercise, resulting in even less energy.

## Help yourself

Millions of people the world over wake up every morning wondering how they'll get through the day ahead. Once a thorough check with your doctor has established that there is no serious underlying illness to cause your lack of energy, the cure is often to be found in your own hands, and self-help can be remarkably successful. All the energy you need comes from what you eat and drink. But choosing the right food is crucial to maintaining health and vitality. Fatigue is exacerbated by a poor diet. When you're tired and lethargic generally, shopping, cooking and planning meals become daunting chores. Snack meals of bread and cheese, sandwiches and tea and biscuits that replace healthy eating will further deplete nutritional reserves and start another downward spiral.

In this chapter you will find simple but energizing recipes that use the best of the high-octane superfoods. Beans and barley in soups; potatoes, rice, eggs and blood-nourishing beetroot; fish, beef and lamb for strength-building protein; herbs, spices and special juices... each recipe is designed to provide the winning combination of instant and long-term energy release to lift you out of the trough of fatigue and keep you going at peak performance levels. All those who feel they haven't got the energy to cope with life will benefit from the recipes in the following pages.

# energy checklist

- Try to refuse all refined carbohydrates. White sugar, white flour and processed foods made with them – cakes, biscuits, packet puddings etc. – are a heavy tax on your digestion, using up energy you can ill afford to spare. These are high-glycaemic-index (GI) foods, which may give you an instant lift but will leave you with a terrible blood-sugar deficit soon afterwards. They also trigger the release of enormous quantities of insulin, and excessive consumption is the first step on the road to type 2 diabetes.
- Fats in excess are a similar drain on the body's resources. Hidden fats are found in processed foods and in most fast foods.
- Alcohol has the most pernicious effect of destroying the B vitamins that are particularly needed for stamina and for the health of your nervous system in general.
- Caffeine inhibits the uptake of iron – a crucial mineral – when consumed at the same time as sources of this nutrient. If you drink tea or coffee, don't do so with meals featuring good sources of iron such as eggs, wholegrain cereals and meat.
- Red meat itself, though supplying valuable iron, is hard work for your digestive system. You're better off getting your iron from other sources for the time being.
- High-energy drinks, marketed as giving energy to the listless, are rich in glucose. They may give you a deceptive lift, but they contain nothing of real value to help combat fatigue at the root of the problem.

## vital statistics

Eggs are rich in protein, vitamin B12, iron and lecithin. They are also a good source of zinc and vitamins A, D and E. Not only are they energy-giving foods, but they also help protect against cancer and heart disease.

# a breakfast salad

It's Sunday morning. You've just come back from your workout and you deserve this muscle-building treat. Although it's rich in muscular protein, this isn't the healthiest salad of all time – but it tastes great. Yes, there is some fat in it, but 'low fat' doesn't have to mean 'no fat'. Eat this brunch dish with some good wholemeal toast and a glass of fresh orange juice, and its good points more than outweigh the bad.

**baby spinach leaves** 1 large bag
**unsalted butter** 10g (¼oz)
**lean back bacon** 8 rashers
**free-range eggs** 4

**1** Wash and dry the spinach leaves – even if they're 'ready-washed'. Spread the leaves over 4 plates.

**2** Melt the butter in a frying pan and fry the bacon until crisp.

**3** Meanwhile, poach the eggs.

**4** Break the bacon into bite-sized pieces and sprinkle over the spinach.

**5** Add the poached eggs and trickle any remaining fat in the bacon pan over each plate.

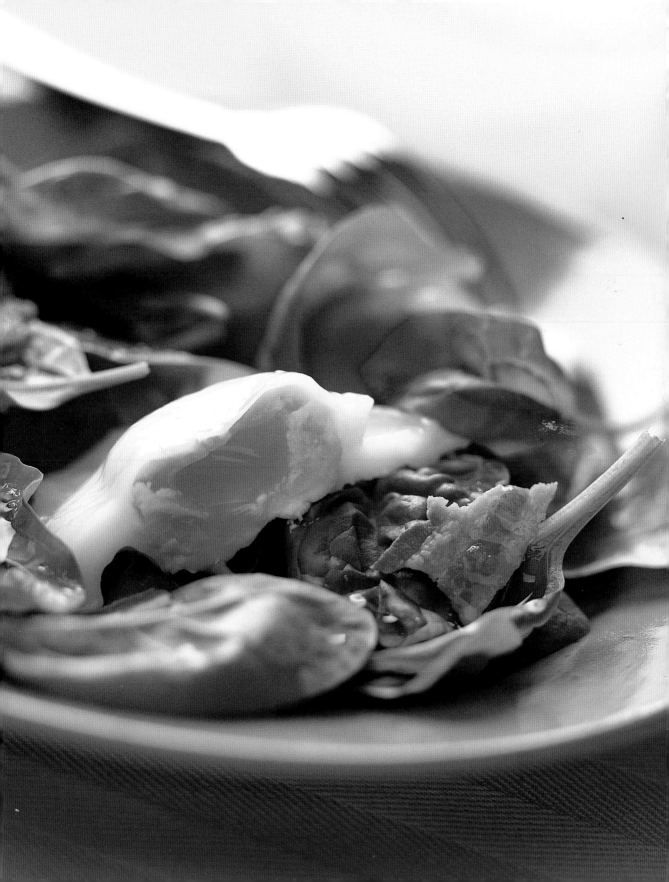

## vital statistics

As well as a mixture of quick- and slow-release energy, this provides loads of protein and plenty of calcium, not to mention some iron, lots of selenium, folic acid and 10 per cent of the recommended daily requirement of vitamin E.

# welsh rarebit

A good Welsh rarebit is a traditional and tasty teatime treat. Some of the best cheesemakers in England, Ireland, Scotland and Wales send their organic farmhouse produce to the famous Neal's Yard Dairy in London's Covent Garden, so get some if you can. Serve with a simple green salad for a wonderful quick and healthy supper.

**sourdough or wholemeal bread** 4 slices

**butter** for spreading

**sharp fruit chutney** 4 heaped tsp

**lancashire or cheshire farmhouse cheese** 90g (3¼oz)

**1** Preheat the grill to high.

**2** Lightly toast the bread on both sides and spread thinly with the butter.

**3** Spread each slice with a heaped teaspoon of chutney. Slice the cheese finely, then crumble on the top of each slice; pile it high and make sure it comes to the edges.

**4** Place under the grill until the cheese is melted.

This delicious dish provides a fifth of the recommended daily requirement of protein, lots of potassium, a quarter of daily iodine and a good supply of folic acid, vitamin C and betacarotene. The sustaining, slow-release energy is good for the entire body, and with just one egg per portion, you needn't worry about cholesterol.

# free-range spanish omelette

The combination of the deep, rich yellow of the eggs and the vivid red of the pepper makes this dish a visual delight as well as a taste sensation. Its roots lie in the peasant cooking of Spain, and, like most peasant food throughout the world, it's delicious, cheap and highly nourishing.

**extra-virgin olive oil** 4 tbsp

**potato** 1 large, peeled and diced

**onion** 1, thinly sliced

**red pepper** ½, cored, deseeded and cut into thin strips

**courgette** 1, thinly sliced

**black pepper** freshly ground, to taste

**free-range eggs** 4, well beaten

**1** Preheat the grill to high.

**2** Heat the oil in a large, heavy-based frying pan and fry the potato for 5 minutes, stirring. Turn the heat down, add the onion and cook for another 5 minutes.

**3** Add the red pepper and cook for 4 minutes, then add the courgette and cook for another 3 minutes, until the vegetables are tender but the onion is not browned.

**4** Add black pepper to taste to the eggs and pour into the pan; turn the heat down and stir thoroughly. Leave the omelette to cook very slowly. As it starts to set, the edge will curl away from the pan.

**5** Give the pan a good shake occasionally to keep the omelette moving, and as soon as the underside starts to brown, remove from the heat and place under the grill for 2–3 minutes to finish cooking.

**6** Hold a large plate over the frying pan and turn upside down. The omelette should drop out, all in one piece!

## vital statistics

This really is a high-power dish, offering brain-boosting protein from the fish and slow-release energy from the potatoes. It's also rich in essential fatty acids, zinc and selenium, and very low in saturated fats. Sage provides thujone, flavonoids and bitters, so it acts as a tonic herb and hormone booster. Marjoram supplies eugenol, which stimulates the metabolism.

# smart sage fish cakes

These delightfully light fish cakes are quick, easy to make, nutritious and inexpensive. The delicate taste of tuna is enhanced by the combination of sage and marjoram, making these a smart choice for everyone – particularly when served with a fresh green salad. These fish cakes are also excellent served cold, and they make a good carbohydrate/protein boost for athletes.

**extra-virgin olive oil**
about 150ml (¼ pint)

**onion** 1, very finely chopped

**tuna** 250g can, drained and flaked

**potatoes** 250g (9oz), cooked, roughly mashed and cooled

**marjoram** 1 tsp finely chopped fresh or ½ tsp dried

**sage** 1 tsp finely chopped fresh or ½ tsp dried

**free-range eggs** 2, beaten

1 Heat 1 tablespoon of the oil in a frying pan and sauté the onion gently. Leave to cool, then mix thoroughly with the tuna.

2 Add the mashed potatoes and herbs, and mix well.

3 Add half the beaten egg and mix again.

4 Form the mixture into 8 flat cakes.

5 Dip each cake in the remaining beaten egg.

6 Heat the remaining oil in the frying pan and shallow-fry the fish cakes gently for 7 minutes on each side.

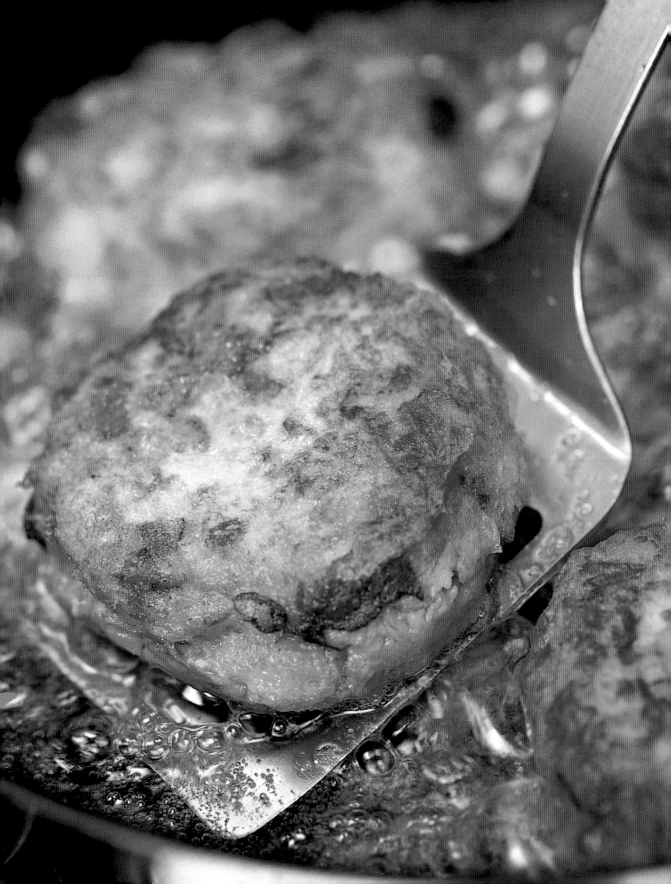

## vital statistics

This dish provides calcium from the two cheeses; protein, fibre and vitamins galore from the vegetables; extra iron and carotenoids from the dandelion leaves; heart-boosting lycopene from the tomatoes and the stimulating volatile oils from marjoram.

# aubergine and courgette layer

A non-meat dish with the power punch of a mule, yet just reading the recipe conjures up images of lazy, sun-drenched lunches in Spain, Portugal, Italy or southern France. The unique flavour and texture of aubergine, the giant, misshapen tomatoes and the ever-present smell of marjoram make this the perfect winter pick-me-up. It's delicious hot or cold, and even your most carnivorous friends won't notice the absence of meat.

**aubergines** 2

**sea salt** 1–2 pinches, to taste

**extra-virgin olive oil** 150ml (¼ pint)

**red onions** 2, finely chopped

**garlic** 3 cloves, finely chopped

**courgettes** 6 large

**buffalo mozzarella cheese** 450g (1lb)

**beef tomatoes** 4

**bay leaves** 3, finely crushed

**marjoram** 3 tbsp finely chopped

**dandelion leaves** 1 tbsp chopped

**raclette cheese** 6 tbsp grated

**1** Preheat the oven to 200°C/400°F/gas mark 6.

**2** Peel and slice the aubergines. Sprinkle both sides with salt, spread out on an oiled baking sheet and bake for 10 minutes.

**3** Meanwhile, heat the oil in a frying pan and sweat the onions and garlic gently for 10 minutes.

**4** Cut the courgettes, mozzarella and tomatoes into medium-sized slices.

**5** Transfer the onion mixture to an ovenproof dish. Layer with the aubergines, tomatoes, courgettes and mozzarella, finishing with a mozzarella layer on the top.

**6** Mix the bay leaves, marjoram, dandelion leaves and raclette together and sprinkle over the mozzarella layer.

**7** Cover with foil and bake in the oven for 50 minutes.

**8** Remove the foil and bake for a further 10 minutes.

## vital statistics

This dish is a good source of protein, fibre, folic acid and energy, together with useful amounts of vitamins A and C.

# pasta with raw courgette

Pasta is good at any time. Wholemeal pasta contains fibre and B vitamins, so choose your favourite – preferably organic. For the best quality and flavour of Parmesan, again opt for organic; nearly all organic cheeses are made by small traditional cheesemakers. Combined with the fresh, clean flavours of courgette, this dish provides a delicious and healthy, easy-to-cook meal.

**extra-virgin olive oil** 1 tsp
**sea salt** 2 pinches
**spaghettini** 450g (1lb)
**courgettes** 200g (7oz), finely grated
**butter** 10g (¼oz)
**parmesan cheese** 2 tbsp freshly grated
**black pepper** freshly ground, to taste

**1** Add the oil and salt to a large saucepan of water and bring to the boil.

**2** Add the pasta, stir for a few seconds to avoid sticking and cook according to the packet instructions until al dente.

**3** Meanwhile, fill a heatproof serving dish with boiling water to warm it.

**4** When the pasta is cooked, drain. Empty the water from the serving dish; put in the pasta, add the courgettes, butter, Parmesan and black pepper to taste and mix thoroughly.

## vital statistics

A feast of power-boosting iron comes from the liver, together with protein, vitamin B12 and a massive dose of vitamin A. This dish also provides a day's dose of vitamin C from the lime juice, all brilliantly absorbed thanks to the phytochemicals in wild chicory. Note to expectant mothers: avoid this dish due to its high vitamin A content.

# lively chicory liver

The pink calves' liver contrasts beautifully with the bright green of the limes and the colours of wild chicory and blackened sage to make this dish as appealing to the eye as it is to the taste buds. Crisp, fried sage leaves are a perfect foil for the melt-in-the-mouth consistency of calves' liver – and the iron the latter provides (enhanced by the wild chicory) makes this a power dish extraordinaire.

**sunflower oil** 6 tbsp
**sage leaves** 16
**unsalted butter** 75g (2³/₄oz)
**calves' liver** 4 thin slices, organic
**wild chicory leaves** 4 tsp
**limes** 2, halved

**1** Heat the oil in a frying pan and fry the sage leaves for about 1 minute or until crisp.

**2** Drain the leaves on kitchen paper and keep warm.

**3** Wipe the frying pan out. Melt the butter in the pan. Add the liver, sprinkle with the chicory leaves and cook for 1 minute on each side.

**4** Serve scattered with the sage leaves, with the lime halves on the side.

## vital statistics

A good source of protein, fibre, folic acid and energy, together with useful amounts of vitamins A and C.

# cheese and bread pudding

This savoury bread pudding takes a few minutes to make and half an hour to cook, and it is another high-energy lunch or light evening meal. You can vary the flavour by trying any variety of hard organic farmhouse cheese.

**butter** 60g (2¼oz)

**wholemeal bread** 4 slices, crusts removed

**shallots** 3, finely chopped

**mature Cheddar or Gruyère cheese** 175g (6oz), grated

**free-range eggs** 4

**milk** 600ml (1 pint)

**black pepper** freshly ground, to taste

**paprika** ¼ tsp

**tomatoes** 2, thinly sliced

**1** Preheat the oven to. 200°C/400°F/gas mark 6.

**2** Use some of the butter to grease a pie dish. Spread the rest on the bread and cut into small squares. Place a layer in the dish.

**3** Make another layer with the shallots, then add the cheese and top with more of the bread.

**4** Beat the eggs, milk and black pepper (to taste) together, then pour the mixture into the dish. Sprinkle with the paprika.

**5** Cover with the tomato slices and bake for about 30 minutes until brown on top.

## vital statistics

Lamb is chock-full of protein and B vitamins, both of which are great energy boosters, and iron, which is essential for the production of red blood cells.

# malaysian muscle salad

Although it's a salad, this wonderful rack-of-lamb dish is substantial enough to be a meal in itself. Its huge muscle- and blood-building benefits come from the protein and iron in the meat. You also get the delicious flavour of peanut butter, the betacarotene in the mixed leaves, the natural plant hormones from the soy sauce and the digestive benefits of fresh coriander.

**extra-virgin olive oil** 4 tbsp
**turmeric** 1 tsp
**ground cloves** 1 tsp
**rack of lamb** 1 (8 chops)
**mixed salad leaves** 1 large bag
**crunchy peanut butter** 2 tbsp
**garlic** 2 cloves, finely chopped
**soy sauce** 2 tsp
**tamari** 1 tsp
**fresh coriander leaves** 1 tbsp
roughly chopped

**1** Preheat the oven to maximum temperature.

**2** Mix 2 tablespoons of the oil thoroughly with the turmeric and cloves, and rub all over the lamb. Put the lamb into a roasting dish and cook in the oven for exactly 20 minutes.

**3** Remove the lamb from the oven, cover loosely with foil and leave to rest for 15 minutes.

**4** Meanwhile, wash and dry the mixed salad leaves.

**5** Combine the peanut butter, garlic, soy sauce and tamari with the remaining oil in a food processor or blender.

**6** Make a mound of the mixed salad leaves on a large serving platter.

**7** Separate the lamb chops and place them against the mound in a circle, with all the bones pointing upwards.

**8** Sprinkle with the chopped coriander leaves and serve with the sauce in a separate dish.

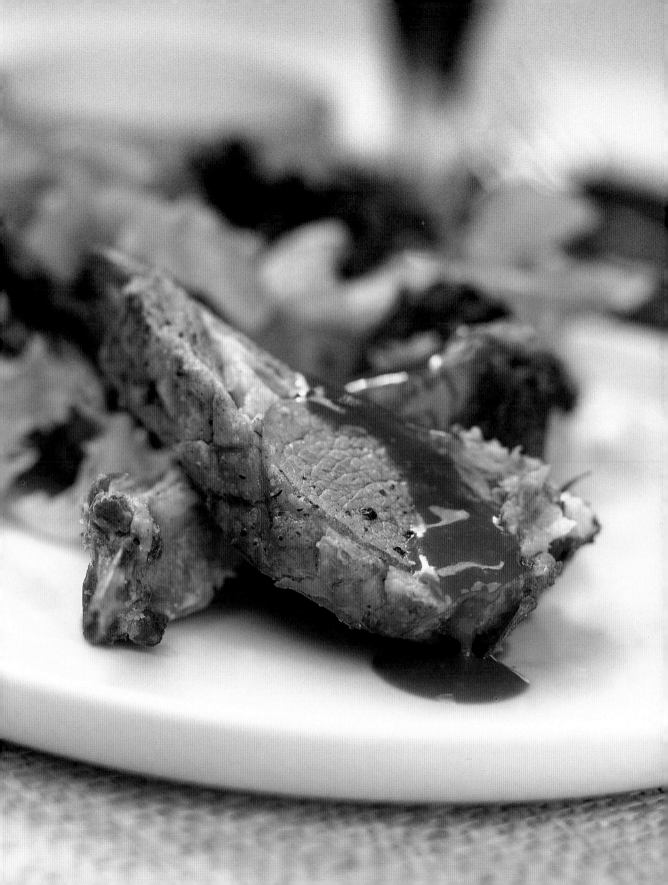

## vital statistics

Bursting with minerals and betacarotene from the root vegetables, and fibre, protein and other important carotenoids from the spinach or chard. Rosemary's borneol, apigenin and rosmarinic acid produce tonic and anti-inflammatory properties, and stimulate mental powers. Added stimulation comes from the cineol and laurenolide present in bay leaves.

# robust rosemary lamb

Super-charged power radiates from this lovely lamb dish, and even though it takes a few hours to cook, the preparation couldn't be simpler. The classic flavour of rosemary enhances the rest of the power nutrients contained in the vegetables and meat.

**extra-virgin olive oil** about 6 tbsp

**onion** 1 large, chopped

**garlic** 2 cloves, chopped

**lamb** 4 chops or 8 cutlets, most of the fat removed

**sea salt and black pepper** freshly ground, to taste

**carrots** 2 large, peeled and diced

**turnips** 4 baby, peeled and sliced

**fennel** 1 bulb, cut into chunks

**bay leaves** 4

**rosemary** 1 large sprig

**herb or vegetable stock** 850ml (1½ pints) – see page 396

**spinach or Swiss chard** 500g (1lb 2oz)

**1** Preheat the oven to 200°C/400°F/gas mark 6.

**2** Heat the oil in a frying pan and sweat the onion and garlic gently until softened. Remove from the pan.

**3** Season the lamb with salt and pepper and fry in the oil, browning it all over.

**4** Transfer to a large, flameproof casserole dish along with the onion and garlic.

**5** Add the vegetables, bay leaves, rosemary and stock to the casserole.

**6** Bring gently to the boil, adding more water if necessary, then cook, uncovered, in the oven for 2 hours, checking the stock level occasionally.

**7** Half an hour before the dish is ready, tear the spinach or Swiss chard into shreds, then add to the casserole, making sure that the leaves are covered with the stock.

## vital statistics

Rich in iron, B vitamins – especially B12 – and plenty of good energy calories from the rice. Volatile oils are provided by pennyroyal, particularly pulegone, menthol and limonene. Pennyroyal also contains bitter phytochemicals, which stimulate gastric juices and improve the digestion of meat.

# mediterranean steak

A power-packed dish sure to please even the fussiest carnivore. Steak isn't a principal part of the Mediterranean diet, but when they do it, it's a veritable feast. Here, the flavours of the marinade and meat blend seamlessly with the garlic, sage, parsley and marjoram in the rice. It's made all the more interesting by the addition of the pungent, minty pennyroyal – but use it sparingly. This hardy perennial grows well in a pot.

**beef** 4 fillet steaks, preferably organic

**red wine** 300ml (½ pint)

**bay leaves** 2

**onion** 1, chopped

**garlic** 2 cloves, chopped

**extra-virgin olive oil** 8 tbsp

**arborio rice** 225–250g (8–9oz)

**mixed herbs** 1 tbsp each sage, parsley and marjoram chopped

**fresh pennyroyal** 1 small pinch

**vegetable stock** 500ml (18fl oz) – *see* page 396 or use a good stock cube or bouillon powder

**1** Marinate the steaks in the wine with the bay leaves, half the onion, half the garlic and half the oil for 1 hour in the refrigerator.

**2** Heat the remaining oil in a saucepan and sweat the rest of the onion and garlic gently until softened.

**3** Add the rice and stir until coated in the oil.

**4** Mix the herbs and pennyroyal into the stock.

**5** Add the stock a ladleful at a time to the rice. Simmer until each addition is absorbed before adding the next.

**6** Add the wine marinade, minus the bay leaves, to the rice. Cook until it is absorbed and the rice is tender but with a little bite.

**7** Meanwhile, grill or fry the steaks for 5–6 minutes on each side, depending on preference.

## vital statistics

This comforting dish provides plenty of protein, fibre, calcium, potassium and vitamin B12, together with useful amounts of iron, zinc, iodine and vitamin E.

# mother's yorkshire pudding, with apples

Here's a dessert that tastes good and does you good – a sweet you can eat without feeling guilty. It is quite substantial, however, so save it as a partner for a fairly light meal. As well as loads of energy, this delicious recipe supplies heart-protective pectin, which helps reduce cholesterol. It also offers digestive benefits from the volatile oils present in cloves and cinnamon.

**crisp dessert apples** 450g (1lb), peeled, cored and sliced

**seedless raisins** 30g (1oz)

**lemon juice** 1 tbsp

**soft brown sugar** 30g (1oz)

**cloves** 2

**ground cinnamon** 1 tsp

**batter**

**wholemeal flour** 175g (6oz)

**plain white flour** 60g (2¼oz)

**soft brown sugar** 90g (3¼oz)

**free-range eggs** 2

**milk** 600ml (1 pint)

1 Preheat the oven to 170°C/325°F/gas mark 3.

2 Layer the apples on the bottom of a lightly greased ovenproof dish.

3 Add the raisins, lemon juice, sugar and cloves, and sprinkle with the cinnamon.

4 Mix all the batter ingredients together in a bowl, beating thoroughly, and pour over the top.

5 Bake for 1 hour.

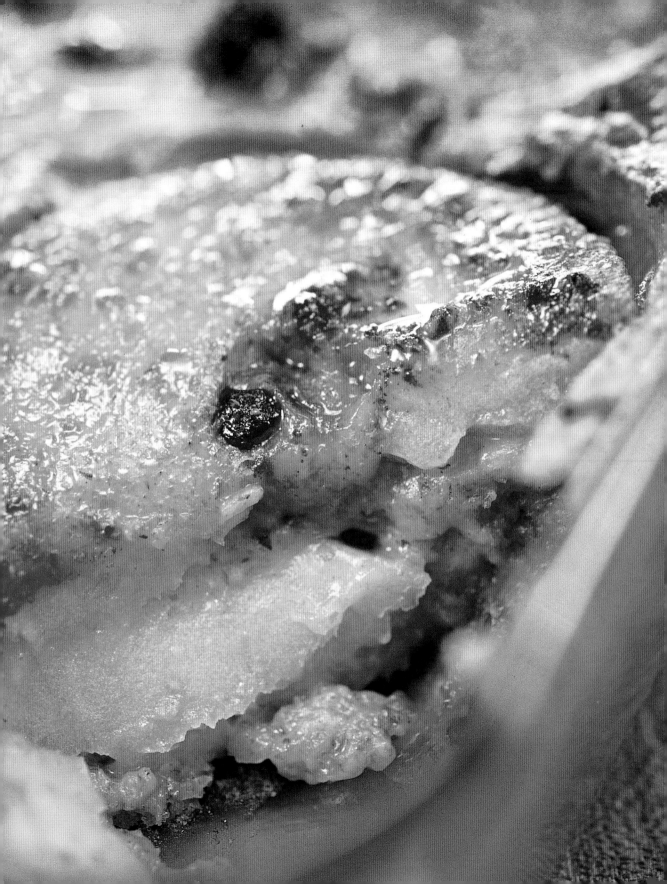

## vital statistics

Ideal for a nutritional energy boost, since beans and potatoes supply masses of slow-release energy. Carrots are also rich in immune-boosting vitamin A.

# vegetable and bean soup

In the middle of winter, you not only need the warming properties of this typical peasant soup, but you'll also benefit from the antibacterial effects of the garlic and onion. A bowlful of this delicious combination will keep you going when you have to shovel the snow away from your door.

**extra-virgin olive oil** 4 tbsp

**onion** 1 large, very finely chopped

**garlic** 2 cloves, very finely chopped

**courgettes** 2 large, grated

**new potatoes** 4, scrubbed and grated just before use (otherwise they'll discolour)

**carrot** 1 large, trimmed and peeled unless organic, grated

**vegetable stock** 1.4 litres (2½ pints) – *see* page 396 or use a good stock cube or bouillon powder

**flageolet beans** 2 x 240g cans (drained weight), rinsed

**1** Heat the oil in a large saucepan and sweat the onion and garlic gently for about 5 minutes.

**2** Add the grated vegetables and cook for 5 minutes, stirring continuously and adding a little more oil to the pan if necessary.

**3** Pour in the stock and simmer for 10 minutes.

**4** Whizz the mixture in a food processor or blender – or use a hand blender – until smooth.

**5** Return to the pan.

**6** Add the beans to the pan, bring back to a simmer and heat gently for 5 minutes.

## vital statistics

This soup provides plenty of vital nutrients. Pot barley is rich in fibre, calcium, potassium and B vitamins.

# thick barley and vegetable soup

Barley is a staple food in the Middle East, and in ancient Rome it was used in soups to feed the gladiators. Sadly, these days it's mostly ignored in Western cooking. Whole pot barley is used here, available in most supermarkets and health-food stores – it is a real winter tonic. In contrast, the polished, refined pearl barley provides only calories.

**extra-virgin olive oil** 2 tbsp

**onion** 1 large, finely chopped

**carrot** 1 large, trimmed and peeled unless organic, finely cubed

**leek** 1 large, very finely diced

**vegetable stock** 1 litre (1³/4 pints) – *see* page 396 or use a good stock cube or bouillon powder

**bay leaves** 3

**pot barley** 5 tbsp

**parsley** 1 large handful, chopped

**1** Heat the oil in a large saucepan and sweat the onion, carrot and leek gently for 5 minutes.

**2** Add the stock and bay leaves.

**3** Bring to the boil and add the barley.

**4** Turn the heat down and simmer for about 1 hour.

**5** Remove the bay leaves.

**6** Serve with the parsley sprinkled on top.

## vital statistics

A soup that provides all-round nutrition. Chickpeas are rich in calcium, while the beef in the sausages provides protein, iron and B vitamins, all of which nourish the nervous system.

# chickpea and spicy beef sausage soup

This is the perfect soup to choose if you're suffering from SAD (the winter blues), because it helps improve everything from circulation to mood. The combination of chickpeas and spicy sausage protects your bones during the dark days of winter, improves blood flow and promotes balanced blood-sugar levels – lifting the spirits as well as treating the taste buds.

**extra-virgin olive oil** 3 tbsp

**onion** 1 large, finely chopped

**garlic** 1 large clove, finely chopped

**fennel** ½ bulb, finely chopped

**spicy beef sausage** 300g (10½oz), cut into chunks

**beef stock** 1.2 litres (2 pints) – *see* page 397 or use a good stock cube or bouillon powder

**chickpeas** 2 x 240g cans (drained weight), rinsed

**1** Heat the oil in a large saucepan and sweat the onion, garlic and fennel gently until softened.

**2** Add the sausage.

**3** Pour in the stock and chickpeas and simmer until tender – about 15 minutes.

**4** Remove 4 tablespoons of the chickpeas and whizz the rest of the mixture in a food processor or blender – or use a hand blender – until smooth.

**5** Return to the pan and heat until boiling.

**6** Serve with the whole chickpeas floating on top.

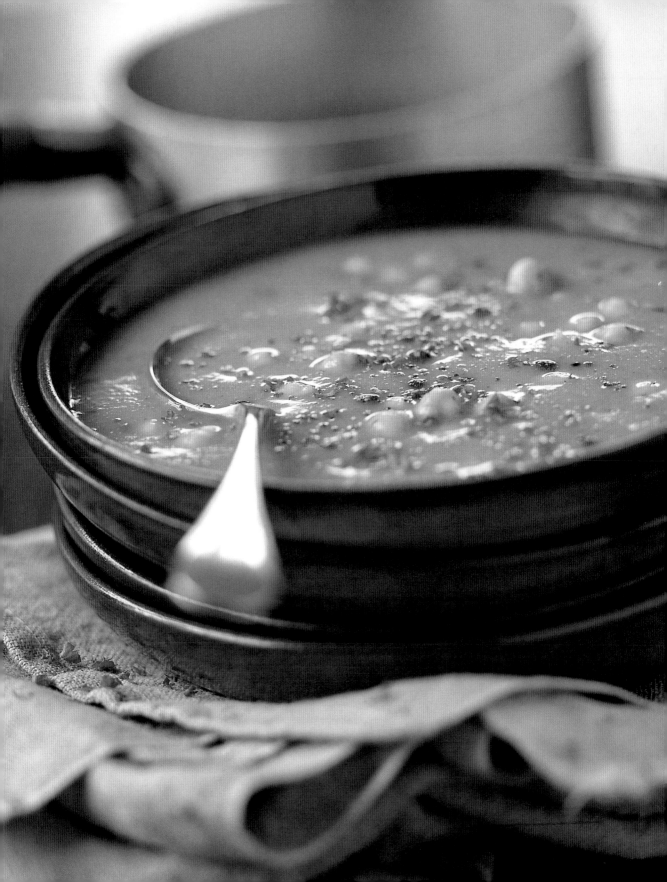

## vital statistics

This soup will help fight off winter depression. Butter beans and broad beans contain fibre, protein, minerals and natural plant hormones, which help to elevate mood.

# spanish bean and chorizo soup

Good neighbours can make an enormous difference to your quality of life. My wife, Sally, and I are blessed with the best. Denzil lived for some years in Spain and passed this recipe on to his wife, Vee, who often arrives on our doorstep with a steaming pan of this fabulous taste of Spanish sun to chase away the winter blues.

**extra-virgin olive oil** 2 tbsp

**onion** 1, finely chopped

**garlic** 2 cloves, finely chopped

**plain flour** 1 tbsp

**ham stock** 1.2 litres (2 pints) – *see* page 397 or use a good stock cube or bouillon powder

**butter beans** 450g can, rinsed

**broad beans** 100g (3½oz)

**thin chorizo sausage** 250g (9oz), finely cubed

**1** Heat the oil in a large saucepan and sweat the onion and garlic gently for about 10 minutes until softened.

**2** Stir in the flour and cook, stirring continuously, for about 5 minutes.

**3** Pour in the stock very slowly, stirring until the flour takes up the liquid completely.

**4** Add the butter beans and broad beans.

**5** Simmer until the beans are almost tender – about 10 minutes.

**6** Add the chorizo and heat through.

Root vegetables are an abundant source of minerals, carotenoids and other phytochemicals. Although most of the vitamin C is lost during the prolonged cooking, nearly all the other nutrients end up in the soup, together with the immune-boosting and antiviral components from the chicken.

# chicken yum-yum

This may look like a soup, smell like a soup and taste like a soup – that's because it is a soup, and what could be more of a pick-me-up than a mug full of this crystal-clear, energizing, warming and immune-boosting chicken broth? In different locations around the world, from traditional Jewish villages in frozen Siberia to the steamy humidity of the Far East, the burning heat of India or the plains of China, chicken broth functions like Jupiter: the bringer of jollity.

**chicken quarter** 1 (not a breast)
**leek** 1, quartered
**fennel** 1 bulb, quartered
**carrot** 1, sliced lengthways
**onion** 1, unpeeled and halved
**mixed summer herbs** 1 large handful
**cold water** 850ml (1½ pints)

**1** Trim any fat off the chicken quarter, then put it into a large saucepan.

**2** Add the vegetables, herbs and water.

**3** Bring to the boil, then turn the heat down and simmer, covered, for 40 minutes.

**4** Strain off the chicken and vegetables.

**5** Serve the yum-yum immediately.

This can be kept in the refrigerator for up to 3 days. If you do this, skim off any residue of cold fat and heat on the hob or in a microwave before serving.

A soup tailor-made for warmth and energy. Split peas are rich in fibre and minerals, while sausage supplies vital protein.

# dutch pea soup with smoked sausage

Redolent of those wonderful Dutch paintings of frozen winter scenes, this is another of the great peasant recipes of Europe. Split peas give this soup its unique character and its consistency of thick porridge. A bowlful with a chunk of bread and a crisp winter salad is all you need for a nourishing lunch or supper. My dear Dutch friend Henri van der Zee has a pea soup party on his birthday every year – but don't wait a year before you try this recipe.

**split green peas** 300g (10½oz)

**unsalted butter** 40g (1½oz)

**smoked back bacon** 200g (7oz), finely chopped

**onion** 1, coarsely chopped

**ham stock** 1.4 litres (2½ pints) – *see* page 397 or use a good stock cube or bouillon powder

**smoked sausage** 500g (1lb 2oz), rind removed and cut into chunks

**1** Soak the peas in plenty of cold water overnight.

**2** Melt the butter in a large saucepan and sauté the bacon gently for 2 minutes.

**3** Add the onion and sauté for 4 minutes.

**4** Stir in the drained soaked peas, add the stock and bring to the boil. Turn the heat down and simmer, covered, for 1–2 hours until the peas are tender.

**5** Mix in the smoked sausage and simmer for another 10–15 minutes.

This robust soup can also be served cold, with any fat skimmed from the top.

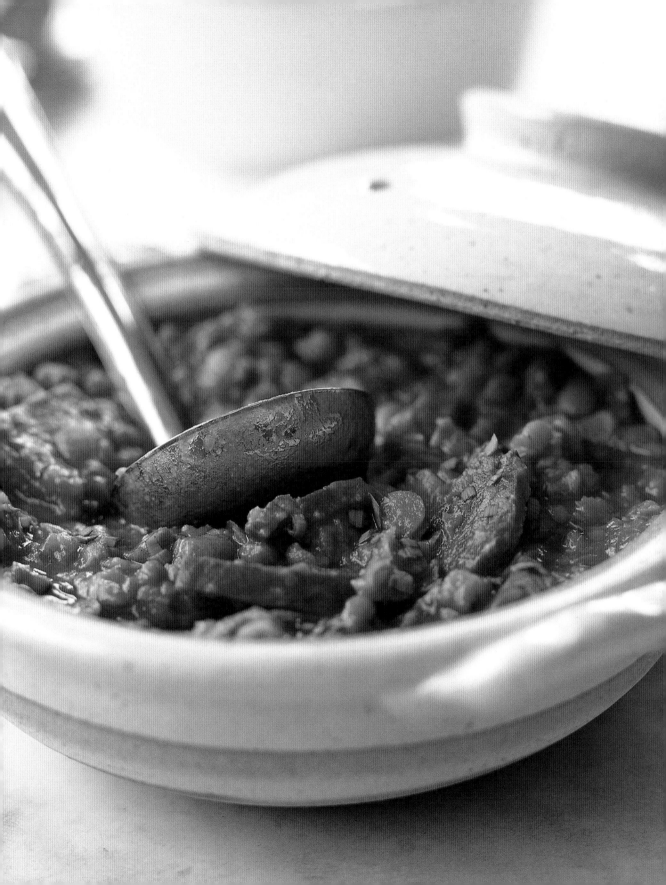

## vital statistics

This soup contains lots of potassium, half the daily requirement of vitamin C, useful amounts of iron, zinc, selenium, iodine, folic acid and betacarotene, and a healthy contribution of fibre.

# leek and potato soup

Potatoes are at their healthiest and most nutritious when eaten with their skins – something you can do safely only by using organic produce. As well as providing high levels of energy, leeks make this soup a useful treatment for gout, arthritis, rheumatism, chest infections and sore throats.

**butter** 60g (2¼oz)

**garlic** 1 clove, chopped

**leeks** 2, chopped

**small new potatoes** 375g (13oz), scrubbed

**onion** 1 large, sliced

**vegetable stock** 850ml (1½ pints)

**parsley** 2 tbsp finely chopped

**black pepper** freshly ground, to taste

**double cream** 150ml (¼ pint)

**1** Melt the butter in a large saucepan and sweat the garlic gently for 2 minutes.

**2** Add the leeks, potatoes and onion and cook over a medium heat for 10 minutes.

**3** Add the stock and simmer for 20 minutes or until the vegetables are tender.

**4** Whizz in a food processor or blender – or use a hand blender – until smooth, then finish by adding the parsley, black pepper to taste and cream.

## vital statistics

This broth is a good source of protein. It is also low in fat and contains plenty of fibre, calcium, potassium, trace minerals and vitamins A, B and C.

# celtic broth

If ever there was a liquid mixture of health and energy, this is it. Oats provide slow-release energy, as well as a good dose of soluble fibre, which reduces cholesterol levels. Broccoli is packed with heart- and circulatory-protective nutrients in addition to cancer-fighting agents.

**extra-virgin olive oil** 1 tbsp
**spring onions** 5, chopped
**broccoli florets** 450g (1lb)
**porridge oats** 60g (2¼oz)
**vegetable stock and semi-skimmed milk** half and half
mix to make 1 litre (1¾ pints)
**black pepper** freshly ground, to taste
**nutmeg** freshly grated, to taste
**fromage frais** 1 tbsp
**chives** 1 tbsp chopped

**1** Heat the oil in a large saucepan and sauté the spring onions gently until softened. Add the broccoli florets and cook, stirring, for 2 minutes. Add the oats and cook, stirring, for 2 minutes.

**2** Slowly add the stock and milk, and stir. Cover and simmer gently for 12 minutes.

**3** Add black pepper and nutmeg to taste, then serve with a swirl of fromage frais and a sprinkling of chopped chives.

# shepherds' watch

In 1949, Louis DeGouy, chef at the Waldorf Astoria in New York for 30 years, wrote in *The Soup Book*: 'It breathes reassurance, it offers consolation; after a weary day it promotes sociability. There is nothing like a bowl of hot soup, its wisp of aromatic steam teasing the nostrils into quivering anticipation.' How true of this comforting, nourishing and sustaining dish. But is it a soup or a stew? I don't think it matters.

**lamb fillet** 350g (12oz), finely cut along the grain into 1cm (½in) dice

**onion** 1, very finely chopped

**ground cumin** 1 tsp

**rapeseed oil** 2 tbsp

**tomato purée** 1 tbsp

**lamb stock** 1.4 litres (2½ pints) – *see* page 397 or use a good stock cube or bouillon powder

**turnip** 1, peeled and diced

**celery** 3 sticks, sliced

**potato** 1 large, peeled and diced

1 Put the lamb, onion and cumin into a frying pan with the oil, and cook, stirring continuously, until the lamb is just pink – about 5 minutes (or longer if you prefer your meat well done).

2 Add the tomato purée and stir well. Set aside.

3 Pour the stock into a large saucepan. Tip in the turnip, celery and potato and bring to the boil. Turn the heat down and simmer until the vegetables are cooked – about 15 minutes.

4 Smash the vegetables roughly with a potato masher.

5 Add the lamb mixture and heat through gently.

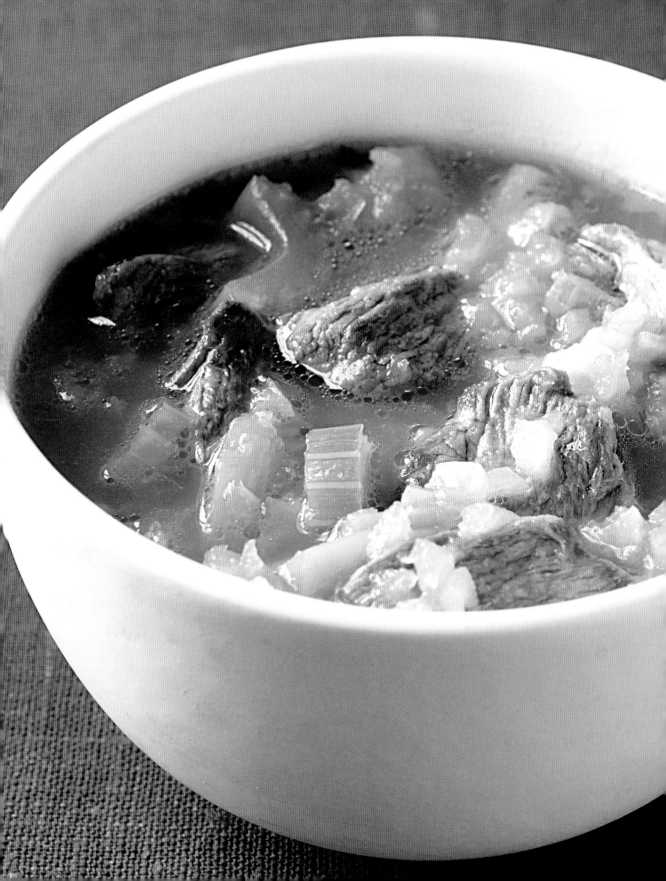

## vital statistics

Super-rich in potassium and vitamin A, this is a detoxifying juice, thanks to the parsley it contains. Both parsley and mint have a healing effect on the entire digestive system, and they are calming to the central nervous system. Melon juice also overflows with healing betacarotenes and is exceptionally curative and cooling.

# the red-eye special

Taken the overnight plane? Been burning the midnight oil? Had a night on the tiles? Whatever the reason, the next day can be hell – but it needn't be. While the Red-Eye Special won't work miracles, it comes pretty close. The ingredients in this superjuice were popular with ancient Greeks and Romans, who knew that the natural oils in parsley and mint soothe the stomach and calm jangly nerves. With clear eyes, no headache and no puffiness or gritty skin, you'll get through the day in better shape than you ever imagined possible.

**mint** 6 sprigs
**spinach leaves** 6
**yellow-fleshed melon** 1, peeled and deseeded
**parsley** 1 handful of sprigs

**1** Put all the ingredients through a juicer.

## vital statistics

This juice is super-rich in vitamins A, C and E, folic acid and potassium, iron and magnesium. Low in calories, it is the perfect start to the day for weight watchers. It also gets a five-star rating for peak power of mind and body, and it is delicious, calming and mildly diuretic to boot. As a final bonus, this superjuice contains lycopene, one of the most powerful natural antioxidants, which protects specifically against heart disease.

# mediterranean muscle

Throughout the southern Mediterranean, the combination of tomatoes and basil is inseparable, not only for taste, but also for the wonderful mixture of aromas. This superjuice is another variation on the theme. Designed for mind and body, it's rich in minerals to give renewed vigour to tired muscles, and contains essential oils from the basil that act specifically on tired minds. Serve with a dash of Worcestershire sauce and some black pepper as a finishing touch.

**plum tomatoes** 4 large ripe

**carrot** 1, trimmed and peeled unless organic

**celery** 1 stick, with leaves

**basil** 1 handful

**lemon** ½

**1** Put the tomatoes, carrot, celery and basil through a juicer.

**2** Squeeze the juice from the lemon into the mixture and stir.

## vital statistics

This vitality drink provides a double dose of betacarotene and potassium from the carrots and kiwi fruit, along with extra magnesium and plenty of vitamin C. The spinach adds extra carotenoids and a powerful boost of cancer-fighting plant chemicals. The coriander contains heart- and circulatory-protective coumarins, and an effective antiseptic essential oil called linalol.

# a punch of power

Here's another super-vitality juice with plenty of essential nutrients and some surprisingly potent natural phytochemicals from the coriander and spinach. It makes an excellent drink for physically active people, since it provides a boost of instant energy from the natural sugars in the carrots and kiwi fruit. It is also a good source of potassium – so important for muscle performance.

**carrots** 4, trimmed and peeled unless organic
**kiwi fruit** 1, unpeeled
**fresh coriander** 1 small handful, with stalks
**baby spinach leaves** 1 handful

**1** Put all the ingredients through a juicer, reserving a few coriander leaves, if desired.

**2** Mix well and serve with the coriander leaves, if reserved, on top.

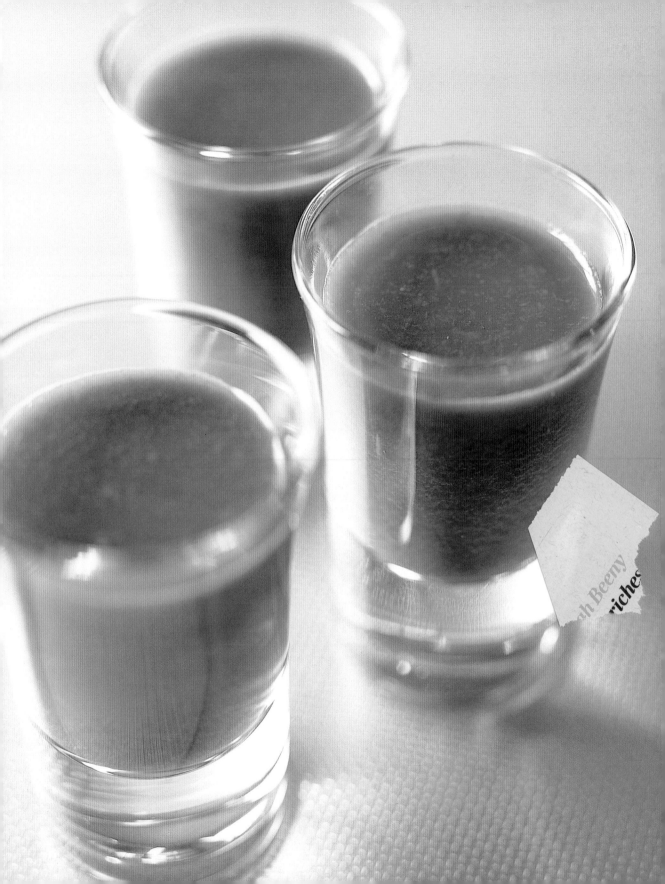

## vital statistics

This superjuice is bursting with good stuff. It is super-rich in vitamins A, C and E, potassium and vitamin B6. It also contains some calcium and traces of other B vitamins. With just under 300 calories a glass, it's a good quick-energy source. In addition, horseradish contains the natural substance sinigrin, a powerful antibiotic that also protects against infections.

# horse power

It may sound simple, but this classic apple-and-carrot mixture spiked with fresh horseradish is fuel for any bucking bronco. As well as the instant energy derived from the natural sugars in the carrots and apples, it features a whole new dimension courtesy of the horseradish. You'll get very little juice and lots of pulp from 85g (3oz) horseradish, but what you do get is instant stimulation of the circulation. With the blood coursing through your veins, you'll be ready for anything.

**carrots** 4, trimmed and peeled unless organic
**apples** 2, unpeeled, uncored and quartered
**fresh horseradish** 85g (3oz)

**1** Put all the ingredients through a juicer.

## vital statistics

This juice is super-rich in iron, vitamin C, folic acid, betacarotene and other carotenoids. The vitamin C makes the iron it contains all the more easily absorbed by the body, while its betacarotene and other carotenoids protect against cancers. All this, plus its instant supply of natural sugars, makes Pumping Iron the perfect juice for serious exercisers, body builders, vegetarians and women planning pregnancy.

# pumping iron

Here's a power pumping iron tonic in a glass for those dull, grey days when you just can't seem to charge up the batteries. It's all too easy to dismiss cucumber as nothing more than water. While its nutritional content is very low, it is nonetheless regarded as an important healing vegetable in natural medicine – which explains why it appears in lots more recipes. Here, cucumber's cool, refreshing flavour contrasts superbly with the astringency of beetroot, spinach and watercress.

**apples** 2, unpeeled, uncored and quartered
**raw beetroot** 1 small, unpeeled, with leaves
**cucumber** 1, halved lengthways
**spinach leaves** 1 handful
**watercress** 1 handful

**1** Put all the ingredients through a juicer.

## vital statistics

Apricots are a wonderful health-giving fruit, long prized by the Hunza peoples living in Himalayan mountain villages. The Hunza's legendary fitness, vitality and longevity are attributed to their consumption of fresh and dried apricots throughout the year. This fruit offers a perfect balance of instant and slow-release energy, and is a huge source of vitality-boosting betacarotene, essential for immunity, and healthy skin and eyesight.

# apricot delight

The thick consistency of this wonderful drink is more reminiscent of nectars than juices. Fortunately, unlike the commercial varieties, there's no added sugar here – just the wonderful flavour of apricots, redolent of summertime but available all year round.

**ready-to-eat dried apricots** 12
**cold water** 500ml (18fl oz)

**1** Snip each of the dried apricots into half the size of a small fingernail.

**2** Reserving 6 pieces, put the rest into a saucepan and cover with the water.

**3** Bring to the boil, then turn the heat down and simmer gently for 15 minutes.

**4** Leave to cool slightly before whizzing in a blender or food processor until smooth.

**5** Reheat and serve, with the reserved apricot pieces on top.

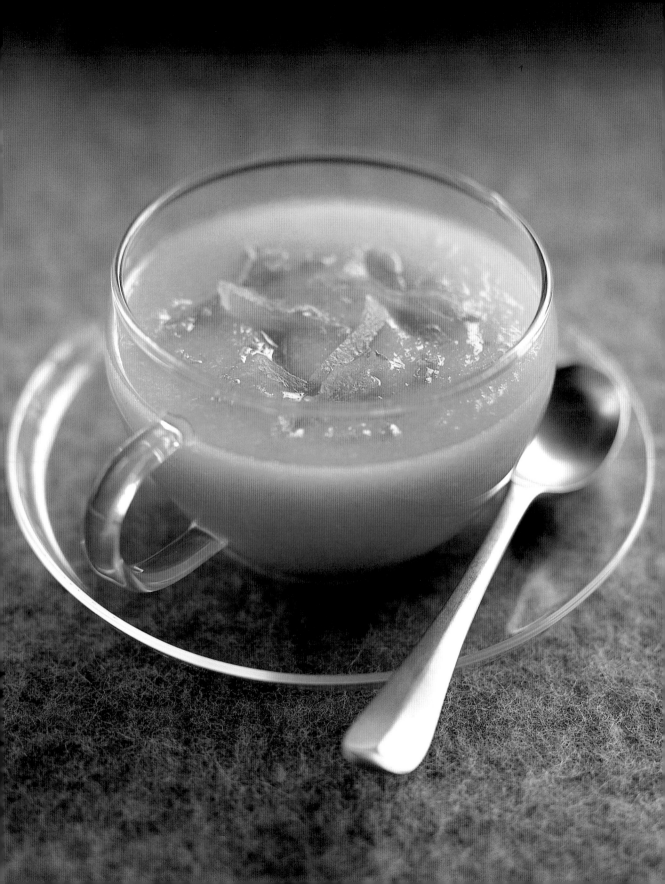

## vital statistics

Guavas and mangoes are rich in betacarotene, vitamin C, natural sugars and protective antioxidants. The banana contains large amounts of potassium, which is important to prevent cramp during sustained muscular activity. This juice also helps maintain a high level of mental activity over long periods of time. The guarana adds the age-old wisdom of rainforest Indian medicine to this modern-day vitality drink.

# guava delight

This smoothie is the ideal combination of instant and slow-release energy, with the added sting in the tail of the Brazilian rainforest herb known as guarana. Whether you're sitting in a high-powered meeting, working at your computer or going off to play a weekend game of football or tennis, this is the way to give your vitality a healthy boost. All the tropical fruits are rich in natural sugars for an instant lift, while the banana provides some protein and lots of complex carbohydrates for a more gradual release of usable energy.

**guava** 1, peeled
**mango** 1, peeled and stoned
**banana** 1, peeled
**guarana powder** 5g (1 tsp)

**1** Put the guava and mango through a juicer.

**2** Whizz the banana with the juice in a blender or food processor until smooth.

**3** Add the guarana and whizz again.

**4** Chill before serving.

## vital statistics

This juice is rich in vitamins A and C. Used for centuries as a diuretic in India, melon helps get rid of morning puffiness. Melons also contain adenosine, which makes blood less sticky, thus reducing the risk of blood clots and heart attack. Mango is a super-rich source of instant energy and nutrients. The vitamin A content of melon and mango juice is a boost to the immune system and helps protect the body from cancer.

# melon and mango tango

Just smelling this wonderful juice first thing in the morning awakens the brain, opens the eyes and quickens the blood. Quick and easy to make, this cool, refreshing drink will kick-start your metabolism and help shrug off that early-morning sluggishness. One glass, and you'll be running at full power throughout the day.

**mango** 1, peeled and stoned
**cantaloupe, ogen or muskmelon** ½, peeled and deseeded

**1** Put the ingredients through a juicer.

## vital statistics

The protein and plant lignins in the peanuts provide slow-release energy and help reduce cholesterol and insulin levels. Add the banana for more slow-release energy and lots of potassium to prevent cramp during exercise, and you've got the basis of this great vitality drink. The rest of the fruit provides vitamin C and soluble fibre, while the crème fraîche gives you calcium and B vitamins. A delicious feast of nutrients.

# wake-up call

This combination of quick- and slow-release energy, essential nutrients, protein and fibre is a great early-morning starter or before-sport booster for your vitality. Most women I know think peanut butter is one of the greatest sins, since it must be fattening. This is far from the truth. Peanut butter helps in any weight-loss plan, as it provides slow-release energies that prevent a fall in blood sugar and a craving for sweet things. Furthermore, because peanuts are broken down very slowly into energy-giving sugars, the nuts and peanut butter help protect against adult-onset diabetes.

**apples** 2, unpeeled, cored and quartered
**pear** 1, unpeeled, cored and quartered
**bananas** 2, peeled
**smooth peanut butter** 1 heaped tbsp
**crème fraîche** 150ml (¼ pint)
**ground cinnamon** 1 tsp

**1** Put the apples and pear through a juicer.

**2** Put the resulting juice with the bananas, peanut butter and crème fraîche into a blender or food processor and whizz until smooth.

**3** Serve with the cinnamon sprinkled on top.

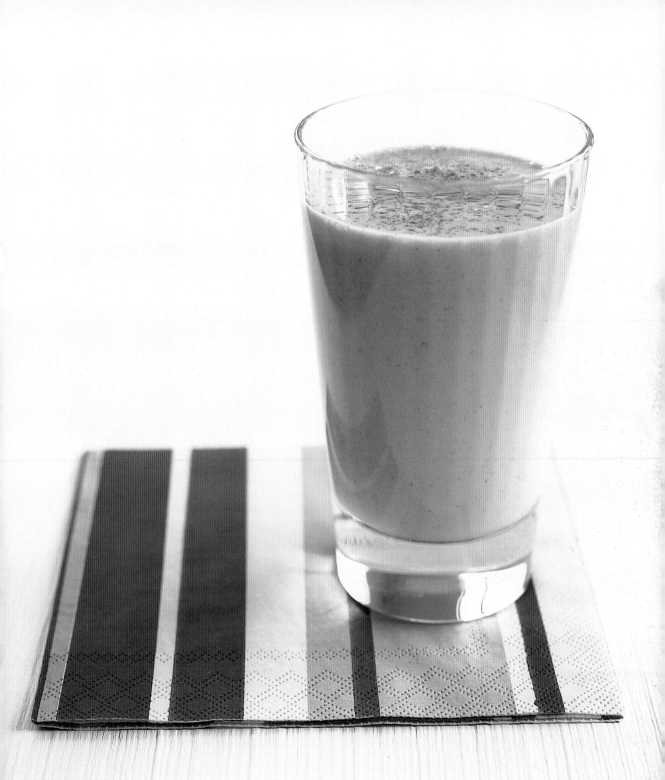

This juice is rich in potassium, pectin (soluble fibre) and natural healing enzymes. It contains vitamin C, calcium and traces of B vitamins. The tannins, powerful flavones and other aromatic compounds harboured in grapes combine to make them energizing and cancer-fighting – all this in a superjuice that tastes as great as it smells!

# peak performer

Never underestimate the power of pears! Few people realize the nutritional value that may be found in a ripe pear of any variety – and the juice adds a unique flavour to this recipe. Even just sniffing its wonderful aroma helps set the stage for a real 'feel-good' day. If you're feeling a bit sluggish, then the soluble fibre found in the pears and apples – together with the rich supply of natural sugars in grapes and pineapple – is just the thing to aid digestion and provide instant energy.

**black or white seedless grapes** 12

**pears** 4, unpeeled, uncored and quartered

**apples** 2, unpeeled, uncored and quartered

**pineapple** 2 slices, peeled and cored

**1** Put all the ingredients through a juicer.

## vital statistics

This punch is super-rich in vitamins A, C, E and B6 and folic acid, magnesium and potassium. It also contains some calcium and iron. The soluble fibre in apples and natural oils in mint have a wonderful effect on the entire digestive system, since they are soothing and provide a gentle laxative effect.

# green apple power punch

A zappy cleanser to start your day, the Green Apple Power Punch is ideal for stimulating the digestive system and replacing lost minerals following physical activity – on or off the sports field. Take this on an empty stomach and don't eat or drink anything else for half an hour to allow its natural fruit sugars do their work.

**sorrel leaves** 6

**dessert apples** 2 large Granny Smiths, unpeeled, uncored and quartered

**lime** 1, peeled (unless key lime) and halved

**mint** 1 sprig

**parsley** 1 handful of sprigs

**1** Put all the ingredients through a juicer.

# lychee, buttermilk and honey

If you've only ever had canned lychees in syrup in your local Chinese restaurant, then this smoothie will be a revelation. Fresh lychees are a totally different taste sensation. They have the most delicate flavour and are also a useful source of nutrients. Using buttermilk rather than yogurt or ordinary milk provides a different texture, as well as an unusual taste, to this energy-giving recipe.

**lychees** 10, peeled and stoned
**buttermilk** 125ml (4fl oz)
**runny honey** 3 tbsp
**redcurrants** 2 sprigs, to serve

1 Put the lychees into a blender or food processor and whizz until puréed.

2 Add the buttermilk and honey, and whizz again.

3 Remove the redcurrants from the sprigs and scatter them on top of the smoothie to serve.

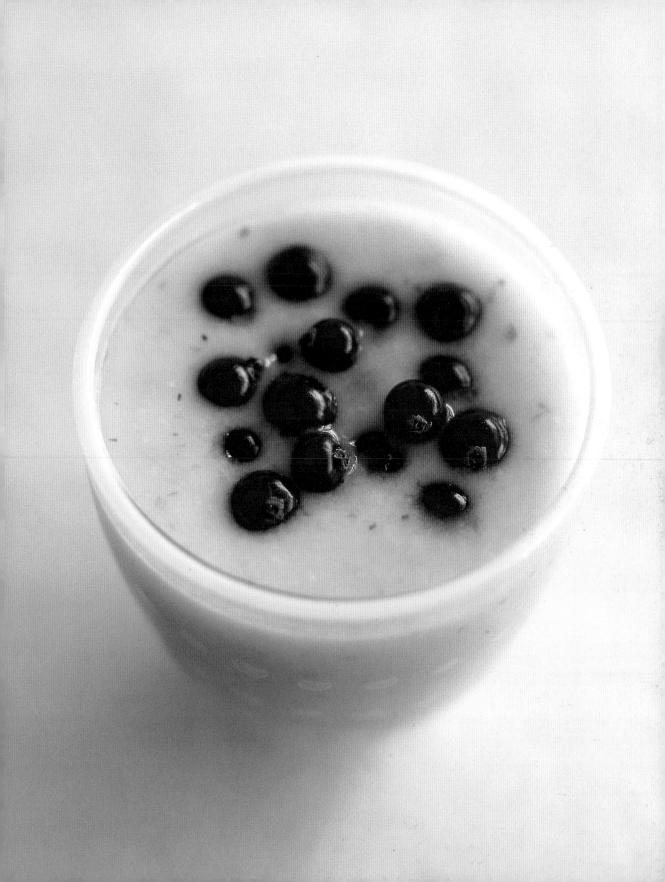

Papayas are rich in vitamin C, and they provide flavonoids, betacarotene and a surprisingly high amount of the essential mineral magnesium. The natural gingerols and zingiberenes in ginger boost the circulatory system and give an almost instant lift to your vitality.

# papaya and ginger refresher

If you want to 'ginger up' your vitality, then this is the drink for you. The ginger accentuates the delicious flavour of the papaya but also adds its own distinctive boost to this drink. This is a wonderful recipe for a lazy Sunday morning when you read the papers, and just the thing to have before your weekly treat of a real English breakfast. The digestive enzyme papain in the papaya is a great aid to the digestion of high-protein foods.

**papayas** 3, peeled and deseeded
**ground ginger** ½ tsp

1 Put the papayas into a blender or food processor with the ginger and whizz until smooth.

2 Dilute with water to your desired consistency.

3 Chill well before serving.

Live yogurt is an excellent source of calcium for strong and healthy bones, and the best source of the probiotic bacteria responsible for producing the essential B vitamins that nourish the nervous system and banish anxiety, stress and fatigue. Add the slow-release calories, the zinc from the pumpkin seeds and the mood-enhancing benefits of allspice, and you've got a great recipe for improved vitality.

# spiced smoothie

One of the most common causes of chronic fatigue is a deficiency of zinc, a mineral that is often in short supply in the convenience-food diet so many of us live on today. The extra zinc supplied by pumpkin seeds is often the first step on the road to feeling more vital and healthy. Lack of vitality is often caused by poor resistance and repeated infections such as flu, sore throats, coughs and colds. Regular consumption of live yogurt is a tremendous boost to the immune system, thanks to the beneficial bacteria it contains.

**natural live bio-yogurt** 300ml (½ pint)

**tahini** 1 tbsp

**ground allspice** ½ tsp

**milk** a little (optional), for thinning

**ice cubes**

**pumpkin seeds** 1 tsp

**1** Put the yogurt, tahini and allspice into a blender or food processor and whizz until combined.

**2** Thin with milk to your desired consistency.

**3** Serve over ice cubes with the pumpkin seeds scattered on top.

## vital statistics

It's the circulatory-enhancing effect of the zingiberenes and gingerols that make ginger such a powerful stimulant. The hotness of this spice is offset by the coolness of the yogurt, which supplies valuable quantities of calcium, some protein, B vitamins and the important probiotic bacteria that are so essential for immunity and good digestion. Add the mint, which is the best of all natural digestive aids, and you have a cooling and revitalizing smoothie.

# ginger it up

This spicy variation on the traditional Indian lassi will give an instant lift to anybody's flagging vitality. The stimulating effects of ginger, the beneficial bacteria in the yogurt and the digestive benefits of mint all work together to give your vitality a welcome lift just when you need one.

**natural live bio-yogurt** 250ml (9fl oz)

**fresh root ginger** 4cm (1½in) piece, peeled and grated

**mint** about 10 leaves, plus 4 small sprigs, to garnish

**sparkling mineral water** chilled, to taste

**1** Put the yogurt, ginger and mint leaves into a blender or food processor and whizz until smooth.

**2** Mix with the chilled sparkling mineral water to your desired consistency.

**3** Pour into glasses and serve with the mint sprigs floating on top.

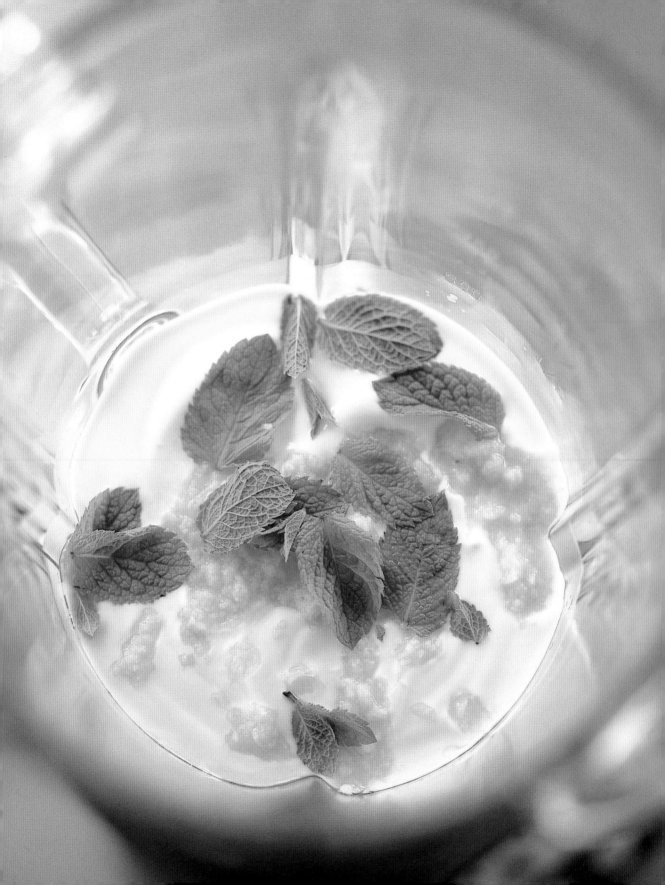

## vital statistics

For anyone who can't tolerate dairy milk, this recipe is just as good a vitality booster if you make it with soya milk. Dates are a key to the benefits of this drink and have been part of man's staple diet since 3000BC. Some varieties are an extremely rich source of iron, particularly Gondela from Sudan and Khidri from Riyadh. All dates are vitality foods thanks to their ease of digestion and instant energy.

# desert-island juice

Drinks made from milk have long been associated with growth, health and vitality. Milk is an excellent source of calcium, protein, B vitamins and energy from its natural lactose (milk sugar). It is, for most people, one of the most easily digestible of all foods. There are those who have an intolerance to lactose, and others have an allergy to milk protein. But for everyone else, milk – mixed here with health-boosting dates – is a great vitality drink.

**ready-to-eat dried dates** 8, stoned
**milk** 200ml (⅓ pint)
**coconut milk** 200ml (⅓ pint), or the equivalent in coconut cream diluted with hot water to the consistency of milk – about 4 heaped tsp

1 Cut the dates into 8 pieces each. Put into a small heatproof bowl and just cover with freshly boiled water.

2 Leave to soak for 10 minutes.

3 Purée the dates, with the water, in a small blender until completely smooth.

4 Heat the milk and coconut milk (or cream mixture).

5 Add the puréed dates.

6 Froth with a whisk or cappuccino wand and serve.

## vital statistics

Prunes are truly a majestic fruit. Hugely prized in France, where they originated, they have their own *appellation contrôlée*, Pruneaux d'Agen, just like the finest of wines. Weight for weight, prunes are by far the richest food source of protective antioxidants, and they provide a massive boost to natural resistance and vitality.

# hot and smooth prune

I've never managed to understand why the prune is the butt of so many jokes. Yes, it does contain a natural chemical called hydroxyphenylisatin that has a mild laxative effect. But prunes are far more than this, and combined here with live yogurt, their juice makes a surprisingly delicious and enjoyable revitalizing drink.

**prune juice** 450ml (16fl oz)
**natural thick-set live bio-yogurt** 2 tbsp

**1** Warm the prune juice gently in a saucepan.

**2** Pour into 2 mugs.

**3** Serve with the yogurt floating on top.

## vital statistics

Few people realize just how revitalizing live yogurt really is. As well as the easily available calories from the natural carbohydrate it contains, the millions of beneficial live bacteria have a profound effect on the immune system, boosting your resistance and enhancing the conversion of food into energy. Peanuts provide health-giving lignans, vitality-boosting monounsaturated fatty acids and a bonus of minerals and fibre.

# peanut-butter surprise

This may sound like a kid's milkshake, but it's great for adults, too. For some reason, to many people the very thought of peanut butter means bad health, piling on the pounds and something not to be eaten by sensible adults. Nothing could be further from the truth – especially if you choose organic, low-salt brands. The vitality boost from this drink comes from the combination of instant and slow-release energy.

**smooth peanut butter** 4 tbsp
**natural runny live bio-yogurt**
300ml (½ pint)
**milk** 150ml (¼ pint)
**runny honey** to serve (optional)

1 Put the peanut butter and about half the yogurt into a blender or food processor and whizz until blended.

2 Pour into a saucepan with the rest of the yogurt and the milk.

3 Warm, stirring continuously, until well combined, but don't boil it or you'll kill the good bacteria.

4 Serve in mugs or heatproof glasses. Drizzle with runny honey, if desired.

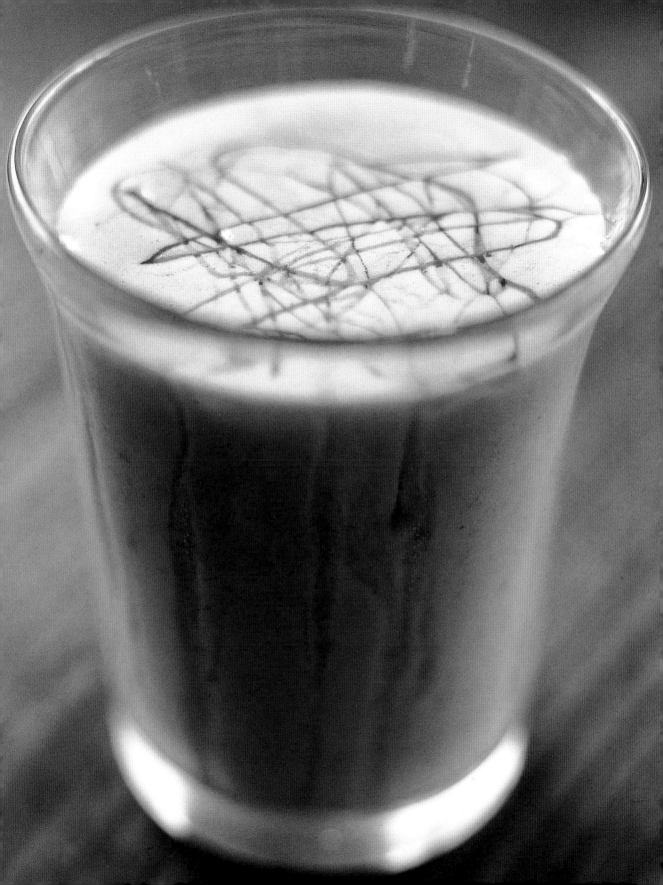

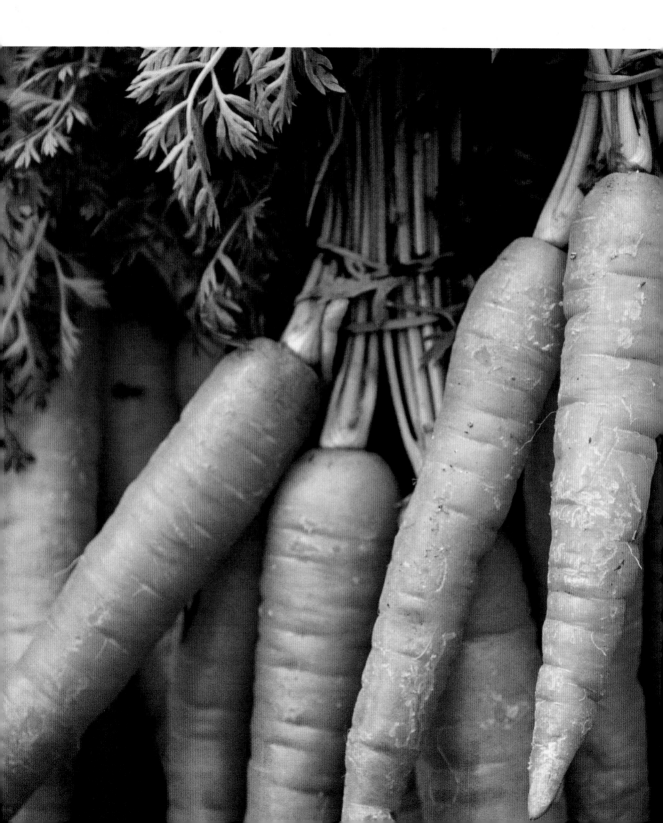

# immunity and protection

**H**ave you ever wondered why someone you know never catches the flu, never goes down with mystery viruses and travels all over the world without getting Delhi belly or Montezuma's revenge? They have a highly effective immune system. How did they get it? Well, it's partly nurture and partly nature. Inheriting the right genes from your parents gets you off to a good start, as does exposure to bacteria at an early age – this kick-starts the immune system and actually strengthens it in the long run. Yet, even with a strong genetic background, it is vital to eat a healthy diet rich in all the vitamins and minerals that help build strong immunity.

The body has its own natural defence mechanisms that protect it from infections and against the internal damage created by free radicals. This immune system depends on an adequate consumption of essential vitamins and minerals, a sufficient amount of natural protective plant chemicals and an adequate supply of antioxidants to mop up damaging free radicals.

But in order to function at its optimum level, the immune system also needs to be protected against antinutrients. High intakes of fats, sugars, alcohol, caffeine; exposure to heavy metals such as cadmium, lead and mercury; smoking and general atmospheric pollution... all these can compromise natural immunity and make disease more likely.

## Choose foods wisely

Unfortunately, the human body faces another obstacle to health in the form of food production. Due to modern intensive methods of farming and horticulture, including monocropping, intensive rearing, synthetic fertilizers, insecticides and pesticides, much food may be nutrient-deficient and contaminated with residues. Even a sensible diet of these foods may not supply the optimal nutrient needs of the immune system, so it is important to include regular amounts of high-nutrient foods in your diet. By altering food intake to increase the amount of beneficial nutrients, and choosing organic food whenever you can, it is possible to improve the effectiveness of natural resistance. An adequate consumption of good protein is essential, so opt for fish, poultry, lean meat, low-fat dairy products, cereals and legumes.

A selection of vitamin A- and betacarotene-rich foods should be eaten every day; a deficiency impairs immune responses, but only a small increase in consumption improves them. Carrots, spinach, sweet potatoes, melon and a small portion of liver a week is sufficient. Deficiencies of the vitamin B complex are known to interfere with natural immune responses. White fish, oily fish, poultry, spinach, peas, kidney beans, chickpeas, brown rice and bananas should all be eaten regularly. Citrus fruits and all fresh produce are needed to supply vitamin C, large amounts of which appear to increase levels of immunoglobulin, whereas deficiency causes a delayed reaction of the immune system.

Another reason for including large amounts of oily fish in the diet is their high content of vitamin D, which is also essential for the immune system. They are also rich suppliers of vitamin E, together with olive oil, nuts, avocados and wholegrain cereals.

One of the most common and least recognized nutrient deficiencies that affects the immune system is zinc deficiency. Shellfish, pumpkin seeds, lean beef and, best of all, oysters all contain this mineral. Essential fatty acids present in fish oils and cold-pressed safflower and linseed oils are also vital to the integrity of the body's defences.

Surprising but vital immune boosters are the natural probiotic bacteria that live in your gut – 2kg (4lb 8oz) if you're healthy. These come from fermented foods such as live or bio-yogurts, probiotic yogurt-like drinks or natural supplements. These good bugs not only improve your digestion but have a powerful strengthening effect on your natural defences. You need the good bugs to kill off the bad ones. Don't forget that whenever you are prescribed a course of antibiotics, you must eat live yogurt every day or take one of these probiotic supplements – this is because antibiotics kill the good bugs as well as the bad.

# immunity checklist

- Eat more oily fish for omega-3 fatty acids; poultry and lean meat for protein; spinach, sweet potatoes and carrots for betacarotene; chickpeas and wholegrain cereals for B vitamins and folic acid; olive oil, safflower oil, nuts, seeds and avocados for vitamin E; citrus fruits, cherries and berries for vitamin C and bioflavonoids; and low-fat dairy products for calcium and vitamin D.
- Consume less animal fat, sugar, alcohol, caffeine, highly processed carbohydrates and all processed, prepacked, ready-made foods.

Natural chemicals found in watercress make it specifically protective against lung cancer. Combined with the antibacterial, circulatory and cholesterol-lowering properties of onions, this is a salad that should be eaten regularly – particularly by anyone who smokes.

# green-and-white delight

There's more than visual appeal to this simple but powerfully immunity-boosting salad. Watercress belongs to the same valuable plant family as cabbages, broccoli and Brussels sprouts. It contains some iodine, lots of potassium and the strong mustard oil known as benzyl, which is an effective antibiotic.

**watercress** 1 large bunch
**white onions** 2, thinly sliced
**extra-virgin olive oil** 2 tbsp
**walnut oil** 1 tbsp

**1** Thoroughly wash the watercress – even if it's 'ready-washed'.

**2** Dry and pick off any very thick stalks.

**3** Put the watercress into a bowl, then lay the onion slices on top.

**4** Drizzle with both oil – and enjoy!

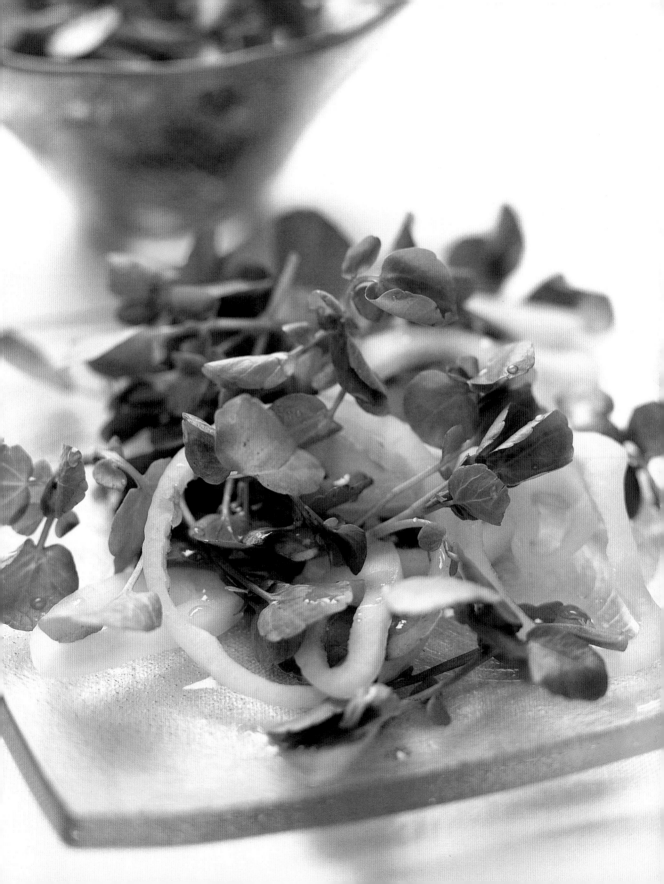

## vital statistics

This salad is packed with the protective isoflavones present in the beans. These natural phyto-oestrogens protect against breast cancer, osteoporosis and the uncomfortable symptoms of the menopause.

# savory fava salad

This instant, inexpensive meal is as full of health benefits as it is of good hearty flavour. All beans burst with nutrients, but the combination of broad beans, known as fava beans throughout the Mediterranean, and kidney beans contains more than most. Generally speaking, fresh is always best, but canned beans are more delicious than other preserved vegetables; just rinse them thoroughly to remove the salt.

**broad beans** about 500g (1lb 2oz), shelled fresh, cooked or canned, rinsed

**kidney beans** 400g can, rinsed

**spring onions** 4, finely chopped

**tomatoes** 3, coarsely chopped

**cucumber** 1, peeled and diced

**savory and thyme** 1 tbsp chopped

**herb vinaigrette** 7 tbsp extra-virgin olive oil, 3 tbsp herbal vinegar (*see* below), a dash of runny honey and Dijon mustard and freshly ground black pepper, whisked together

**crusty wholemeal bread** to serve

**Herbal vinegar**

**cider or white wine vinegar** best-quality

**herb of your choice**

**1** For the herbal vinegar for the vinaigrette, decant the vinegar into a bottle with a largish neck and an airtight stopper. Choose your herb leaves, petals or flowers (I prefer using a single herb), such as dill or fennel (good with fish), mint (wonderful with cold lamb, potato salad and in tabbouleh) or tarragon (brilliant with chicken or fish), or use peeled garlic cloves (which go with almost everything) or coriander seeds (great on bean salads, as here, or in coleslaw). Bruise gently in a mortar with a pestle or the back of a wooden spoon (seeds should be partially crushed). Put in the vinegar, stopper tightly and leave for 3 weeks or so before using.

**2** Put both beans, spring onions, tomatoes, cucumber and herbs into a large bowl.

**3** Add the herb vinaigrette and mix together well, then cover and leave for 30 minutes to allow the flavours to blend together.

**4** Serve with crusty wholemeal bread.

# viva españa bread salad

Nothing could be quicker, easier or more delicious than this typical Spanish salad, which I first ate at a hilltop cantina in the lovely mountain village of Frigiliana, in Andalucía. Followed by fresh fruit and a piece of cheese, it's an instant summer meal bursting with Mediterranean sunshine, but make it using only really ripe tomatoes and stale, coarse wholemeal or country bread.

**extra-virgin olive oil** 3 tbsp
**garlic** 2 cloves, chopped
**bread** 4 thick slices, crusts removed, cubed
**plum tomatoes** 6 ripe, roughly chopped
**red onion** 1, sliced
**lemon juice** 1 tbsp
**coarse sea salt** 1 pinch
**black pepper** freshly ground
**basil leaves** 1 handful, torn

**1** Heat the oil in a frying pan and fry the garlic and bread cubes, stirring, until the bread becomes crispy.

**2** Remove the bread cubes with a slotted spoon and drain on kitchen paper.

**3** Put the bread cubes into a bowl.

**4** Add the tomatoes, onion, lemon juice, salt, plenty of black pepper and the basil.

**5** Toss well and serve.

## vital statistics

All cabbages are rich sources of vitamin C and sulphur, a protective and antibacterial combination, and red cabbage also contains large amounts of betacarotene. The addition of live yogurt means a massive injection of beneficial bacteria, which play a vital role in natural immunity.

# caraway coleslaw

A traditional healing salad with a yogurt twist, this dish combines all the healing powers of cabbage with the digestive benefits of caraway seeds.

**red cabbage** ½ small, finely shredded
**white cabbage** ½ small, finely shredded
**dessert apple** 1 large, unpeeled, cored and coarsely grated
**seedless raisins** 1 handful
**natural live bio-yogurt** 1 small carton (about 125ml/4fl oz)
**unwaxed lemon** juice and grated rind of 1
**caraway seeds** 1 tsp
**black pepper** freshly ground, to taste

**1** Mix both the shredded cabbages with the apple. Add the raisins.

**2** Combine the yogurt with the lemon juice and rind. Mix into the cabbage mixture and stir thoroughly.

**3** Sprinkle the caraway seeds on top, and season with black pepper to taste.

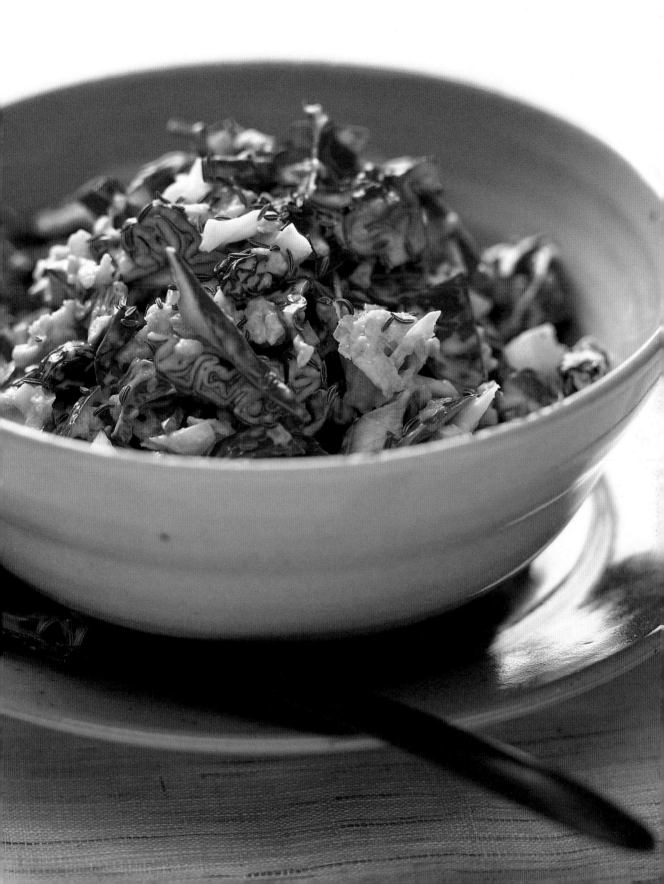

## vital statistics

This dish is rich in heart-protective omega-3 fatty acids from the anchovies and monounsaturated fat from the olive oil and garlic, with the added bonus of vitamin C from the lemon juice, tomatoes and parsley. Lemon balm has strong antiviral properties and is specifically protective against the cold-sore virus. It also helps over-active thyroid conditions.

# pasta melissa

Lemon balm (its Latin name is *Melissa*) is a remarkable herb, traditionally used as a heart relaxer and aid to wound healing. Its volatile oils, flavonoids and tannins also help fight depression, stress and indigestion. Looking at the rest of the ingredients, you might think this recipe can't possibly work, but it does – deliciously. It's one of my favourite quick mid-week suppers.

**anchovy fillets** 2 x 50g cans
**garlic** 2 cloves, chopped
**lemon** juice of 1
**extra-virgin olive oil** 4 tbsp
**spaghetti** 400g (14oz)
**lemon balm** 3 tbsp chopped
**tomatoes** 3 tbsp coarsely chopped
**parsley** 2 tbsp chopped

**1** Put the anchovy fillets, with some oil still clinging to them, into a mortar and crush with a pestle until they break down.

**2** Add the garlic and keep crushing.

**3** Remove to a medium-sized bowl, add the lemon juice and mix well.

**4** Slowly drizzle in the oil and mix well.

**5** Cook the pasta according to the packet instructions until al dente. Drain well.

**6** Stir in the anchovy and oil mixture.

**7** Add the lemon balm and mix again.

**8** Serve sprinkled with the tomato pieces and parsley.

## vital statistics

This dish is immensely rich in lycopene, one of the carotenoid family of natural chemicals that protect against heart disease and prostate cancer. Oregano, the essential Italian herb for all tomato recipes, is full of antibacterial volatile oils, which help ward off coughs, colds and other infections. Finally, the cheese contains valuable protein and masses of calcium.

# hot or cold italian bake

This combination of tomatoes, courgettes (or use thin slices of peeled marrow), oregano and Emmental cheese is equally delicious as a hot supper dish or served warm or cold as a salad to accompany a jacket potato, cold chicken or cold roast beef or lamb.

**extra-virgin olive oil** 2 tbsp

**onion** 1, finely chopped

**garlic** 2 cloves, finely chopped

**chopped tomatoes** 400g can

**courgettes** 4, thinly sliced

**fresh tomatoes** 4, thinly sliced

**oregano leaves** 2 tsp

**black pepper** freshly ground, to taste

**emmental cheese** 85g (3oz), grated

**1** Preheat the oven to 180°C/350°F/gas mark 4.

**2** Heat the oil in a saucepan and sweat the onion and garlic gently until softened but not browned.

**3** Add the canned chopped tomatoes and stir until warmed through.

**4** Tip the contents of the pan into an ovenproof dish and add a layer of courgettes, a layer of tomatoes, a sprinkle of oregano and some black pepper. Repeat until you've used all the tomatoes and courgettes.

**5** Cover with the grated cheese and bake for 30 minutes.

## vital statistics

This dish is low in saturated fats, yet rich in healthy monounsaturated fats and vitamin E. It provides heart, lung and skin protection, some good fibre and plenty of calcium and B vitamins. Oregano is a powerful antibacterial, and the linalool in basil relieves acne.

# mediterranean rarebit

This colourful, tasty Mediterranean treat is a feast for all the senses. The green and red of basil and tomato set against the creamy white cheese make it inviting to the eye, while the pungent, unmistakable odour of oregano and the delicate scent of basil create an explosion of aromas and flavours.

**wholemeal baguette** 1, cut into 2.5cm (1in) slices

**garlic** 2 cloves, halved

**avocado** 1 small, peeled and stoned

**parsley** 1 small bunch, finely chopped

**tomatoes** 3–4, sliced thinly enough to cover each slice of bread

**goats' cheese** sliced as for the tomatoes

**dried oregano** about 2 tsp

**basil leaves** as many as you have slices of bread

**1** Preheat the grill to high.

**2** Toast the bread slices gently on both sides. Rub one side with the cut side of a garlic clove half.

**3** Mash the avocado with the parsley and spread thinly on the toasted bread.

**4** Top the bread with the tomato slices, then the goats' cheese slices.

**5** Sprinkle with oregano.

**6** Place under the grill for about 5 minutes or until the cheese starts to run. Add a basil leaf to each slice and grill for 1 minute only.

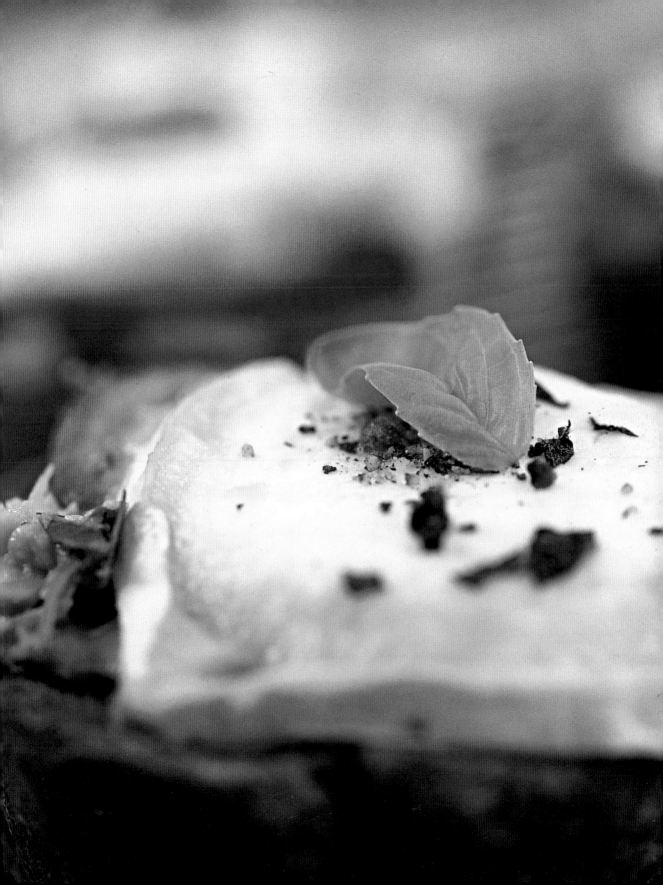

## vital statistics

This dish provides lots of protein, phosphorus, potassium and folic acid, and useful amounts of minerals, B vitamins and vitamin C.

# baked fish with tomato, onion and garlic

This recipe comes from my favourite fishmonger, David Blagdon. In spite of fears about ever more polluted oceans, deep-water fish remains one of the healthiest foods in the world – as long as you don't overcook it. In addition to tasting great, this dish is a healthy choice due to its low fat content, and thanks to the tomatoes, onions and garlic, it helps prevent heart disease into the bargain.

**fresh fish** such as halibut, hake or cod, 4 x 175g (6oz) fillets

**tomatoes** 4, finely chopped

**onion** 1 large, finely chopped

**garlic** 2 cloves, finely chopped

**black pepper** freshly ground, to taste

**extra-virgin olive oil** 2 dessertspoons

**1** Preheat the oven to 200°C/400°F/gas mark 6.

**2** Tear off 4 pieces of foil large enough to make a loose parcel around each fillet.

**3** Mix the tomatoes, onion and garlic together and spread a layer in the centre of each piece of foil. Put the fish on the mixture and sprinkle what's left on top of each fillet. Season with black pepper and a drizzle of the oil.

**4** Wrap each fillet into a loose parcel. Bake in an ovenproof dish for 20 minutes.

# salmon maundy

Chervil, tarragon and chives are three of the strongest protective herbs around, and this simple dish contains them all. It also has real visual appeal, which makes for a great starter or, in more substantial quantities, a perfect light lunch or supper.

**herb vinaigrette** 4 tbsp (*see* page 72)

**chives** 3 tbsp finely snipped

**tarragon leaves** 1 tbsp coarsely chopped

**chervil** 2 tbsp coarsely chopped

**basmati rice** 250g (9oz), cooked, cooled and chilled

**salmon fillet** 250g (9oz), poached and chilled

**tomatoes** 2 large, roughly chopped

**red pepper** 1 large, cored, deseeded and thinly sliced

**black pepper** freshly ground

**1** Mix the herb vinaigrette and most of the herbs together, then pour over the rice.

**2** Flake the salmon, discarding any skin, and stir into the rice along with the tomatoes and red pepper.

**3** Add a generous grind of black pepper and stir again.

**4** Sprinkle with the remaining herbs.

## vital statistics

This meal is rich in protein, B vitamins and the minerals you'd expect from deep-water sea fish. The particular protective value of capers comes from their content of capric acid. This substance increases the flow of gastric juices, which stimulates appetite and makes digestion more efficient, ensuring that all the protective nutrients in the fish are better absorbed.

# caperbility fish

I've never understood why John Dory is probably near the bottom of the list of popular fish. Since being introduced by my neighborhood fishmonger to this extremely ugly but perfectly textured and wonderfully flavoured fish, I have become quite the fan. Enjoy this protective dish.

**john dory** 4 fillets
**butter** 4 generous knobs
**sprigs** 4 sprigs
**dry white wine** 1½ glasses
**capers** 1 tbsp, rinsed
**black pepper** freshly ground

1 Preheat the oven to 180°C/350°F/gas mark 4.

2 Place the fish fillets on a large sheet of foil in an ovenproof dish.

3 Put a knob of butter and a sprig of dill on each fillet.

4 Pour over the wine.

5 Scatter the capers over the fish.

6 Season generously with black pepper.

7 Pull the foil over the fish and secure firmly at the top and sides.

8 Bake for 20 minutes.

## vital statistics

This low-fat, high-protein fish dish is an excellent source of minerals, especially iodine. Low-fat and cholesterol-free, this is a heart- and circulatory-protective meal. Bergamot contains heart-protective and cancer-preventing essential oils, especially limonene and linalyl, which aid digestion and relaxation. Myrtle leaves are generally tonic and antiseptic, and they protect the urinary system from infection.

# earl's fish

The distinctive flavour of bergamot is most commonly associated with Earl Grey tea, but it also combines brilliantly with fish, particularly the blander varieties. Here, it is used in combination with the exotic spiciness of myrtle leaves. This recipe is equally suitable for hake, cod and white tuna – the perfect dish to set before a king, let alone an earl.

**unsalted butter** 60g (2¼oz)
**extra-virgin olive oil** 2 tbsp
**swordfish** 4 steaks
**bergamot leaves** 1 tbsp chopped
**rosé wine** 1 glass
**myrtle leaves** 8 whole
**black pepper** freshly ground, to taste

**1** Melt the butter with the oil in a large frying pan.

**2** Fry the fish with the bergamot leaves for about 12 minutes, turning once, until just crisp on each side.

**3** Remove the fish with a slotted fish slice, leaving the juices in the pan.

**4** Turn the heat up. Add the wine, then the myrtle leaves, and boil briskly for 1 minute.

**5** Pour the sauce over the fish, season with the pepper, and serve.

## vital statistics

The egg noodles in this dish provide carbohydrates and some protein while the garlic and peppers supply antioxidants, carotenoids and vitamin C, making this an instant protector of the heart and immune system. This recipe has the added bonus of the antibacterial and antifungal properties of marigold, the anti-inflammatory oils in fresh coriander and the digestive benefits of tarragon.

# summer noodles

Everyone knows how good it is to wake up in summer with the sun streaming through the windows. This recipe imparts that warm feeling, whatever the weather. Sunny, orange marigold petals combined with the fresh green of tarragon and coriander give an added lease of life to noodles.

**egg noodles** 250g (9oz)

**rapeseed oil** 2 tbsp

**garlic** 2 cloves, chopped

**yellow pepper** 1 large, cored, deseeded and very thinly sliced

**unwaxed lemon** juice and grated rind of ½

**fresh coriander** 1 tbsp chopped

**tarragon** 1 tbsp chopped

**marigold petals** 1 tbsp

**garlic oil** 1 tbsp best-quality shop-bought or *see* page 244 and use a peeled garlic clove in place of the rosemary

**1** Cook the noodles according to the packet instructions until just tender.

**2** Heat the oil in a large wok or frying pan and stir-fry the garlic and yellow pepper for 1 minute.

**3** Add the noodles and stir-fry for 3 minutes.

**4** Stir in the lemon juice and zest and rind and herbs, and continue stir-frying for 1 minute.

**5** Add the garlic oil, mix in thoroughly and serve.

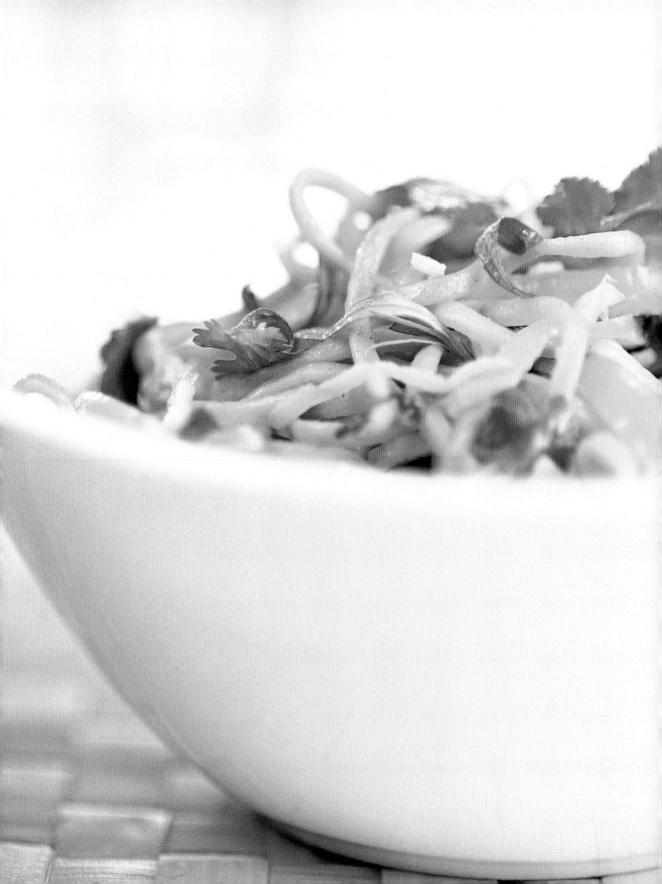

## vital statistics

True peppermint (*Mentha piperita*) is rich in essential oils, especially menthol and menthone. It also contains cancer-fighting limonene and is a valuable source of carotenes. As well as protecting the digestive system, peppermint is a powerful antiviral. The unusual addition of hyssop – rich in many volatile oils, especially hyssopine, and the expectorant marubiine – makes this recipe good protection against coughs, colds and flu.

# posh hyssop hotpot

Adding mint to lamb stems from the days when most sheep were eaten as mutton, and meat was higher in fat than modern cuts. Though the digestive benefits of mint are as important as its flavour, few people think of its medicinal qualities. The unique taste of this recipe also depends on the parsley, lemon juice and spices, which naturally give it even greater nutritional value.

**rapeseed or groundnut oil** 2 tbsp

**scrag end of lamb** 1kg (2lb 4oz), cut into serving pieces

**onion** 1 large, thinly sliced

**vegetable stock** 400ml (14fl oz) – *see* page 396 or use a good stock cube or bouillon powder

**bouquet garni** 1 bunch parsley, mint and hyssop, tied together with string

**lemon** juice of 1

**fresh root ginger** 1 tsp grated

**freshly grated nutmeg and ground cloves** 1 generous pinch each

**1** Preheat the oven to 180°C/350°F/gas mark 4.

**2** Heat the oil in a large, flameproof casserole dish and fry the meat, browning it all over.

**3** Add the onion and fry gently for 2 minutes.

**4** Stir in all the remaining ingredients.

**5** Cover the casserole, transfer to the oven and cook for 2 hours.

## vital statistics

The combination of the sulphurous allicin from garlic and the powerful antiseptic thymol from thyme (it's in the pink mouthwash you get at the dentist) offsets the slightly higher animal-fat content in the beef. Super-rich in protein, betacarotene and lycopene, which offers extra heart protection, this dish is also an excellent source of easily absorbed iron.

# beef gaulloise

While the avoidance of red meat may be of benefit to those suffering from specific illnesses – high blood pressure, gout, raised cholesterol levels or heart disease – modest amounts of best-quality organic lean beef make a valuable contribution to the diet. The typical Gallic flavour of this casserole is redolent of holidays in France; just inhaling its aroma is sure to lift the spirits.

**extra-virgin olive oil** 30ml (1fl oz)

**garlic** 2 cloves, chopped

**lean chuck steak** 750g (1lb 10oz), cubed

**chopped tomatoes** 400g can

**pitted black olives** 75g (2³⁄₄oz)

**red pepper** 1 small, cored, deseeded and thinly sliced

**thyme** 1 sprig fresh or 1 tsp dried

**red wine** 1–2 glasses, to taste

1 Preheat the oven to 150°C/300°F/gas mark 2.

2 Heat the oil in a flameproof casserole dish and sauté the garlic gently.

3 Add the meat and fry until browned all over.

4 Add all of the remaining ingredients, including the juice from the tomatoes and enough red wine to cover the meat.

5 Cover the casserole, transfer to the oven and cook for about 2 hours.

## vital statistics

An apple a day may keep the doctor away, according to the proverb, but in truth it should be two apples, since they will supply sufficient fibre and natural plant chemicals to reduce cholesterol and blood pressure. Add the digestive and antiseptic volatile oils in the mint and the antibacterial properties of cicely for an all-round protective sweet.

# cicely surprise

Nothing could be simpler than this delicious variation on traditional baked apples. The natural combination of mint and apple is enhanced by the intriguing hint of aniseed that is imparted by sweet cicely. Together with the added sweetness and succulence of the honey and butter, these herbs create a beguiling mixture of fragrance and flavour.

**dessert apples** 4
**mint leaves** 8
**sweet cicely leaves** 1 tsp finely chopped
**runny honey** 4 tsp
**butter** 4 very small knobs

**1** Preheat the oven to 180°C/350°F/gas mark 4.

**2** Core the apples and discard each core, but ensure that the bottom of each fruit remains intact.

**3** Place each apple on a large square of foil and fill with mint leaves, a pinch of cicely, a teaspoon of honey and a knob of butter.

**4** Wrap each apple securely in its foil.

**5** Bake in the oven for 20–30 minutes or until soft. (This recipe also works brilliantly on a barbecue.)

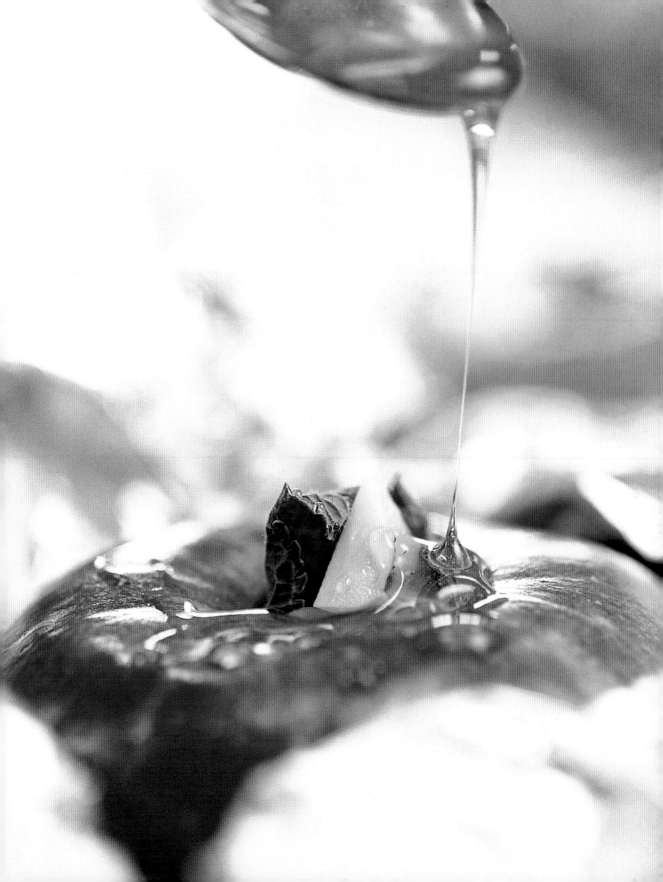

Plenty of calcium and vitamin D from full-fat milk makes this dish a good bone protector. Borage is a useful sick-room herb, because it reduces fevers and is soothing to the whole respiratory tract. It is also mildly diuretic and helps reduce fluid retention.

# moorish rice pudding

A better-than-average rice pudding that not only tastes good, but does you good, too. For a bit of extra dash, sprinkle a few pure, deep-blue borage flowers on top. This wonderful plant was much revered by the Moors in southern Spain, where it originates. Its heath benefits are listed above, however, be aware that it contains a toxic alkaloid and therefore it should not be eaten on a regular basis.

**full-fat milk** 500ml (18fl oz)
**borage leaves** 1 tsp shredded
**coriander seeds** 2 pinches crushed
**pudding rice** 60g (2¼oz)
**dried apricots** 75g (2¾oz), chopped into small pieces
**brown sugar** 1 tbsp

**1** Preheat to 150°C/300°F/gas mark 2.

**2** Put the milk, borage leaves and coriander into a saucepan. Bring slowly to the boil, then turn the heat off and leave until cool.

**3** Strain the milk and pour into an ovenproof dish with the remaining ingredients.

**4** Transfer to the oven and cook for 2 hours, stirring occasionally during the first 45 minutes.

**5** Serve hot or cold.

## vital statistics

Elderflowers are traditionally used for the prevention and treatment of respiratory infections. They are also helpful for catarrh, hayfever and children's ear infections. In combination with mint, they are also useful for the relief of flu and its symptoms. Elder is reputedly a good anti-inflammatory, thanks to its content of ursolic acid, so it also helps relieve arthritis and rheumatism.

# flowery rhubarb delight

Whether you eat the rhubarb hot or cold, the addition of the yogurt sauce makes for a delightful combination. The delicate, scented taste of elderflower contrasts with the more astringent flavour of rhubarb, its acidity tempered beautifully by the creamy yogurt. You can gather elderflowers for free from any hedgerow, but don't plant a tree in your garden unless you want a forest full!

**rhubarb** 750g (1lb 10oz), cut into 2cm (3/4in) pieces

**brown sugar** 2 tbsp, or to taste

**fresh elderflowers** 1 handful, well washed

**natural live bio-yogurt** 600ml carton

**mint leaves** 4 chopped, plus 4 whole to decorate

**ground cinnamon** 1 tsp

**unwaxed lemon** grated rind of ½

**1** Put the rhubarb and sugar into a large saucepan with just enough water to cover.

**2** Tie the elderflowers in a piece of kitchen muslin and add to the rhubarb.

**3** Cover and bring slowly to the boil, then turn the heat down and simmer for 10–15 minutes until cooked, stirring occasionally. Remove the bag of elderflowers.

**4** Whisk the yogurt, chopped mint, cinnamon and lemon rind together.

**5** Serve the rhubarb covered with the flavoured yogurt and decorated with the whole mint leaves.

## vital statistics

This dish is designed for prevention and protection. Cabbage is rich in antibacterial sulphur and cancer-fighting thiocyanates, and potatoes provide vitamin C.

# cabbage soup with gammon

Cabbage has been the medicine of the poor since a pot was first hung over a fire in prehistoric times. Of all the vegetables, cabbage and its relatives must be regarded as among the most important for their medicinal value. This soup also provides a good dose of protein from the gammon and immunity-enhancing carotenoids from the stock.

**gammon** 300g (10½oz), fat removed, cubed

**extra-virgin olive oil** 150ml (¼ pint)

**red onions** 2, finely chopped

**vegetable stock** 1.4 litres (2½ pints) – *see* page 396 or use a good stock cube or bouillon powder

**potatoes** 300g (10½oz), peeled and cubed

**savoy cabbage** 500g (1lb 2oz), finely shredded

**noodles or spaghettini** 200g (7oz)

**Beetroot floaters**

**wholemeal flour** 150g (5½oz)

**free-range egg** 1

**raw beetroot** 100g (3½oz), freshly grated

**fresh horseradish** 1 tsp freshly grated

**black pepper** freshly ground

1 Heat a frying pan and dry-fry the gammon. Set aside.

2 Heat 4 tablespoons of the oil in a saucepan and sweat the onions gently for about 10 minutes until soft.

3 Add the stock and potatoes and simmer until the potatoes are just tender.

4 Meanwhile, for the floaters, beat the flour into the egg and season with black pepper. Squeeze out all the moisture from the beetroot. Mix with the horseradish. Flatten walnut-sized balls to 1cm (½in) thick.

5 Whizz the stock mixture in a food processor or blender – or use a hand blender – until smooth. Return to the pan and bring back to a simmer. Add the cabbage and cook for 5 minutes. Stir in the gammon and noodles or spaghettini and cook for 3–4 minutes until al dente.

6 Meanwhile, coat the floaters in the batter. Shallow-fry gently in the remaining oil for 3 minutes on each side. Serve on the soup.

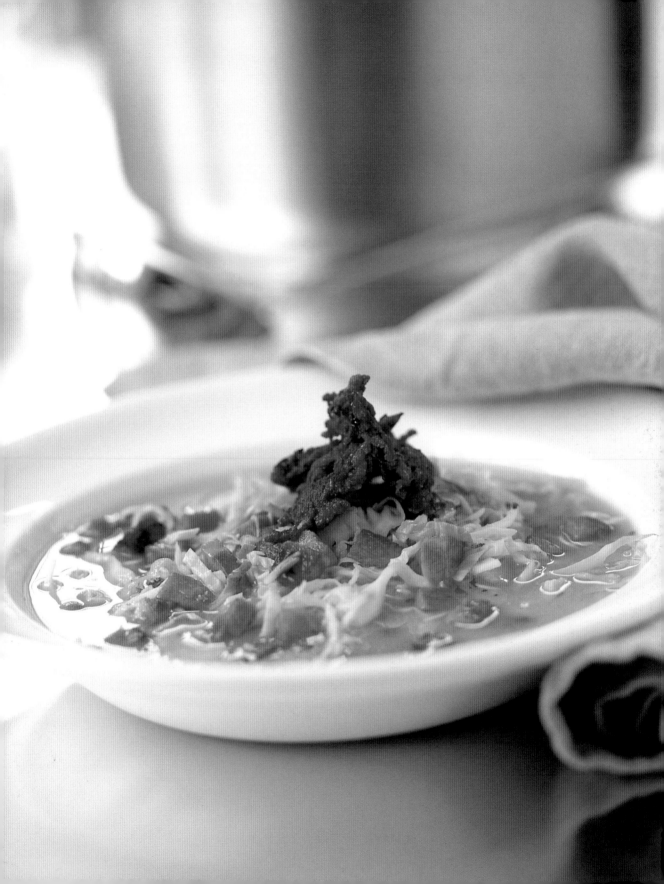

This soup will help protect the lungs and fight chest infections. Onions offer antiviral and antibacterial protection. Parsley, a natural diuretic, aids the natural cleansing process.

# white-onion soup

Onions have a long tradition in folk medicine, particularly for helping the body overcome the effects of chest infections. In this recipe, this healing property is combined with the protective essential oils from bay leaves, thyme and rosemary to make a delicious and health-giving, flavour-packed soup.

**unsalted butter** 55g (2oz)

**white spanish onions** 500g (1lb 2oz), very finely sliced

**plain flour** 3 tbsp

**full-fat milk** 1 litre (1³/₄ pints)

**bay leaves** 4

**peppercorns** 10, slightly crushed

**bouquet garni** 3 sprigs each parsley, thyme and rosemary, tied together with string, or a good commercial bouquet garni bag

**flat-leaf parsley** 1 bunch, finely chopped, to garnish

**1** Melt the butter over a very low heat.

**2** Add the onions. Stir until thoroughly coated, then cover and leave to sweat gently for 10 minutes.

**3** Sift in the flour and cook for another 5 minutes, stirring continuously.

**4** Pour in the milk and add the bay leaves, peppercorns and bouquet garni.

**5** Simmer very gently for about 10 minutes until the onions are quite soft.

**6** Remove the bay leaves and bouquet garni, and strain out the peppercorns.

**7** Serve garnished with the chopped parsley.

## vital statistics

This is a soup to help fight bacteria. Garlic contains powerful antibacterial substances, and oregano adds antiseptic thymol. Eggs provide health-giving B vitamins.

# bread and garlic soup

There are many variations of this soup throughout Spain, and to judge from the number I've tried, every family must have its own favourite recipe. This is mine. If garlic's potency puts you off, take heart: cooking it this way seems to prevent the residual garlic breath, so be brave and give it a try if you want a bowlful of super-immunity.

**olive oil** 5 tbsp

**garlic** 1 head, separated into cloves, finely chopped

**wholemeal breadcrumbs** 85g (3oz)

**vegetable stock** 1.4 litres (2½ pints) – see page 396 or use a good stock cube or bouillon powder

**oregano** ½ handful fresh or 2 generous pinches dried

**free-range eggs** 4, beaten

**Herb croûtons**

**wholemeal breadcrumbs** 85g (3oz)

**soft herbs** such as mint, parsley, sorrel, coriander or basil, 2 tsp finely chopped

**free-range egg** 1 small, beaten

**extra-virgin olive oil** 3 tbsp

**1** Heat the olive oil in a large saucepan and sweat the garlic gently, covered, for 3 minutes.

**2** Add the breadcrumbs, stock and oregano to the pan.

**3** Keep covered and simmer for 2 minutes, adding more stock if the mixture gets too thick.

**4** Add the eggs to the pan and simmer very gently for 2 more minutes.

**5** Meanwhile, for the herb croûtons, mix the breadcrumbs with the soft herbs. Form into balls about the size of an acorn, then flatten slightly. Dip into the beaten egg and drain.

**6** Heat the extra-virgin olive oil in a frying pan until smoking slightly and fry the croûtons until pale golden – about 2 minutes.

**7** Serve the croûtons with the soup.

## vital statistics

There are lots of anti-cancer and immunity-boosting phytochemicals in watercress. Antibacterial properties are found in garlic, and there are wonderful chest- and heart-protective effects from the onion.

# cress and chorizo

The first hospital in the world was built by Hippocrates, who chose a site by a stream flowing with pure spring water just so that he could grow watercress for his patients. In 460BC, this Greek father of modern medicine had already described the protective and immunity-boosting properties of watercress. Combining it with garlic and the chilli in the sausage, makes for an instantly comforting and strengthening soup.

**unsalted butter** 10g (¼oz)

**chorizo sausage** 150g (5½oz), thinly sliced

**onion** 1, thinly sliced

**garlic** 1 large clove, flattened with the blade of a large knife and finely sliced

**plain flour** 1 heaped tbsp

**vegetable stock** 1 litre (1¾ pints) – *see* page 396 or use a good stock cube or bouillon powder

**watercress** 1 large bunch, thick stalks removed

**crème fraîche** about 350ml (12fl oz)

**1** Melt the butter in a large saucepan and fry the chorizo gently until crisp – about 10 minutes. Remove and set aside.

**2** Add the onion and garlic and sauté gently, stirring continuously, until soft and golden.

**3** Sprinkle on the flour, stir well and cook for another 2 minutes, again stirring continuously.

**4** Pour in the stock and bring to the boil, stirring.

**5** Tip in the watercress and crème fraîche, stir well and simmer for 2 minutes.

**6** Whizz in a food processor or blender – or use a hand blender – until smooth.

**7** Tip in the chorizo, stir and leave to stand off the heat for 2 minutes before serving.

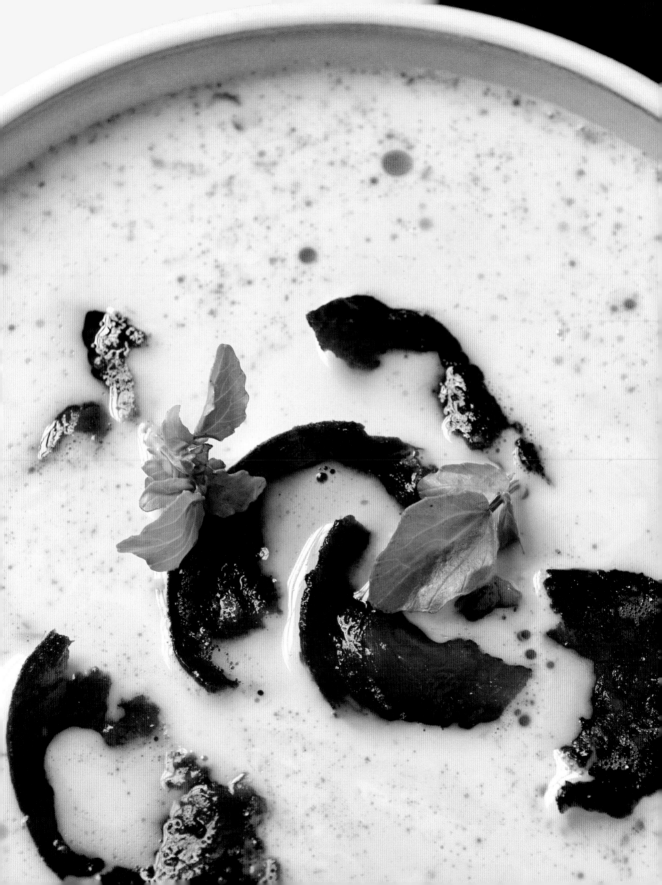

# vital statistics

Watercress contains antibacterial mustard oils, lots of betacarotene and a phytochemical that protects the cells of lung tissue against the carcinogenic effects of smoking.

# creamy watercress soup

In addition to having a wonderful peppery flavour, watercress is one of the most important immunity protectors you can eat. If you are a smoker, eat this soup twice a week, because it may well reduce your chances of lung cancer. There's an additional benefit from the protective probiotic bacteria in live yogurt. It is well known that these 'good bugs' are not only a part of the body's natural defences, but they also release specific chemicals that enhance the effectiveness of the immune system.

**unsalted butter** 100g (3½oz)

**spring onions** 4 large, thinly sliced

**watercress** 1 large bunch or bag – about 350g (12oz)

**vegetable stock** 1 litre (1¾ pints) – *see* page 396 or use a good stock cube or bouillon powder

**bouquet garni** 3 sprigs each parsley, thyme and rosemary, tied together with string, or a good commercial bouquet garni bag

**natural live bio-yogurt** 200ml (⅓ pint)

**herb croûtons** (*see* page 95), to serve

**1** Melt the butter in a large saucepan and sweat the spring onions gently for 3 minutes.

**2** Pull the leaves off any thick watercress stalks; discard the thicker stalks.

**3** Add the watercress to the pan and stir briskly for 1 minute.

**4** Add the stock and bouquet garni.

**5** Simmer for 10 minutes. Remove the bouquet garni.

**6** Whizz in a food processor or blender – or use a hand blender – until smooth. Return to the pan.

**7** Add the yogurt and stir thoroughly.

**8** Serve hot with the herb croûtons.

## vital statistics

This soup provides protection against colds and flu. Root vegetables offer a mineral boost, while beans and peas provide natural plant hormones. Finally, leeks add protective phytochemicals.

# welsh minestrone with rice and leeks

The Roman emperor Nero used to eat leeks every day to protect his voice. It's no wonder that this vegetable is the national emblem of Wales, a nation renowned for its singing. When coughs, colds, flu and sore throats abound, nothing could be better than this thick cornucopia of germ-fighting nutrients. What's more, it tastes terrific.

**extra-virgin olive oil** 3 tbsp

**onions** 3 Welsh or 1 ordinary onion, chopped

**leeks** 2, thinly sliced

**mixed root vegetables** 300g (10½oz), peeled unless organic and finely diced

**vegetable stock** 1.2 litres (2 pints) – *see* page 396 or use a good stock cube or bouillon powder

**long-grain rice** 100g (3½oz)

**peas** 100g (3½oz), fresh or frozen

**green beans** 100g (3½oz), cut into 2cm (¾in) slices

**1** Heat the oil in a large saucepan and sweat the onions and leeks gently for 5 minutes.

**2** Add the diced vegetables and stir until thoroughly coated with oil.

**3** Pour in the stock and rice, and bring to the boil, then turn the heat down and simmer for 15 minutes.

**4** Add the peas and beans and continue simmering until tender.

This soup will strengthen the immune system. Pak choi contains protective thiocyanates and large amounts of betacarotene for good cell health.

# chinese pak choi and chicken

Pak choi is another member of the cabbage family that offers good all-round protection from germs. The good news is that this tasty vegetable is now widely available; it is also easy to prepare. When combined with the immunity-boosting spring onions, garlic and chicken stock in this recipe, it creates a power-packed supersoup that provides a real lift to your system.

**spring onions** 6 large

**rapeseed oil** 4 tbsp

**garlic** 2 cloves, flattened with the blade of a large knife

**chicken stock** 1.2 litres (2 pints) – see page 396 or use a good stock cube or bouillon powder

**chicken breasts** 2, skinned and finely shredded along the grain of the flesh

**pak choi** 4 heads, thick stalks removed and reserved, leaves finely chopped

**chinese noodles or vermicelli** 150g (5½oz) (optional)

**tamari or light soy sauce** 1 tsp

1 Chop the white parts of 4 of the spring onions very finely; cut the others lengthways almost to the root and reserve.

2 Heat the oil very gently in a saucepan and sweat the chopped spring onions and garlic for just 2 minutes.

3 Pour in the stock. Bring slowly to a simmer and remove the garlic.

4 Continuing to simmer, add the chicken and pak choi stalks, and cook for 10 minutes until the chicken is almost tender.

5 Remove the pak choi stalks.

6 Add the pak choi leaves, noodles or vermicelli, if using, and tamari or soy sauce. Simmer for 5 minutes.

7 Serve with the reserved spring onions floating on the top.

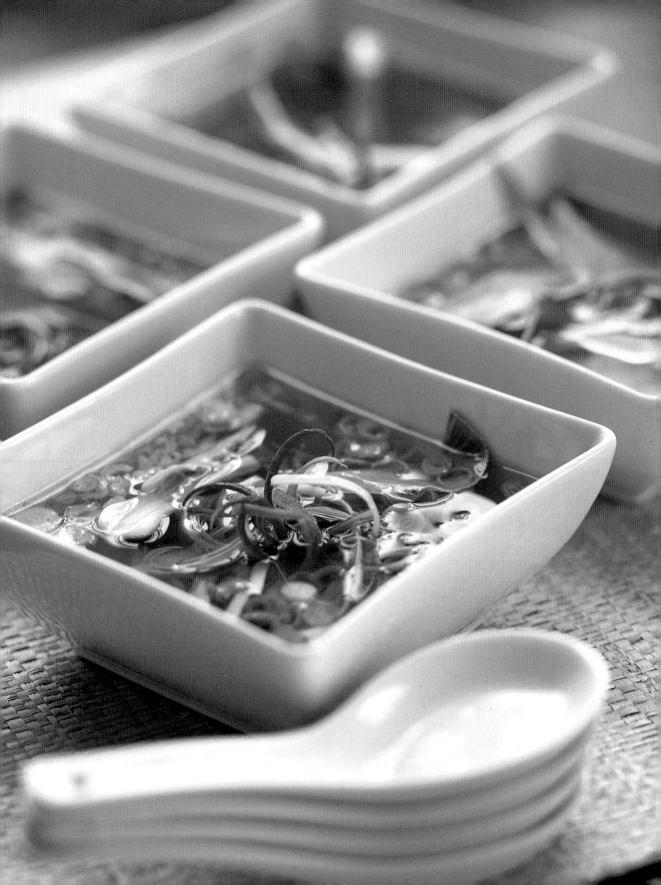

## vital statistics

This soup will aid in the body's continual fight against infection. Chard is an amazing source of betacarotenes, while chillies contain capsaicin, which stimulates the circulation.

# chicken, chilli, chard and noodles

You'll obtain plenty of health benefits here from the traditional immunity-strengthening properties of chicken soup. In addition to the health-promoting benefits of chard and chilli, the egg noodles provide a little iron and easily absorbed energy – always important in the body's fight against infection.

**extra-virgin olive oil** 3 tbsp

**onion** 1 large, very finely chopped

**red chilli** 1 , deseeded and very finely chopped

**chicken stock** 1.2 litres (2 pints) – *see* page 396 or use a good stock cube or bouillon powder

**chard** 150g (5½oz), stalks torn from the leaves

**egg noodles** 250g (9oz)

**1** Heat the oil in a large saucepan and sweat the onion and chilli gently for 5 minutes.

**2** Add the stock and bring to the boil, then turn the heat down and simmer for 10 minutes.

**3** Strain into a clean saucepan.

**4** Slice the chard stalks very thinly, add to the pan and simmer for 10 minutes.

**5** Tear the chard leaves roughly and add to the pan with the noodles.

**6** Simmer until the noodles are tender – usually not more than 3 minutes.

## vital statistics

This soup is great for fortifying general immunity. Duck is rich in body-building protein, protective enzymes and B vitamins, while bay leaves provide cineole and laurenolide, essential oils that help fight respiratory infections.

# duck soup with prunes

Duck, like chicken, is a delicious source of a whole host of vitamins and minerals. The unusual addition of prunes makes this soup an extremely high source of protective antioxidants. The prunes' slight sweetness is balanced by the parsley, thyme and rosemary, which also provide beneficial essential oils.

**duck** 1 cooked carcass, some flesh still attached, but with all the skin and visible fat removed

**bay leaves** 2

**bouquet garni** 3 sprigs each parsley, thyme and rosemary, tied together with string, or a good commercial bouquet garni bag

**onion** 1 large, finely chopped

**carrots** 2 large, trimmed and peeled unless organic, coarsely chopped

**celery** 2 sticks, coarsely chopped

**peppercorns** 10

**vegetable stock** up to 1.4 litres (2½ pints) – see page 396 or use a good stock cube or bouillon powder

**prunes** 200g (7oz), stoned (or dried apricots, if preferred)

**1** Put all of the ingredients, except for the prunes (or apricots), including 1 litre (1¾ pints) of the stock, into a large saucepan.

**2** Bring to the boil, then turn the heat down and simmer for an hour. Strain into a bowl.

**3** Set the duck aside. Discard the bouquet garni and push some of the vegetables through a sieve into the stock, depending on how thick you like the soup. Add the remaining stock at this stage to give the quantity and texture you prefer.

**4** When the duck is cool enough to handle, scrape off the remaining meat and add to the stock.

**5** Chop or snip the prunes (or apricots) into peanut-sized pieces.

**6** Add to the pan and simmer gently for 20 minutes.

## vital statistics

You'll get vitamin C and a high level of protective antioxidants from the raspberries, hugely powerful antibacterial benefits from the manuka honey and bone-building calcium from the milk in this soup.

# raspberry relish

Like all berries, raspberries are at the top of the league table of 'ORAC' foods, the oxygen radical absorbance capacity method of measuring antioxidants in food. These delicious super-antioxidant berries lose very little of their immunity-boosting value through freezing, making this a great year-round taste-of-summer soup. All natural honey has healing properties, but manuka, from New Zealand, is uniquely powerful.

**raspberries** 400g (14oz); frozen fruit will do, defrosted and drained

**milk** 200ml (⅓ pint)

**manuka honey** 2 tbsp

**single cream** 150ml (¼ pint)

**amaretti biscuits** 6, crushed, to serve

1 Put the raspberries, milk, honey and cream into a food processor or blender and whizz until smooth.

2 Leave to chill thoroughly in the refrigerator.

3 Scatter the crushed amaretti biscuits over to serve.

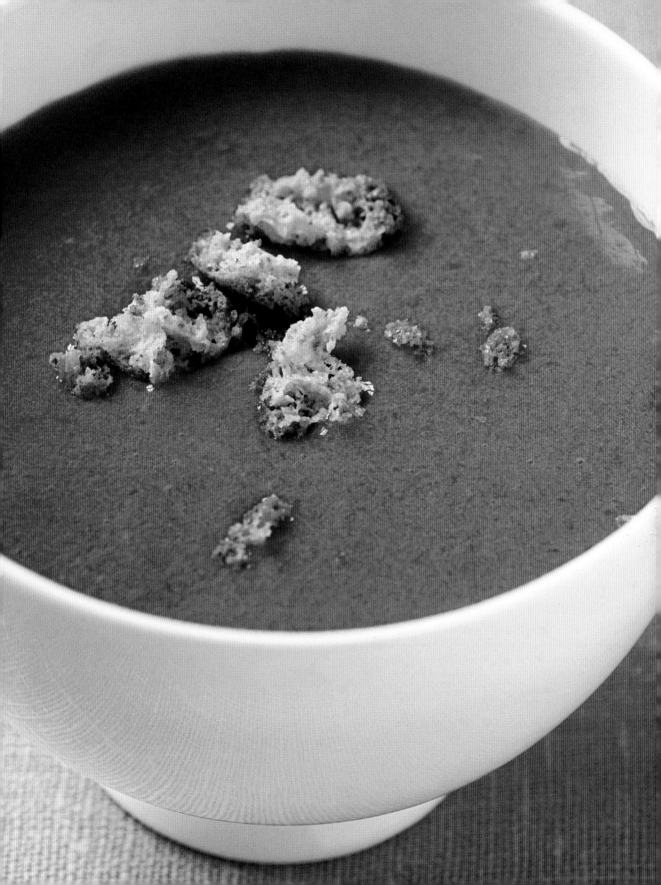

As well as the carotenoids you'd expect from fruit the colour of papayas, there's a special benefit to be gained from the digestive enzyme papain, which they also contain. It improves the efficiency of digestion and helps ensure that the maximum nutritional benefit is extracted from the food you eat. Ground ginger is a surprising immunity booster; the gingerols in this extraordinary root will help 'ginger up' your entire system.

# veggie wake-up call

Mixing sweet papayas with vegetable juice may sound a bit strange, but there's nothing odd about the finished smoothie. Here, you've got multiple benefits to your immune system from some of the healthiest of fruits, the nutrients in the mixed vegetable juice, the spiciness of ginger and the creamy smoothness of a good, natural live yogurt – all this and improved resistance, too.

**papayas** 2, peeled and deseeded
**vegetable juice** 150ml (¼ pint)
**apple juice** 150ml (¼ pint)
**ground ginger** 1 tsp
**natural live bio-yogurt** 50ml (2fl oz)

**1** Put all the ingredients into a blender or food processor and whizz until smooth.

## vital statistics

This juice is super-rich in calcium, magnesium and vitamin C, and rich in folic acid and potassium. It also contains iron and phosphorus. The extra nutrients from the beetroot tops, the cancer-fighting bonus of the nutrients in cabbage and the calming influences of celery make this protective juice a powerful tonic, as well as a bone builder.

# pro-bonus

The earlier women start to build healthy bones, the less likely they are to develop osteoporosis in later life. The superjuice Pro-Bonus is a good source of easily absorbed calcium and magnesium, both of which are essential for bone development. It's a great bone tonic for women throughout their lives – but don't forget that some men also develop osteoporosis, so it's good for them, too.

**apples** 3, unpeeled, uncored and quartered
**celery** 2 sticks, with leaves
**beetroot** 1, with leaves, halved
**cabbage** ½ small round, cut into wedges

**1** Put all the ingredients through a juicer.

The peaches and mangoes in this smoothie provide lots of betacarotene and other carotenoids, which specifically protect the skin and mucous membranes and help boost immunity, while an extra vitamin C boost comes from the lime. The yogurt provides resistance-boosting friendly bacteria that live in the intestine, where they both help destroy unwanted bugs and have a direct effect on the general immune system.

# tango smoothie

This tastes and smells wonderful, and even when fresh peaches are not available, it's pretty good made with canned ones, as long as they're in pure juice or water and not sugar syrup. The unique taste of lime contrasts well with the sweeter, heavier flavours of the other fruits, and when the yogurt is added, the smoothie takes on a wonderful creamy consistency. For a thicker version, try using traditional Greek yogurt or adding some mascarpone cheese or crème fraîche.

**peaches** 2 large, stoned
**mangoes** 2 large, peeled and stoned
**lime** 1
**natural live bio-yogurt** 450ml
(16fl oz)

1 Put the peaches and mangoes through a juicer.

2 Cut 2 or 3 slices from the lime, then squeeze the juice from the rest.

3 Mix all the fruit juices with the yogurt.

4 Serve with the reserved lime slices on top.

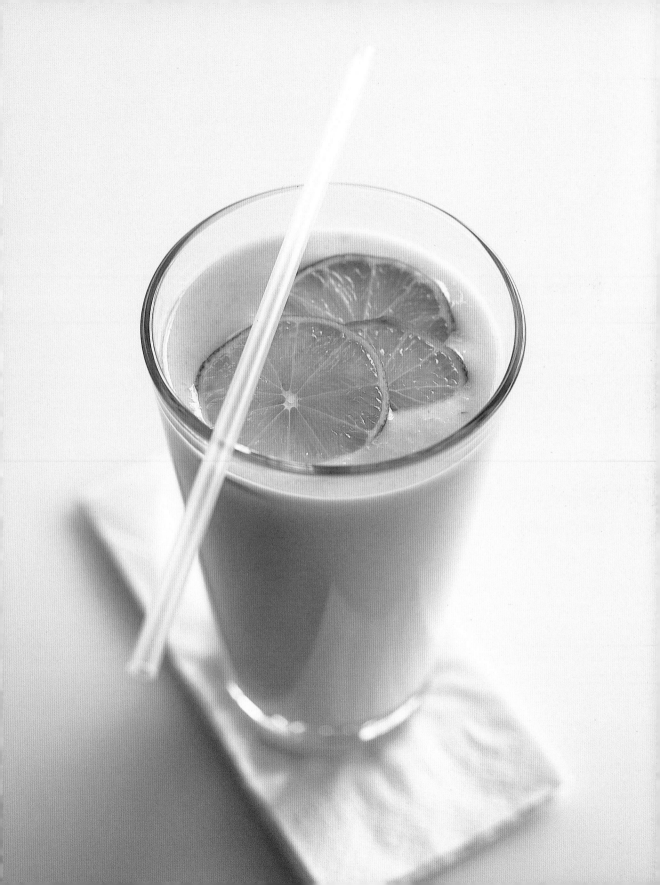

## vital statistics

Huge amounts of vitamin C from the kiwi fruit and orange juice are coupled with betacarotene and a range of other essential carotenoids in this recipe, as well as the cancer-fighting phytochemicals in the sweet potato. The orange juice also provides another group of chemicals called bioflavonoids, which play an important role in the protection of your blood vessels. This mixture is an all-round protector that increases your natural resistance to bugs and degenerative diseases.

# spuds 'r' us

You may never have thought of juicing a sweet potato, but this really is one of the most immunity-building and cancer-preventative foods around. Mixing sweet potatoes with the flavours of kiwi fruit and orange juice makes a delicious combination that tastes better than it sounds and is a powerful protector against short-term infections and long-term disease.

**sweet potato** 1 large, scrubbed
**kiwi fruit** 3, peeled
**orange juice** 300ml (10fl oz) freshly squeezed

1 Put the sweet potato and kiwi fruit through a juicer.
2 Add the orange juice and mix well.

Theobromine from chocolate and myristicin from nutmeg are two plant chemicals that have mood-enhancing properties. Nutmeg also helps sleep and improves digestion, both of which are good for the immune system. Beneficial bacteria in live yogurt produce by-products that are absorbed directly through the intestinal lining and play a very important part in strengthening natural immunity.

# help, i'm a chocoholic!

We all feel happier after eating chocolate, and just being happy gives your immune system a jump-start. But there's more to it than that; chocolate is a source of immunity-boosting phytochemicals. Bananas are nature's miracle fast food, providing energy and essential nutrients that the body needs in order to stay fit and well. The benefits of friendly bacteria, a good dose of your daily requirement of calcium and the mood-enhancing benefits in nutmeg mean you'll soon be back for more of this one.

**banana** 1, peeled and chopped

**natural live bio-yogurt** 400ml (14fl oz)

**chocolate powder** 1 heaped tbsp organic

**nutmeg** 2 small pinches freshly grated

1 Put the banana into a blender or food processor with the yogurt and chocolate powder and whizz until smooth.

2 Serve with the nutmeg sprinkled on top.

This delicious smoothie works just as well if you substitute 6 large strawberries for the banana.

## vital statistics

Plenty of calcium, magnesium, potassium and protein and modest amounts of vitamins B and D come from the coconut and full-fat milk in this drink. Cloves provide aromatic essential oils that are both healing and antibacterial. Even the honey has protective benefits, since it contains traces of natural antibiotics produced by the bees – which is why honey never goes mouldy.

# spiced coconut

Coconut milk is easily available in your local supermarket, so there's no excuse for not trying this exotic, spicy way to protect yourself from all sorts of infections. The heady scents of coconut and cloves are redolent of tropical islands, blue seas and sunshine, and thinking of that is enough to make you feel better on its own. This takes just seconds to prepare, but do take the time to savour the taste and soak up the benefits.

**coconut milk** 300ml (½ pint)
**full-fat milk** 150ml (¼ pint)
**runny honey** 1 tbsp
**ground cloves** 2 tsp, plus a little to serve

**1** Put the coconut milk, ordinary milk, honey and cloves into a blender or food processor and whizz well.

**2** Serve with an extra pinch of ground cloves on each glass.

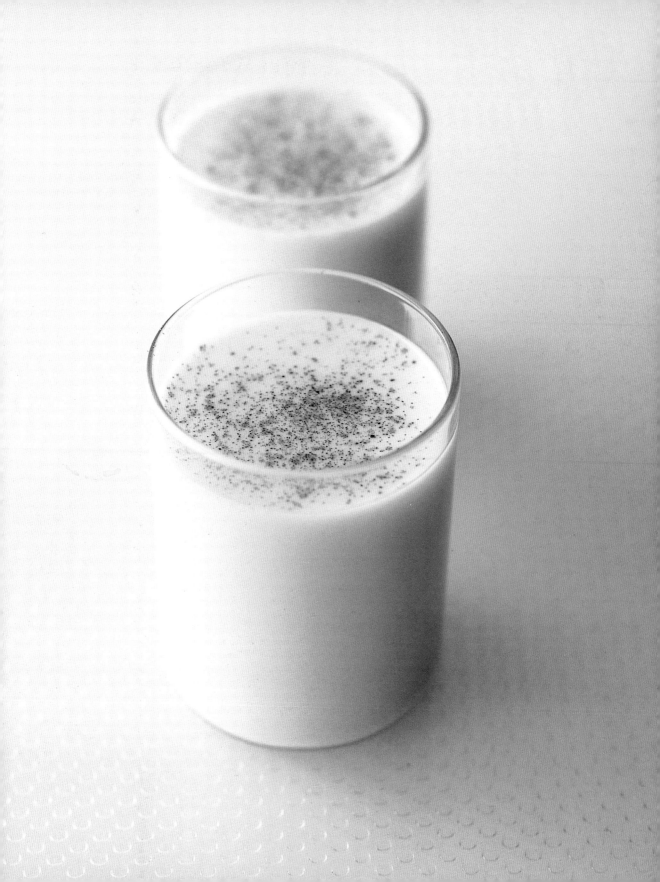

The protective properties of cranberry juice are legendary, and the juice of this amazing berry is both a treatment for and a protector against urinary infections. Star anise is rich in essential oils like estragole and anethole, which improve digestion, protect against flatulence and help the appetite. They also protect against coughs, colds and catarrh.

# cranberry cup

Many people think that hot fruit juices are rather strange, although they have no qualms at all about hot punches or mulled wine. Fruit juices are no different – except, of course, that they don't contain alcohol. Apart from tasting amazingly good, this mixture of cranberry juice and star anise is doubly protective because it's hot. Served cold, the essential oils from the star anise would not be extracted, so you'd get neither the benefit nor much flavour.

**star anise** 4
**cranberry juice** 300ml (½ pint)

**1** Stir the star anise into the cranberry juice in a medium saucepan.

**2** Bring slowly to just under boiling point.

**3** Leave the star anise floating on top to serve.

## vital statistics

The red colouring of beetroot carries specific anti-carcinogens attached to its molecules, and it also more than doubles the amount of oxygen the body cells are able to absorb. This juice will boost natural resistance, protect convalescents from relapse and act as a valuable aid to good digestion. It's a mild liver stimulant, too, so it helps in the digestion of fats. Adding the ginger boosts the circulation and also helps improve digestion.

# gingered-up beetroot

This is another extremely protective drink that sounds a bit bizarre. But before you turn up your nose and turn over the page, try it – you'll be pleasantly surprised. It tastes like slightly spicy, bubbly borscht (the traditional Eastern European beetroot soup). Beneficial to both blood and circulation, this mixture protects against fatigue, loss of concentration and many forms of cancer.

**beetroot juice** 400ml (14fl oz)
**ginger essence** 4 drops
**ginger ale** 100ml (3½fl oz)

**1** Heat the beetroot juice in a medium saucepan until just boiling.

**2** Pour into 2 mugs and add 2 drops of ginger essence to each.

**3** Top up with ginger ale and serve.

## vital statistics

As well as all the B vitamins, minerals and antioxidants in the organic chocolate contained in this drink, there is also calcium and the essential vitamin D in the full-fat milk. The natural bacteria and extra calcium from the fromage frais and the peppermint oil from the mint leaves add extra nutrients and improve digestive absorption, while the almonds are a rich source of protective vitamin E, zinc and selenium.

# aztec dream

To the Aztecs, chocolate was so precious that only royal families were allowed to drink it. It isn't hard to see why; besides its wonderful taste, chocolate contains valuable antioxidants and other protective substances. Here, it is combined with cardamom and star anise, which also protect against chest infections, sore throats and sinus problems, while soya milk's natural plant hormones help strengthen bones – vital protection against osteoporosis. Hot chocolate will never be the same again.

**hot chocolate** 300ml (½ pint) organic dark, prepared according to the packet instructions using half full-fat milk and half soya milk

**cardamom seeds** 4

**ground star anise** a sprinkling

**flaked almonds** 15g (½oz)

**mint** 1 generous handful of leaves, plus 2 sprigs to decorate

**fromage frais** 100g (3½oz)

1 Prepare the chocolate in a saucepan according to the packet instructions, then add the cardamom seeds and ground star anise.

2 Heat the almonds gently in a dry frying pan until they start to brown and crisp.

3 Put the mint leaves and fromage frais into a blender or food processor and whizz until well combined.

4 Pour the hot chocolate into 2 large mugs. Top with the fromage frais, sprinkle with the almonds and add a sprig of mint to each.

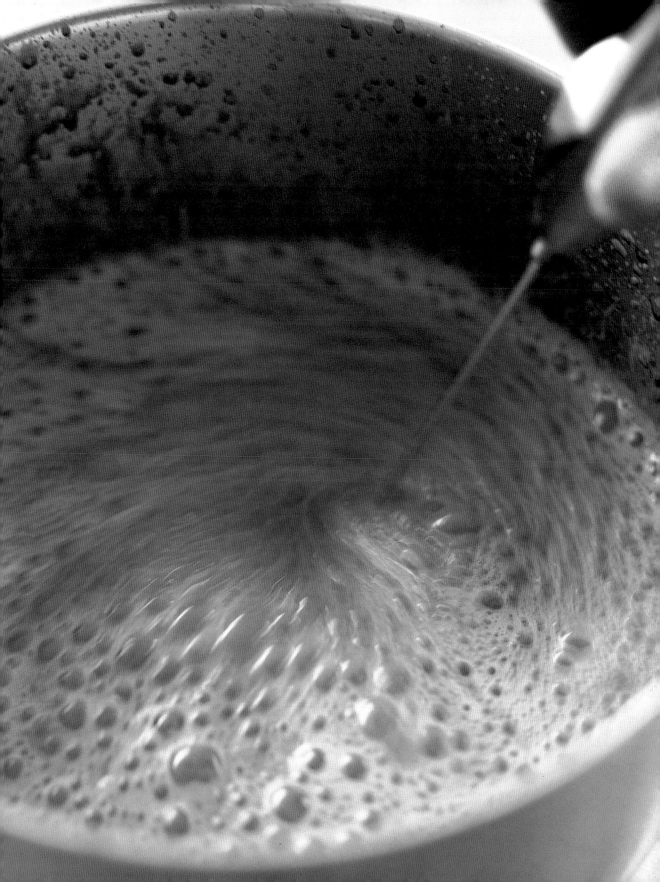

## vital statistics

An average papaya provides twice your daily requirement of vitamin C and a quarter of vitamin A. Both these nutrients are essential for the functioning of your immune system. As a result, the recipe is a super-protector. Additional nutrients from the papaya and apple juices, the immunity-boosting properties of cinnamon and allspice, and the feel-good factor from nutmeg push this drink to the top of the protective list.

# mulled papaya

This is truly super-protection in a glass. Serve it to your friends in a large punch bowl before dinner, and it will give them all a glow of well-being – and that's without any alcohol. You could, of course, always add some white rum if you wanted something a little stronger. Like many tropical fruits, the papaya is rich in protective enzymes and vitamins, and when combined with tropical spices, it provides a huge boost to the immune system.

**cloves** 10

**cinnamon stick** 1, broken into 3 pieces

**demerara sugar** 150g (5½oz)

**papaya juice** 1 litre (1¾ pints)

**apple juice** 1 litre (1¾ pints)

**ground allspice** 1 tsp

**nutmeg** 3 pinches freshly grated

**papaya** 1 small, peeled, deseeded and thinly sliced

**1** Tie the cloves and cinnamon stick in a piece of kitchen muslin.

**2** Put the sugar and juices into a large saucepan.

**3** Add the muslin bag, allspice and nutmeg.

**4** Bring slowly to the boil, then turn the heat down and simmer for 10 minutes.

**5** Remove the muslin bag.

**6** Serve in a punch bowl or other large, heatproof bowl with the papaya slices floating on top.

## vital statistics

Ripe tomatoes are a rich source of the carotenoid lycopene, an essential nutrient that protects against prostate and breast cancers, heart disease and eye problems. Many commercially produced tomatoes are harvested early and artificially ripened, so they contain less of this nutrient. However, very ripe tomatoes are used for canning and juicing; the lycopene content is also concentrated by the processing. This guarantees optimum intake.

# hot bloody mary

It's not often that any form of processing increases the protective value of fresh produce, but this is definitely true of tomatoes. This juice is hugely protective against prostate and breast cancers, and it also helps prevent age-related macular degeneration (AMD), the most common cause of blindness in the elderly. With or without the vodka, this is a really delicious drink with huge health benefits.

**tomato juice** 300ml (½ pint)
**tabasco sauce** 2 dashes
**vodka** 2 small measures (about 1 tbsp)
**cinnamon sticks** 2

**1** Warm the tomato juice and pour it into 2 decorative, heatproof glasses.

**2** Add the Tabasco sauce and vodka.

**3** Serve immediately, with the cinnamon sticks for stirring.

## vital statistics

Using quality chocolate with a minimum cocoa solid content of 70 per cent, you'll get a reasonable amount of the natural chemical theobromine, which triggers the release of good-mood chemicals from the brain. Evidence shows that feeling happy and positive gives a substantial boost to the immune system and helps protect the body against infection and disease. The calcium from the milk gives added protection against osteoporosis.

# hot, hot chocolate

Isn't it great to discover that one of your favourite foods – which you always thought of as sinful and unhealthy – is suddenly considered good for you? That's certainly the case with chocolate, as long as you stick to modest quantities and use the best possible quality. Not only does chocolate contain feel-good chemicals that lift your mood, it's also a rich source of protective antioxidants. So it's official: you can enjoy this drink with a clear conscience.

**chocolate powder** 1 heaped tsp organic
**full-fat jersey milk** 300ml (½ pint)
**cinnamon stick** 1cm (½in) piece

**1** Mix the chocolate powder with 2 teaspoons of the milk in a mug.

**2** Bring the rest of the milk to the boil in a saucepan.

**3** Pour into the mug containing the chocolate mixture.

**4** Stir and serve with the cinnamon stick floating on top.

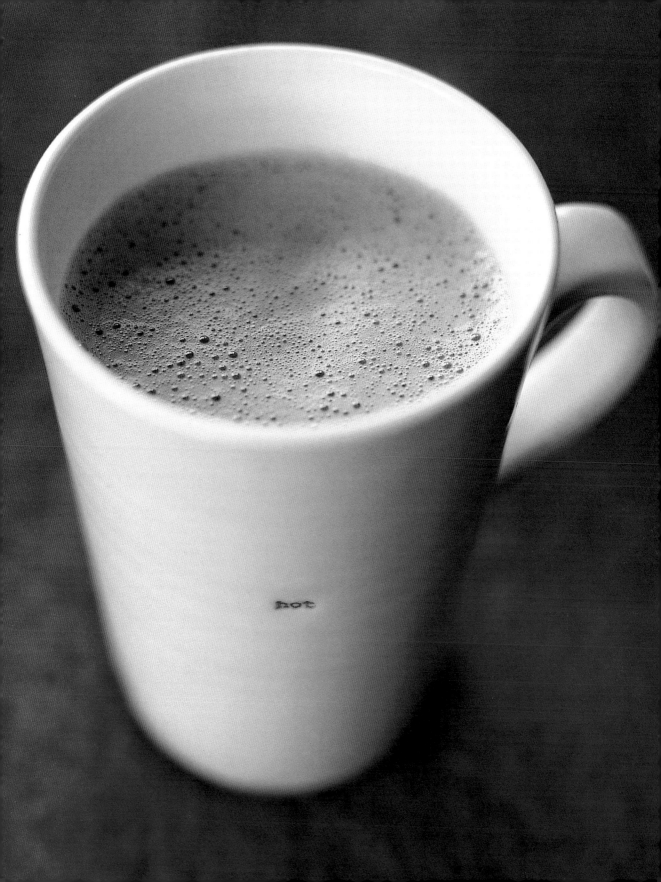

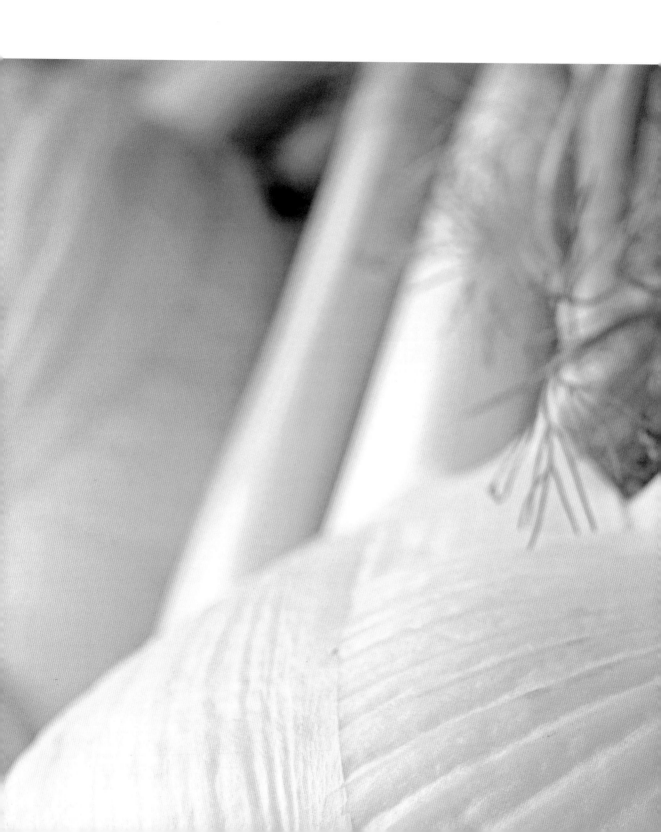

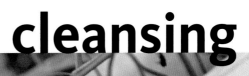

# cleansing

The body has an amazing system for cleansing itself. The main organs involved are the liver and kidneys, so all cleansing regimes must focus on doing everything to improve their efficiency. Of course, the body's largest single organ is the skin, and one of its major functions is the elimination of waste products. All the dietary advice below applies in equal measure to a successful skin-cleansing regime. Yet there's no reason to become a food freak – after all, life is for enjoying. This means sharing a drink with friends or indulging in the occasional 'death by chocolate'. The simple answer is to give your system an occasional rest and spring-clean by using the recipes in this cleansing section and following the simple dietary advice below.

## The kidneys

Some serious illnesses affect the kidneys' ability to do their cleaning-up job. High blood pressure, tuberculosis, repeated infections and kidney stones can all damage these complex and delicate organs. Severe injuries can also be a problem. As we age, the kidneys can become less efficient at getting rid of waste products, and this can be aggravated by the long-term use of many prescribed medicines. To stimulate kidney function, dandelion leaves, parsley, radishes, leeks and their cooking water and parsley tea should be regulars in your diet. Most important of all is to drink plenty of water to reduce the risk of stones and infection.

Anyone with a tendency to kidney stones should avoid spinach, beetroot, rhubarb and chocolate, which all contain oxalic acid, as well as coffee, tea and cocoa, which contain irritating caffeine and large amounts of potassium.

The kidneys are amazingly efficient. Next time you eat asparagus, just see how long it takes before your urine develops the distinctive smell it produces. If your cleansing system is working properly, your urine should be a pale-straw colour, odourless and sterile. If the colour darkens, you're not drinking enough. If it remains dark after a litre (1¾ pints) of water, see your doctor, since this could be a sign of an underlying problem.

## The liver

Think of the liver as the body's sewage plant: it's there to filter out all the unwanted and toxic rubbish and waste. But if you abuse your liver or, unfortunately, you develop some form of liver disease, it very soon becomes inefficient and unable to cope. Keep a healthy liver by eating more globe artichokes for the liver-cleansing cynarin they contain; oily fish, rabbit and game, which are very low in saturated fat; Brussels sprouts, red cabbage and chickpeas for vitamin B12 and folic acid. The special fibre in oats is also very important to improve the elimination of fats that can damage the liver. You should eat less red meat and fewer high-sugar foods, and drink fewer caffeine-containing drinks and sweet fizzy drinks. Avoid alcohol completely.

The huge increase of binge drinking among young people is a great concern, since this will inevitably lead to liver damage and a breakdown in the body's cleansing processes later in life. An early sign of liver malfunction is a yellowing, spotty skin, and I'm constantly amazed at how many young women who spend fortunes on clothes, make-up and hair are happy to spend even bigger fortunes every weekend on binge drinking, which is guaranteed to make them look prematurely old.

## Foods for thought

There are two more powerful weapons in your cleansing programme: juices and raw foods. You'll find lots of salads, herbal teas and juices in this chapter, as well as healthy recipes you'll be happy to serve to friends without them having any idea that they're eating a 'cleansing' meal. Here, you'll find some of the great old wives' favourites, such as French onion soup, traditionally enjoyed after a night on the tiles in Paris.

There's even food for free, with a great soup made out of stinging nettles that helps cleanse the kidneys, digestive system and skin. Pick a few days each month to eat from this chapter – or why not do a whole week before the festive binge at Christmas?

# cleansing checklist

- Eat more celery, parsley, watercress, fennel, dandelion, peppers, mint, citrus juices, fish, prunes, brown rice and wholegrain cereals, and drink more water.
- Eat fewer foods with E numbers, refined carbohydrates, less white bread, less of most commercial breakfast cereals, less animal protein, coffee, alcohol, sweets, chocolates and high-fat, -salt and -sugar snacks and convenience foods.

## vital statistics

The fibre and vitamin C in oranges, together with the red onion in this salad, improve digestive function and aid the elimination of cholesterol.

# florence fennel salad

This salad is guaranteed to help any cleansing programme, thanks largely to the natural plant chemicals provided by fennel (the bulb's 'proper name' is Florence fennel). Among others, this delicious bulb contains essential oils called anethole and fenchone, which are mildly diuretic and thus help the body get rid of excess fluid. In addition, fennel is very good news for women, because its beneficial oils play an important part in maintaining hormone balance.

**oranges** 2, peeled and white pith removed, thinly sliced

**fennel** 1 large bulb, sliced as thinly as possible

**red onion** 1 large, sliced

**orange** juice of 1

**balsamic vinegar** 2 tsp

**mint sprigs** to garnish

**1** Put a layer of orange slices on to each of 4 plates.

**2** Cover the oranges with the fennel.

**3** Sprinkle the onion on top of the fennel.

**4** Mix the orange juice with the vinegar and drizzle the dressing over each plate.

**5** Garnish with the sprigs of mint.

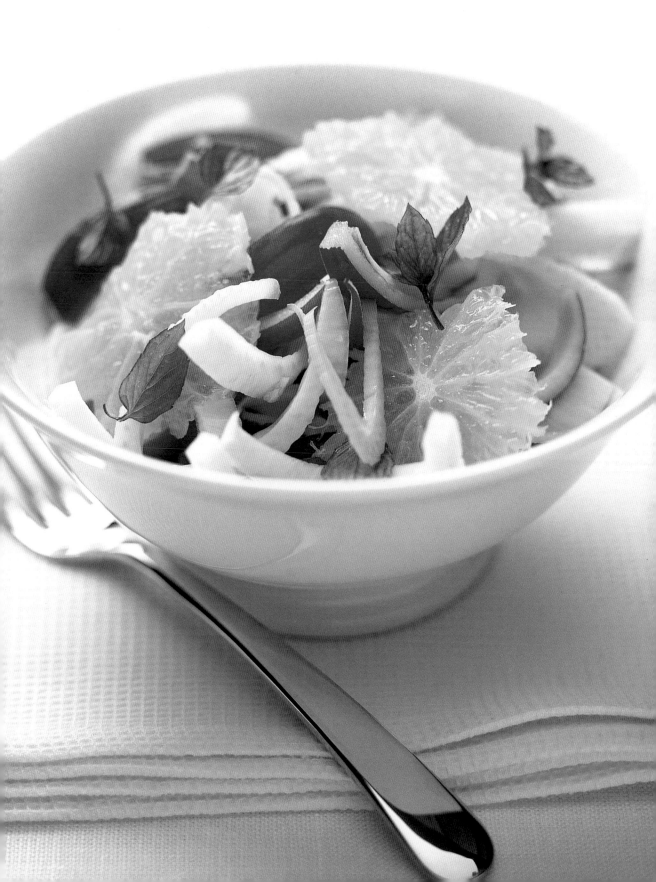

This salad combines the cleansing properties of apples with the diuretic effect of celery and the high-fibre content of raisins. It's rich in iron, vitamin C, pectin, potassium and essential oils.

# granny's cleanser

It's hardly surprising that a lot of old wives' tales turn out to be true. After all, many of them refer to practices that have been in use for hundreds of years, and if they didn't work at all, they wouldn't stand the test of time.

**apples** 2 large Granny Smiths, unpeeled and cored

**lemon** juice of 1

**celery** 2 sticks, preferably with leaves

**seedless raisins** 2 tbsp

**natural live bio-yogurt** 1 small carton (about 125ml/4fl oz)

**cider vinegar** 1 tbsp

**extra-virgin olive oil** 3 tbsp

**runny honey** 1 tsp

**1** Cut the apples into small wedges and put them into a salad bowl. Add half the lemon juice and mix thoroughly to prevent browning.

**2** Slice the celery into 1cm (½in) chunks, chop the leaves and add to the apple pieces.

**3** Add the raisins.

**4** Mix the yogurt, vinegar, oil, honey and remaining lemon juice together.

**5** Add to the salad and toss lightly.

Dandelion has diuretic qualities, hence it has a powerful cleansing action. In addition, it is rich in iron, which you'll absorb all the better thanks to the vitamin C in the lemon juice.

# dandelion delight

This recipe is rich in iron – and effective for fluid loss. In the north of England, the country name for dandelion is 'wet-the-bed', and in France it's called *pis en lit* – which means exactly the same thing. In most French street markets you can buy these delicious leaves alongside all the other salad ingredients.

**dandelion leaves** 1 generous bunch

**lamb's lettuce** 1 generous bunch

**baby spinach leaves** 2 handfuls

**extra-virgin olive oil** 2 tbsp

**lemon** juice of ½

1 Put all the leaves into a large salad bowl.

2 Pour on the oil.

3 Squeeze the lemon juice over the top.

4 Toss thoroughly so that every leaf is well coated.

# red, hot and healthy

Served on a white plate, this salad looks absolutely stunning, but it's got more than simple eye appeal. Radishes are one of the great traditional foods for stimulating the liver and gall bladder. They increase the production of bile, which in turn helps with the digestion of fat in the diet. They're also a great source of potassium, calcium and sulphur, making this salad a good, all-round, hot little number.

**radicchio** 1 good-sized head

**radishes** 12

**red peppers** 2, preferably dark, pointed ones

**cooked beetroot** 4 small

**salad dressing** 4 tbsp (*see* page 182)

**chives** 1 bunch, finely chopped

**1** Separate the radicchio into its individual leaves.

**2** Slice the radishes.

**3** Slice the red peppers into rounds, discarding all the seeds.

**4** Cut the beetroot into julienne-style strips.

**5** Arrange the radicchio leaves in a bowl. Add the red-pepper slices, then the beetroot strips and then the radish slices.

**6** Drizzle with the dressing and sprinkle with the chopped chives.

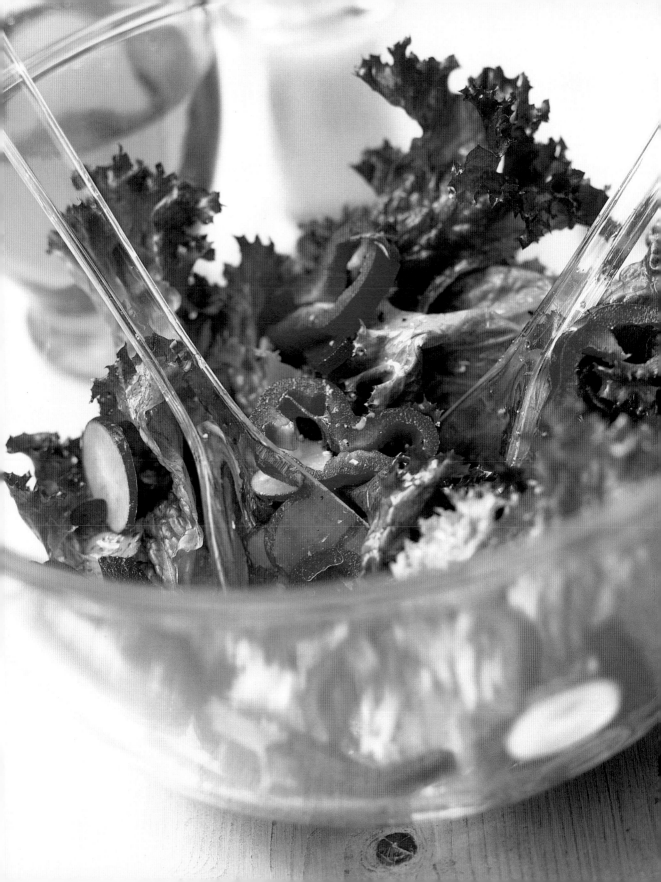

## vital statistics

The vitamin C from the oranges in this salad improves the absorption of iron from the chicory and watercress, which is also a great source of natural protective chemicals. It aids digestion, too.

# bittersweet treat

Chicory and all the curly endives are members of the same family of wonderful winter salad vegetables. They are all descendants of wild chicory, which has a long history in traditional herbalism as a cleanser and detoxifier. In medieval times, it was used as one of the most important late winter/early spring tonic plants to give the body a stimulating spring-clean. This salad offers a wonderful combination of flavours, thanks to the sweetness of the orange, which offsets the bitter chicory.

**chicory** 2 bulbs

**watercress** 1 large bunch

**lime** juice of 1

**rapeseed oil** 1 tbsp

**oranges** 2 large, peeled and white pith removed, thinly sliced

**black pepper** freshly ground, to taste

**1** Separate the chicory leaves, then chop them into bite-sized pieces.

**2** Wash the watercress – even if it's 'ready-washed'.

**3** Whisk the lime juice into the oil.

**4** Lay the orange slices on a serving plate and cover them with the chicory leaves. Pile the watercress in the centre.

**5** Drizzle with the dressing and season to taste with black pepper.

## vital statistics

Apples are a traditional remedy for joint diseases, and watermelon is a traditional cooling fruit that also has mild eliminative benefits.

# waterfall salad

As you'll guess from its name, this is another strongly diuretic recipe. It's great for all women who suffer uncomfortable fluid retention and swelling of ankles, fingers and breasts around period time. This is also a valuable dish for anyone suffering with gout or arthritis, because the celery and celery seeds specifically increase the elimination of uric acid, the chemical that aggravates inflamed joints.

**dessert apples** 2 sweet
**raspberry vinegar** 1 tbsp
**watermelon** 1 chunk
**chicory** 1 bulb
**celery** 2 sticks, preferably with leaves
**celery seeds** 1 tsp
**walnut oil** 1 tbsp

**1** Core and dice the apples, then put them into a salad bowl. Pour over the vinegar and mix thoroughly to prevent browning.

**2** Peel and deseed the watermelon. Cut into cubes.

**3** Slice the chicory into rounds.

**4** Coarsely chop the celery and celery leaves.

**5** Add everything to the bowl of apples, along with the celery seeds, and mix gently.

**6** Pour in the oil and mix again.

## vital statistics

The vitamin C and betacarotenes from the peppers, the essential oil fenchone from fennel, phytonutrients in the aubergine and all the cleansing properties of onions make this a fantastic salad.

# slow-cooked salad

This salad is a delicious mixture of skin-friendly Mediterranean vegetables cooked on the barbecue. However, you don't have to go out into the garden when it's snowing, because this works just as well on a griddle or grill pan, or in a built-in stove-top griddle, if you're lucky enough to have one.

**courgettes** 3, sliced lengthways

**aubergine** 1 large, sliced crossways

**fennel** 1 large bulb, cut into bite-sized chunks

**red pepper** 1, cored, deseeded and cut into bite-sized chunks

**yellow pepper** 1, cored, deseeded and cut into bite-sized chunks

**broccoli** 1 head, broken into florets

**red onion** 1, cut into wedges

**white onion** 1, cut into wedges

**extra-virgin olive oil** 3 tbsp, plus a little extra for frying the garlic

**rosemary** 2 large sprigs

**garlic** 2 cloves, finely chopped

**manchego cheese** 115g (4oz) (if you can't find it, Parmesan will do), shaved into wafer-thin shavings

**1** Heat the barbecue, grill or griddle pan.

**2** Lightly brush all the vegetables with the oil. Place them on the heat, and do not touch them: they won't stick unless you move them about.

**3** Cut the rosemary into 5cm (2in) lengths and put it on top of the vegetables.

**4** Turn the vegetables when they are ready – about 3–4 minutes.

**5** While the vegetables are cooking, put the garlic into a small frying pan with a little oil and cook gently until crisp and slightly golden. Do not overheat – it will burn and taste bitter. Drain on kitchen paper.

**6** When all the vegetables are slightly charred on the outside and tender in the middle, serve sprinkled with the garlic and the shavings of cheese.

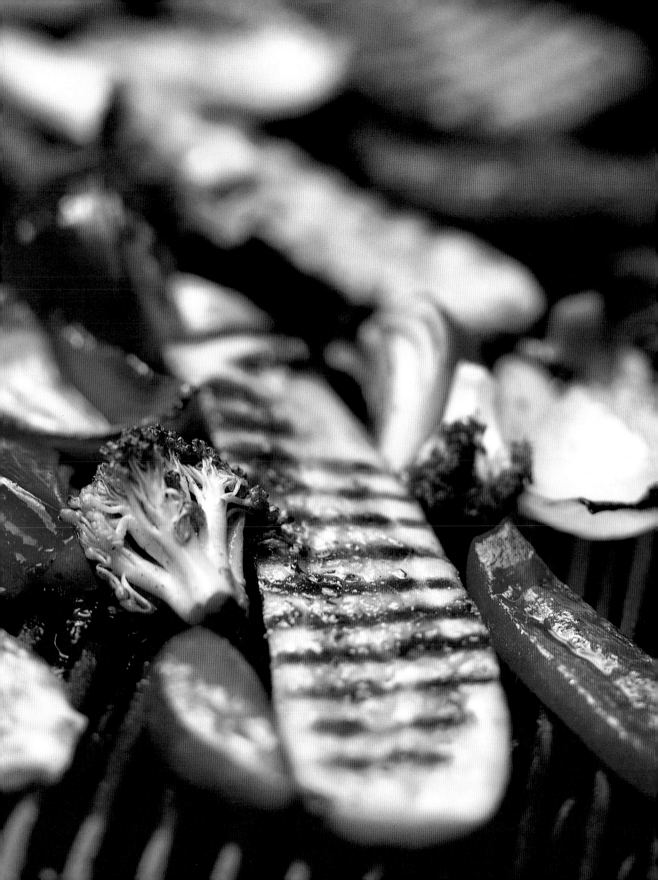

## vital statistics

This is a super-cleansing recipe. Cynarin from artichokes detoxifies the liver, while parsley provides a diuretic effect. The ultimate purifying benefits of garlic, the slow-release sugar, inulin (also from the artichokes), and the calming properties of basil give this dish additional health-enhancing qualities.

# basil's brush

The complex flavours of basil, chives and garlic are the perfect way to bring out the unique taste of artichoke hearts. Most of the recipes in this book are for fresh produce, but unless you're an expert – or have the whole day to spare – preparing a pile of fresh artichoke hearts is a thankless task. Save yourself trouble by buying the best-quality canned ones you can find. Serve with good, coarse bread for mopping up the sauce.

**white wine** 450ml (16fl oz)

**garlic** 6 cloves, chopped

**parsley** 225g (8oz), chopped

**chives** 125g (4½oz), chopped

**plum tomatoes** 3 large, chopped

**extra-virgin olive oil** 125ml (4fl oz)

**artichoke hearts** 2 x 350g cans, drained

**basil leaves** 5 tbsp snipped

**1** Boil the wine with the garlic in a large saucepan for about 3 minutes.

**2** Add the parsley and chives to the pan.

**3** Add the tomatoes, oil and artichokes, and simmer until the artichokes are soft – about 15 minutes.

**4** Just before serving, stir in the basil.

## vital statistics

Unpeeled courgettes are a valuable source of betacarotene, essential for the skin during any cleansing programme. Parsley provides calcium as well as diuretic volatile oils, which speed fluid elimination. Chives enjoy the cleansing and detoxing properties of their relatives, garlic and onions, though with a less strident flavour.

# chervil courgette bake

Give this dish to the most dedicated meat eaters, then let them tell you vegetarian food is boring! Apart from its cleansing benefits, it's a truly tongue-tingling mixture of flavours, especially the delicate overtones of aniseed from the chervil. Chervil's blood-purifying properties are part of ancient herbal folklore: it has been regarded as a traditional spring tonic for centuries.

**garlic** 1 clove, peeled

**mixed herbs** such as coriander, chervil, chives and parsley, 4 tbsp fresh, succulent chopped leaves

**plum tomatoes** 300g (10½oz) plump, skinned, deseeded and diced

**courgettes** 8 small, halved lengthways and deseeded

**extra-virgin olive oil** 3 tbsp

**lemon** ½, thinly sliced

**sea salt and black pepper** freshly ground, to taste

**1** Preheat the oven to 200°C/400°F/gas mark 6.

**2** Rub an ovenproof dish with the garlic, then stir in the chopped herbs and tomatoes.

**3** Arrange the courgette halves on top of the tomatoes and herbs, then pour over the oil. Cover with the slices of lemon.

**4** Season to taste with salt and pepper, cover with foil and bake for about 20 minutes, until the courgettes are soft but not mushy.

## vital statistics

Fish provides easily digested protein and a rich supply of minerals, including iodine. Juniper is rich in the diuretic and anti-inflammatory volatile oils myrcene, sabinene, pinene and limonene. The sulphur compounds in garlic and Welsh onion fight bacteria and fungal diseases, while the diuretic benefits of parsley add to this dish's cleansing properties.

# juniper fish

The traditional use of juniper as a diuretic and anti-inflammatory is one reason for its inclusion in this recipe; its strong, tangy flavours and those of Welsh onions and garlic are another. Together, these herbs perfectly complement the tender white flesh of the sea bass, making this a mouthwatering way to cleanse the system.

**welsh onion** 2 tbsp green leaves, finely chopped

**garlic** 3 cloves, crushed

**juniper berries** 1 tbsp, lightly crushed

**parsley** 2 tbsp chopped

**white wine** 700ml (1¼ pints)

**sea bass** 2 whole, cleaned and scaled

**extra-virgin olive oil** for brushing

**lemon** 1, sliced

1 Preheat the oven to 220°C/425°F/gas mark 7.

2 Mix the Welsh onion, garlic, herbs and wine together.

3 Lay the fish in a large baking dish and brush with oil.

4 Pour the wine and herb mixture over the fish.

5 Cover with the slices of lemon.

6 Bake for about 30 minutes, basting frequently.

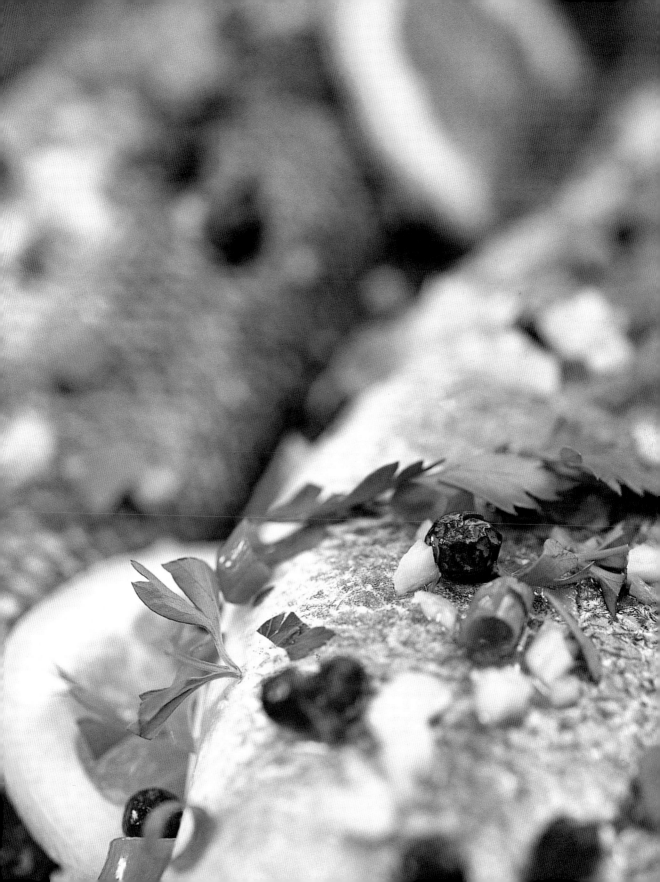

## vital statistics

This dish is a good source of protein, fibre, potassium, iron, selenium and folic acid. It also provides more than the daily requirement of vitamin E, as well as modest amounts of A and C. The high fibre content stimulates the digestive system, making this a great detox recipe.

# aubergine and bulgur stir-fry

If you're trying to reduce your blood pressure, then aubergines are a must, because they reduce the amount of fat circulating in the arteries. Bulgur wheat, sometimes known as cracked wheat, is often used in place of rice in the Middle East. It's highly nutritious and has a unique nutty flavour. This dish is also great cold, particularly if you add a generous amount of chopped flat-leaf parsley.

**bulgur wheat** 250g (9oz)

**cold water** 475ml (17fl oz)

**extra-virgin olive oil** 6 tbsp, plus a little extra

**onions** 2, thinly sliced

**aubergines** 2 large, cubed

**ground coriander** 3 tsp

**ground cumin** 3 tsp

**flaked almonds** 150g (5½oz)

**seedless raisins** 100g (3½oz)

**sea salt** 1 pinch

**black pepper** freshly ground, to taste

**1** Simmer the bulgur wheat in a large saucepan covered with the water for 10 minutes or until most or all of the water has been absorbed and the grains are tender. Drain if necessary.

**2** Heat the oil and fry the onions until brown. Add the aubergines and sauté, stirring frequently, until brown (add extra oil if necessary, since the aubergine acts like a sponge). Add the spices to the pan and cook for 1 minute, stirring continuously.

**3** Turn the heat down, add the flaked almonds and raisins and brown slightly. Stir the cooked bulgur wheat into the vegetables, add a little extra oil and sauté for 1 minute to heat through. Season with the salt and black pepper and serve immediately.

## vital statistics

This dish provides 9g of protein, lots of carbohydrates, fibre, plenty of potassium and valuable amounts of iron, zinc, copper, selenium, iodine, vitamin B6, folic acid and vitamin A. It's a great detoxifier, because it stimulates digestive function.

# mushrooms with egg and buckwheat

Unlike other cereals, buckwheat doesn't contain gluten, the sticky protein present in cereal grains. However, it is rich in rutin, a substance that strengthens the tiniest blood vessels in the circulatory system. This is a really satisfying and cleansing dish, with the added bonus of the beneficial live bacteria from the yogurt. You can find buckwheat at most health-food shops and also in some supermarkets.

**wholegrain buckwheat** 225g (8oz)

**free-range egg** 1 large

**butter** 60g (2¼oz)

**sea salt** 1 pinch

**boiling water** 450ml (16fl oz)

**onion** 1 large, finely chopped

**extra-virgin olive oil** 1 tbsp

**mushrooms** 225g (8oz), thinly sliced

**fresh coriander leaves** 1 tbsp chopped

**black pepper** freshly ground, to taste

**natural low-fat live bio-yogurt** 1 small carton (about 125ml/4fl oz)

1 Preheat the oven to 180°C/350°F/gas mark 4.

2 Boil the buckwheat for 15 minutes until soft.

3 Beat the egg in a large bowl and add the cooked buckwheat, stirring thoroughly. Transfer the mixture to a dry, non-stick frying pan and stir slowly over a low heat until toasted and dry.

4 Use a little of the butter to grease an ovenproof dish. Put in the buckwheat mixture, the rest of the butter, the salt and boiling water. Bake for 20 minutes.

5 While the buckwheat bakes, sweat the onion in the oil until soft but not browned. Add the mushrooms and cook for another 5 minutes. Add the coriander and black pepper to taste, stirring continuously.

6 When the buckwheat is done, stir in the onion and mushroom mixture, add the yogurt and serve hot.

## vital statistics

This dish provides half the minimum daily requirement of protein, more than 10 per cent of the calcium, a third of the iron and selenium and a little of all the B vitamins.

# organic sicilian chicken

Here's a quick recipe that spares you the antibiotics and chemical residues that will almost certainly be present in non-organic poultry. The antiseptic properties of thyme and the cancer-fighting effects of essential oils in the lemon make this dish exceptionally healthy as well as cleansing.

**wholemeal flour** 3 tbsp
**dried thyme** 2 tsp
**sea salt and black pepper** freshly ground, to taste
**chicken thighs** 8 organic
**milk** 100ml (3½fl oz)
**extra-virgin olive oil** 4 tbsp
**lemon** juice of 1

**1** Preheat the oven to 190°C/375°F/gas mark 5.

**2** Mix the flour, thyme and seasoning together. Dip the chicken thighs in the milk, then coat thoroughly with the flour mixture; set aside.

**3** Heat the oil in a frying pan and fry the chicken on all sides until golden brown. Transfer to a wire rack set over a baking sheet.

**4** Pour the lemon juice over the chicken thighs and bake for 15 minutes. It can be served hot or cold.

This is a protein-rich cleansing dish that is also highly protective, thanks to the antioxidants in the root vegetables. Swedes and carrots are particularly rich in betacarotene, and the apple provides the cholesterol-lowering fibre pectin. Catmint offers many volatile oils, particularly citronellol, geraniol, thymol and lactones, which help lower temperature, making this dish ideal for those recovering from coughs, colds and flu.

# catmint chicken

One of the simplest main courses ever: all the vegetables cook with the meat, while the apples, cider and herbs give the most delicious flavour to the vegetables, particularly the potatoes. Catmint, also known as catnip, is rich in purifying volatile oils. As a cleansing herb for humans, it's definitely the cat's meow!

**chicken portions** 4, preferably free-range

**root vegetables** about 450g (1lb) of your favourites, but including potatoes, cubed

**cooking apple** 1 Bramley, peeled, cored and cubed

**rosemary** 1 large sprig

**catmint** 3 large sprigs

**cider** 600ml (1 pint)

1 Preheat the oven to 200°C/400°F/gas mark 6.

2 Put all the ingredients into a large casserole dish.

3 Cover and cook in the oven for 2 hours. Enjoy!

This dish provides large amounts of protein, phosphorus and potassium, as well as lots of selenium. It's a low-fat, heart-friendly dish (only 1g of saturated fat per 100g) that stimulates the circulation and provides slow-release energy.

# grilled paprika chicken

This is a super-easy and very quick recipe that exploits the wonderful texture and flavour of organic chicken. The garlic and paprika give this dish the unmistakable tang of Hungary and combine the detoxifying properties of garlic with the circulatory stimulus of paprika.

**extra-virgin olive oil** 2 tbsp

**unwaxed lemon** juice and grated rind of 1 large

**garlic** 2 cloves, flattened with the blade of a large knife

**paprika** 1 generous tsp

**black pepper** freshly ground, to taste

**chicken breasts** 4 organic, skinned and cut into large cubes

**1** Combine the oil, lemon juice and rind, garlic, paprika and black pepper in a shallow dish. Put the chicken cubes into the marinade, stir well to make sure that they are all coated and cover. Leave in the refrigerator for 30 minutes, but spoon the marinade over the chicken at least twice during that time.

**2** Preheat the grill to high.

**3** Brush the rack of a grill pan with oil. Lift the chicken pieces out of the marinade with a slotted spoon, place them on the rack and cook them under the grill for 10 minutes, turning and basting them with the marinade occasionally, but not for the last few minutes of cooking.

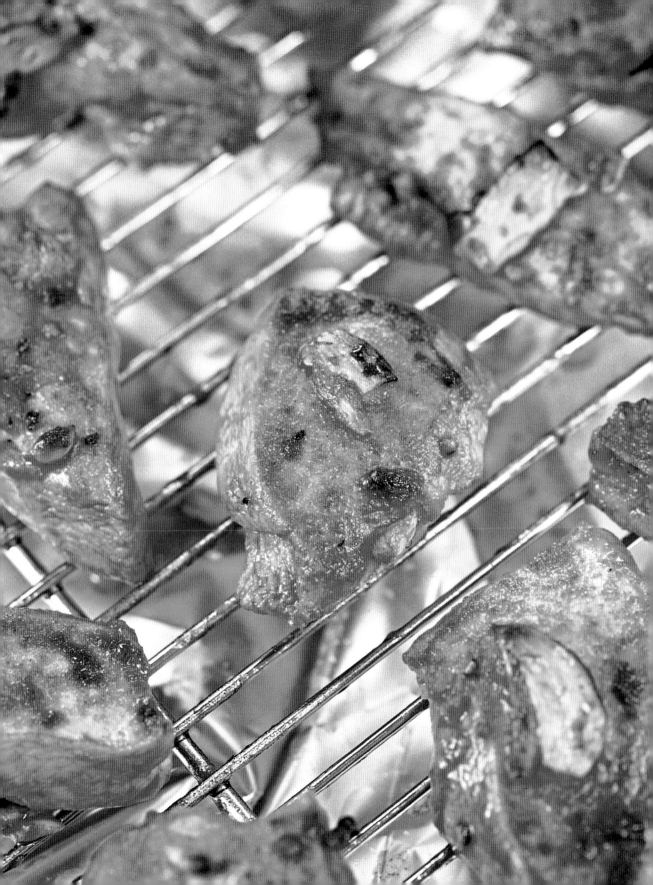

The antiseptic and antibacterial essential oils thymol (from thyme) and linalool, terpinene and eugenol (from marjoram) combine with the detoxing properties of chives to make this a quick-and-easy inclusion in your cleansing regime.

# nutty herb noodles

Simple, delicious and economical, this is a great supper dish at any time, in spite of its cleansing and detoxifying ingredients. You certainly don't have to be ill to enjoy it, but its high energy content also makes it a perfect food for convalescents.

**noodles** 450g (1lb)

**extra-virgin olive oil** 3 tbsp

**cooked chicken or ham** 225g (8oz), cubed or shredded

**pine nuts** 50g (1³/₄oz)

**mixed herbs** such as marjoram, basil, thyme and chives, 2 tbsp finely chopped

**parmesan cheese** 3 tbsp freshly grated

1 Cook the noodles according to the packet instructions until just tender.

2 Meanwhile, heat the oil in a frying pan and gently sauté the chicken or ham pieces.

3 Toast the pine nuts in a separate, dry frying pan for 2 minutes.

4 When ready, drain the noodles and add to the meat mixture with the pine nuts.

5 Stir in the herbs, and serve with the Parmesan.

## vital statistics

Pork is an excellent source of protein, iron and B vitamins. Onions help lower cholesterol, while fennel's volatile oils anethole and fenchone stimulate the liver and the digestive tract. The pinenes, borneol and carvacrol in winter or summer savory help fight infections, and as an added bonus, summer savory also helps prevent flatulence.

# fennel fillet

Low-fat, high-protein organic pork makes Fennel Fillet a healthy addition to your menu collection. Add the cholesterol-lowering and antibacterial effect of onions and the purifying properties of fennel, and you have a cleansing, liver-stimulating and anti-inflammatory meal that – thanks to the unusual combination of fennel and savory in the creamy sauce – tastes terrific, too.

**extra-virgin olive oil** 3 tbsp

**pork fillets** 1kg (2lb 4oz), lean organic

**onion** 1 small, finely chopped

**plain flour** 1 tbsp

**white wine** 150ml (5fl oz)

**natural live bio-yogurt or crème fraîche** 200ml (⅓ pint)

**fennel and savory** 1 tsp each finely chopped

**1** Heat the oil in a frying pan and brown the pork fillets on both sides over a high heat.

**2** Turn the heat down, cover and cook through – about 20 minutes.

**3** Remove the meat, keep warm and pour off all but 3 tablespoons of the fat.

**4** Add the onion and sweat gently until softened. Blend in the flour and add the wine.

**5** Cook, stirring continuously, until thickened. Add the yogurt or crème fraîche, then the herbs.

**6** Pour the mixture over the meat and serve.

## vital statistics

As with all treats, these are a bit naughty, but the protein, vitamins and fibre in the flour and the tremendous calming effect of lavender make them a far better alternative to sleeping pills or tranquillizers. Just making these delicious nibbles is therapeutic, since the aromatic oils pervade your kitchen.

# anise peaches

Few desserts can be enjoyed as part of a cleansing regime, but this one certainly fits the bill, because its flavours are as good as its cleansing properties. The surprising combination of catmint and anise brings out the subtle flavours of the peaches, resulting in a seemingly indulgent but nonetheless health-giving dish.

**caster sugar** 5 tbsp
**cold water** 300ml (½ pint)
**star anise** 3
**peaches** 4 large, peeled, stoned and sliced
**catmint** 4 sprigs, to decorate

**1** Heat the sugar with the water in a saucepan over a low heat until the sugar has dissolved.

**2** Add the star anise and simmer gently for 7 minutes.

**3** Add the peaches and continue simmering for 10–12 minutes.

**4** Remove the peaches and place in a ceramic heatproof dish large enough to contain them in a single layer. Boil the liquid in the saucepan until it is reduced by half.

**5** Pour over the peaches and serve decorated with the sprigs of catmint.

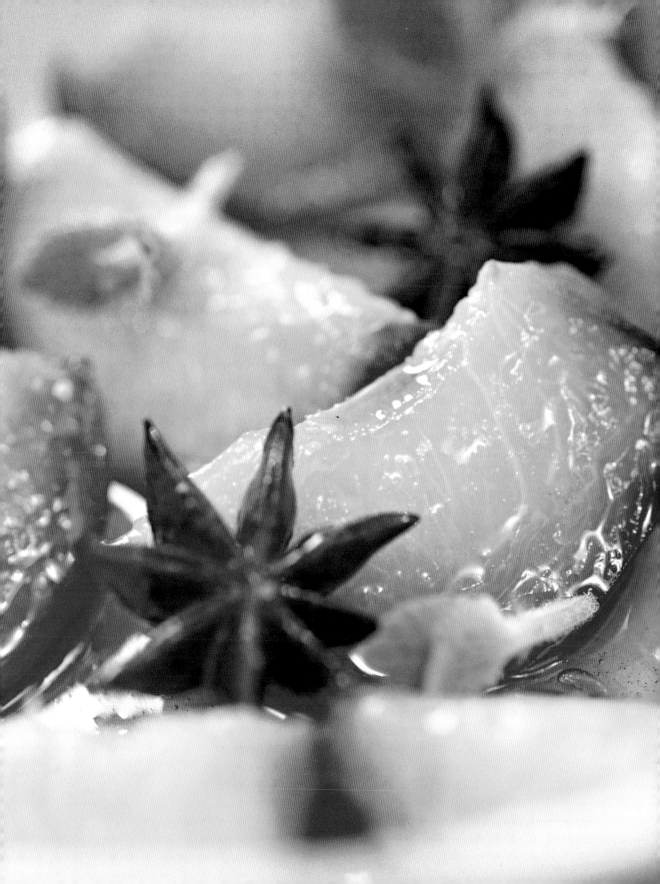

## vital statistics

Cherries are super-rich in vitamin C, potassium, magnesium and a host of cancer-fighting phytochemicals. When combined with lemon verbena's volatile oils – limonene, geraniol and citral – they make a valuable addition to any cleansing regime, gently calming the digestion and pepping up the nervous system.

# verbena delight

This exquisite variation on the classic Provençal *clafouti* is all the more delicious due to the combination of the slightly acidic cherries and the sweet, lemon-scented fragrance of verbena. This recipe also works well with any fresh stone fruits, such as plums, peaches and apricots.

**cherries** 500g (1lb 2oz), stoned

**lemon verbena** 3 tbsp finely chopped

**free-range eggs** 4

**caster sugar** 60g (2¼oz)

**plain flour** 50g (1¾oz)

**crème fraîche or cream** 300ml (10fl oz)

**brandy** 3 tbsp

**1** Preheat the oven to 180°C/350°F/gas mark 4.

**2** Put the cherries into a buttered gratin dish. Sprinkle over the lemon verbena.

**3** Whisk the eggs in a bowl, stir in the sugar, then slowly beat in the flour.

**4** Add the crème fraîche or cream and brandy; stir until well mixed.

**5** Pour the egg mixture over the cherries and verbena, and bake for 30 minutes.

## vital statistics

This dessert provides useful amounts of protein, fibre, selenium, iodine, vitamin B12, folic acid and vitamins A, C and E. Ellagic acid from the apples is cancer-fighting, while pectin is an excellent digestive aid.

# villandry apple flans

Villandry is one of my favourite food shops in London and must be one of the best in the country. Rosie, the proprietor's wife, gave me this recipe, since it's one I love to eat at their restaurant. Made with luscious organic apples and free-range organic eggs, it's a scrumptious, indulgent yet healthy treat.

**caster sugar** 200g (7oz)
**cold water** 75ml (2½fl oz)
**dessert apples** 1.25kg (2lb 12oz), peeled and chopped
**granulated sugar** 2 tbsp
**unwaxed lemon** grated rind of 1
**free-range eggs** 5, plus 2 yolks
**crème fraîche** to serve

**1** Preheat the oven to 180°C/350°F/gas mark 4.

**2** Heat the caster sugar with the water in a heavy-based saucepan over a low heat, stirring lightly, until dissolved. Turn the heat up and cook, without stirring, until the syrup turns a light caramel colour – watch closely to avoid burning. Quickly pour the caramel into 6 ramekins, brushing it around the sides.

**3** Cook the apples in a separate saucepan until soft. Add the granulated sugar and lemon rind. Beat the eggs and yolks lightly, then add them to the apple mixture.

**4** Fill the ramekins with the apple mixture. Transfer to a roasting tin half-filled with hot water, cover with foil and bake for 40 minutes, until puffed and firm. Turn out on to plates and serve with crème fraîche.

This soup contains iron, potassium, folic acid, carotenoids and vitamin C. Dandelion is a powerful diuretic and a rich source of coumarins, relieving fluid retention and high blood pressure. Sorrel is a traditional herbalists' detox plant, whose tannins and volatile oils are good for the skin. Salad burnet aids digestion, and its delicate flavour is perfect in soups and salads.

# wonderful weed soup

Gardeners might have other ideas, but a 'weed' is really just a plant growing where it's not wanted. In this recipe, you'll want as many edible weeds as you can find, because they're nutritious as well as having therapeutic and cleansing benefits. The same basic method will work for all delicate, leafy herbs, preserving their flavours as well as their attractive green colour.

**mixed 'weeds'** such as dandelion, nettles, sorrel, rocket and salad burnet, 90g (3¼oz), stalks removed, well washed

**unsalted butter** 40g (1½oz)

**extra-virgin olive oil** 2 tbsp

**onion** 1 small, chopped

**potatoes** 175g (6oz)

**herb or vegetable stock** 1 litre (1¾ pints) – *see* page 396 or use a good stock cube or bouillon powder

**crème fraîche** 225ml (8fl oz)

1  Purée the 'weed' leaves in a food processor or blender. Add the butter and purée again; set aside.

2  Heat the oil in a saucepan and sweat the onion gently until soft. Add the potatoes and cook gently until golden.

3  Add the stock and simmer until the potatoes are soft. Stir in the crème fraîche and purée again.

4  Just before serving, whisk in the puréed leaves.

## vital statistics

This soup is very low in fat and provides 10 per cent of the recommended daily amount of iron, as well as modest amounts of iodine, selenium, folic acid and vitamin A.

# watercress soup

Like cabbage, broccoli and Brussels sprouts, watercress is a brassica – which means it contains natural antibiotics and cancer-fighting phytochemicals. It's also a great cleansing vegetable, specifically known to be protective against lung cancer. Besides tasting great hot, this dish is equally delicious as a cold summer soup.

**garlic** 2 cloves

**extra-virgin olive oil** 1 tbsp

**onion** 1 large, finely chopped

**curry powder** 1 tsp

**watercress** 4 bunches, with stalks

**vegetable stock** 850ml (1½ pints) – *see* page 396 or use a good stock cube or bouillon powder

**black pepper** freshly ground, to taste

**natural low-fat live bio-yogurt** 1 small carton (about 125ml/4fl oz)

**1** Chop the garlic and leave to stand for 10 minutes before cooking. Heat the oil in a large, heavy-based saucepan and cook the onion over a moderate heat until soft and translucent but not browned.

**2** Add the garlic and cook for 1 minute. Add the curry powder and cook for 1 minute, stirring continuously.

**3** Turn the heat down, add the watercress and cook, stirring, until wilted – around 2–3 minutes.

**4** Add the stock and black pepper and simmer for 10 minutes. Whizz in a food processor or blender – or use a hand blender – until smooth. Pour the soup into serving bowls and add a spoonful of yogurt to each.

## vital statistics

Rhubarb, an underrated medicinal plant, has been valued as a cleanser since the Middle Ages. Strawberries, very rich in vitamin C and with some well-absorbed iron, are also rich in antioxidants that can help delay the effects of ageing.

# face-mask special

Helena Rubinstein famously said that women shouldn't put anything on their faces that they wouldn't put into their mouths. This unusual cold soup is a perfect example; it's bursting with vitamin C and healing phytochemicals from the fruit, as well as essential oils from the spices. It also offers a gentle boost to the circulation from the small amount of alcohol. You probably could put it on your skin, but it will do more good, and give you much more pleasure, if you eat it.

**rhubarb** 450g (1lb), sliced

**strawberries** 225g (8oz), hulled, plus a few chopped to decorate

**orange juice** 450ml (16fl oz)

**cinnamon stick** 5cm (2in) piece

**star anise** 2 (optional)

**caster sugar** 50g (1³/₄oz)

**grand marnier** 3 tbsp (optional)

**mascarpone cheese** 4 tbsp

**1** Put the rhubarb, most of the strawberries, orange juice, cinnamon stick and star anise, if using, into a large saucepan.

**2** Bring to the boil and cook until the rhubarb is tender – about 10–15 minutes.

**3** Remove the cinnamon stick and star anise.

**4** Add the sugar and stir until it dissolves.

**5** Whizz in a food processor or blender until smooth, strain into a large bowl and stir in the Grand Marnier, if using.

**6** Refrigerate until really cold.

**7** Serve with a dollop of mascarpone in each bowl and scatter with a few strawberry pieces.

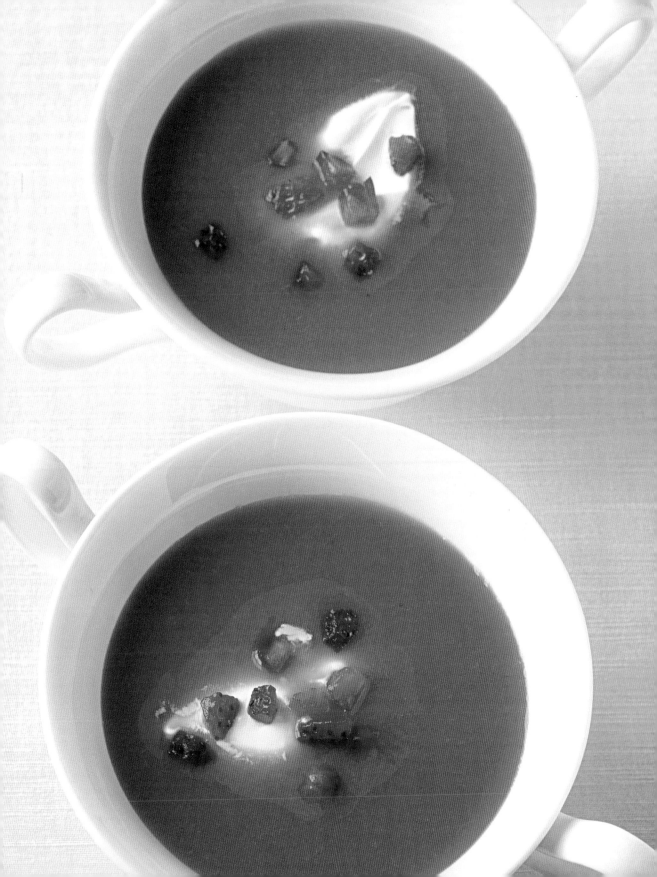

This classic soup provides a quarter of your daily recommended amount of protein, lots of fibre and important amounts of calcium, magnesium, potassium, selenium and folic acid.

# french onion soup

Enjoy the legendary benefits of onions now! Onions are powerfully antibiotic and protect against infections, giving this soup the power to detoxify and cleanse. They also lower cholesterol levels and reduce the risk of blood clots. What more could anyone ask for?

**extra-virgin olive oil** 1 tbsp

**onions** 3 large, sliced

**potato** 1, peeled and diced

**vegetable stock** 850ml (1½ pints) – *see* page 396 or use a good stock cube or bouillon powder

**black pepper** freshly ground, to taste

**thyme** 1 sprig

**lemon juice** 2 tsp, freshly squeezed

Optional

**wholemeal french bread** 8 slices

**gruyère cheese** 115g (4oz), coarsely grated

**1** Heat the oil in a large, heavy-based saucepan and sweat the onions until they just start to turn brown.

**2** Add the potato, stock, black pepper, thyme and lemon juice and bring to the boil, then turn the heat down and simmer gently for 20 minutes.

**3** To enjoy this soup as they do in France, float 2 slices of wholemeal French bread on the top of each serving, sprinkle with grated Gruyère and place under a grill preheated to high until the cheese melts.

The pumpkin in this colourful soup gives a boost of betacarotene and folic acid, while the nasturtium flowers are rich in antibacterial mustard oils. It is perfect for those who want to lift and rejuvenate their complexion.

# pumpkin soup with nasturtium flowers

How sad that the wonderful flavour and nutritional value of pumpkins only emerges for Halloween – and even then, they're wasted as decorative jack-o'-lanterns. Yet pumpkins are perfect as a healthy alternative to stodgier winter foods, and in this soup they help counteract the dehydrating effects of central heating. Topped with nasturtium flowers, this is one dish that looks as delicious as it tastes.

**unsalted butter** 25g (1oz)

**extra-virgin olive oil** 2 tbsp

**white onions** 2 large, finely chopped

**garlic** 2 cloves, finely chopped

**curry powder or paste** 3 tsp

**vegetable stock** 1 litre (1¾ pints) – *see* page 396 or use a good stock cube or bouillon powder

**pumpkin** 1kg (2lb 4oz) (or squash or courgettes) peeled, deseeded and cubed

**crème fraîche** 4 tbsp

**nasturtium flowers** 4 (use chive flowers if unavailable)

**1** Melt the butter with the oil and sweat the onions and garlic gently until soft.

**2** Add the curry powder or paste and cook for 2 minutes, stirring continuously.

**3** Pour in the stock and bring to the boil.

**4** Add the pumpkin (or squash or courgettes) to the stock and simmer until just tender.

**5** Whizz in a food processor or blender – or use a hand blender – until smooth.

**6** Stir in the crème fraîche and mix thoroughly.

**7** Serve with the nasturtium flowers (or chive flowers) on top.

## vital statistics

Fennel contains the natural plant chemicals anethole and fenchone. Although it's traditionally been used for the treatment of colic in children, it has a diuretic effect that makes it a useful cleanser. Both apples and pears are rich in the soluble fibre pectin, which improves digestion and bowel function. Apples are a uniquely rich source of ellagic acid, another cleansing phytochemical.

# fantastic fennel

The liquorice-like flavour of fennel, combined with the sweetness of apples and pears, imparts a delicious and unusual flavour to this drink. Apples have traditionally been used by natural practitioners as a cleansing and detoxifying food, because they have the ability to remove toxic substances from the system. Fennel is a mild diuretic and an extremely good digestive aid; it also has a balancing effect on female hormones.

**carrot** 1, trimmed and peeled unless organic

**apples** 2 large, unpeeled, uncored and quartered

**pears** 2, unpeeled and uncored

**fennel** 1 bulb

**1** Put all the ingredients through a juicer and mix well. Strain if necessary.

## vital statistics

This juice is rich in vitamins A and C, folic acid and potassium, and contains a good amount of iron. Its cleansing power is due to the influence fennel and chicory exert on liver and kidney functions – perfect for easing the bloating that can accompany periods. For menopausal women, its phyto-oestrogens act as a natural 'hormone replacement therapy' to help prevent bone loss and subsequent osteoporosis.

# women's wonder

When 'that time of the month' rolls around, it's time to down a glassful of this superjuice. Women's Wonder is a powerful cleanser and, thanks to the fennel, contains phyto-oestrogens (plant hormones) that help regulate periods and bring some relief from PMS and menopausal symptoms. While this juice has been designed with women in mind, it's fine for men, too!

**apples** 2, unpeeled, uncored and quartered
**carrots** 2, trimmed and peeled unless organic
**chicory** 1 head
**fennel** ½ bulb

**1** Put all the ingredients through a juicer.

## vital statistics

Vitamin E is provided by the avocado in this drink and is essential for maintaining the healthy structure of blood vessels. The gingerols and zingiberene from the ginger are the natural ingredients that stimulate the circulation. Add to this the cleansing properties of the sulphur compounds in garlic and the high concentration of citric acid in lemon juice, and you have a tasty and satisfying smoothie.

# avo go

This combination of juice and smoothie gets many of its cleansing properties from the pear. Pears are rich in pectin, a soluble fibre that not only improves the body's elimination of cholesterol but also helps stimulate the large bowel and prevent constipation. Ginger has a specific cleansing effect through its stimulation of the peripheral circulation and overall improvement of blood flow. This helps remove waste material so that it can be transported to the kidneys and excreted in urine. The live bacteria in the yogurt improve bowel function and elimination, and the overall cleansing effect of lemon juice rounds everything off.

**pear** 1 large, unpeeled and uncored

**garlic** 1 clove, chopped

**fresh root ginger** 1cm (½in) piece, peeled and finely grated

**natural live bio-yogurt** 50ml (2fl oz)

**avocado** 1 ripe

**lemon** ½

1 Put the pear through a juicer. Pour the juice into a blender or food processor.

2 Add the garlic and ginger to the blender or food processor, pour in the yogurt and whizz briefly.

3 Halve and stone the avocado. Scoop out the flesh and add to the blender or food processor.

4 Squeeze the lemon half and pour in the juice.

5 Whizz briefly until smooth.

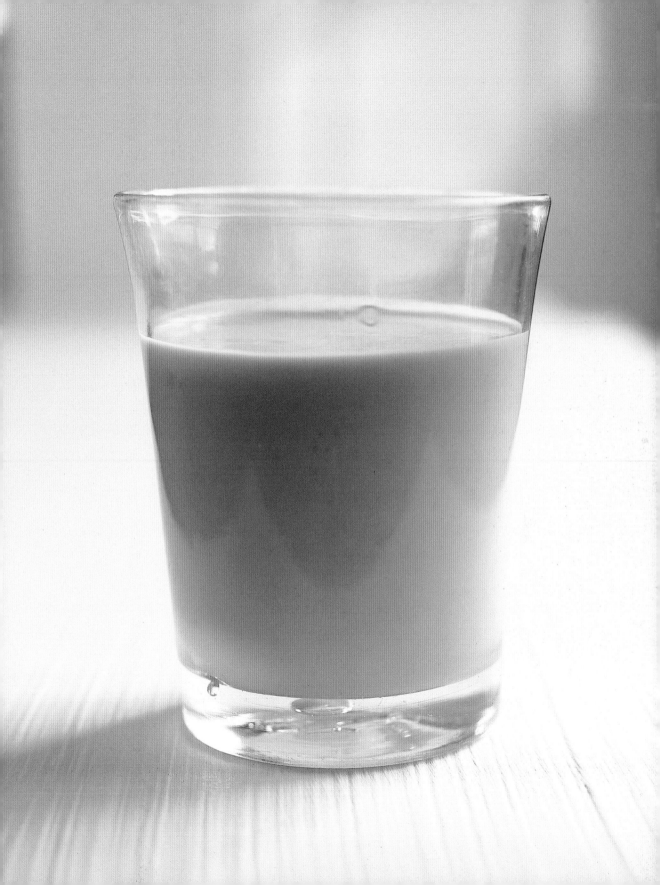

This juice is rich in vitamins A and C, as well as fibre. Ginger is one of the most versatile and valuable of spices. The ancient Greeks used it for digestive problems and as an antidote to poisoning, while medieval herbalists highly valued its warming properties. It also provides an invigorating lift.

# ginger spice

Ginger Spice is a gentle cleanser that benefits from the powerful volatile oils zingiberene and gingerol present in the ginger, as well as offering the cleansing and digestive benefits of carrot, apple and orange. This juice has powerful antiseptic and anti-inflammatory properties and is perfect to use at the onset of a cold or fever, or immediately after a bout of food poisoning.

**carrots** 2, trimmed and peeled unless organic

**apple** 1, unpeeled, uncored and quartered

**orange** 1, peeled but leaving white pith in place

**fresh root ginger** 25g (1oz), peeled and sliced

**1** Put all the ingredients through a juicer.

## vital statistics

Melon provides folic acid, potassium and a little vitamin A, C and B, but it is renowned in folklore as a cleansing fruit. The cancer-fighting phytochemicals, large amounts of folic acid and the eye-protective carotenoids lutein and xeaxanthine all come from spinach, while sage provides plant hormones and the powerfully antiseptic thujone.

# popeye's secret

Popeye's belief that spinach is a great source of muscle-building iron is, unfortunately, not true. There is lots of iron in spinach, but your body can extract hardly any of it due to the oxalic acid that is also present in spinach leaves. However, this wonderful vegetable is a very rich source of other nutrients that are especially good for the eyes. Mixed here with diuretic parsley, cleansing melon and antibacterial sage, it makes a cleansing and healing drink.

**honeydew melon** 1, peeled, deseeded and cubed

**baby spinach leaves** 1 handful

**sage leaves** 4

**flat-leaf parsley** 2 sprigs

**1** Put the melon, spinach and sage leaves into a blender or food processor and whizz until smooth.

**2** Tear the leaves off the parsley stalks, chop them finely and scatter over the juice.

## vital statistics

Cucumber has a gentle diuretic effect. Mint provides menthol and menthone, natural phytochemicals that are both antiseptic and cleansing, and also act as a potent digestive. Using natural sea salt means you get small quantities of iodine, which helps improve thyroid function. This, in turn, stimulates the whole metabolic process and increases eliminative functions.

# cucumber and mint slush

This refreshing, cooling slush is almost tzatziki without the yogurt. Cucumber isn't rich in nutrients, since it's made up mostly of water, but it has long been used as a cleanser – both externally for the skin and internally. It's really the mint that provides the major cleansing benefit, because it is one of the most effective of all digestive aids; its detoxing properties also help relieve headaches and migraine. You'll hardly ever see salt added to any of my recipes, but in this instance it does enhance the flavour and helps boost the metabolism.

**cucumber** 1 large, peeled and deseeded
**mint** 4 large sprigs, plus 2 extra to garnish
**sea salt** scant 1 tsp
**crushed ice**

**1** Put the cucumber into a blender or food processor with the mint and salt and whizz until smooth, adding a little water if the consistency is too thick.

**2** Chill thoroughly.

**3** Serve poured over the crushed ice, garnished with the extra sprigs of mint.

## vital statistics

This juice is rich in vitamin C, soluble fibre and natural sugars. It contains antioxidant bioflavonoids and potassium. The pith of lemons is rich in limonene, believed to have anti-cancer properties. For this reason, when making the Lemon Express, it's best to peel the lemon first, leaving on the white pith, and then put it through your juicer, rather than using a citrus-fruit juicer that leaves all the helpful pith behind.

# lemon express

Grapes are one of nature's great cleansers. Because of their high natural sugar content, they should always feature in any detox regime. If you're cleansing your digestive system and reducing food consumption, the extra sugar will keep your energy levels up. The combination of grapes, soluble fibre in the apples and the gentle diuretic effect of the lemon makes this juice particularly effective.

**apples** 3, unpeeled, uncored and quartered
**lemon** 1, unpeeled if thin-skinned or peeled but leaving white pith in place
**white seedless grapes** 115g (4oz)

**1** Put all the ingredients through a juicer.

## vital statistics

This drink is rich in vitamin C: one glass provides four times the amount you need for a day. Most of the vitamin C comes from the rosehip, but elderflowers are a rich source, too. Nasturtiums are rich in the cleansing essential oils myrosin and spilanthol, which also boost immunity. The delicate flavour of lavender belies its potent therapeutic benefits as a cleansing and protective herb.

# two-flower treat

People imagine nasty things when it comes to cleansing regimes. Nothing could be further from the truth with this wonderful mixture of elderflowers and nasturtiums. Elderflowers contain cleansing natural chemicals such as tannins and rutin. They're also surprisingly rich in the essential fatty acids that are nature's own anti-inflammatories. The peppery flavour of the nasturtium flowers is the result of the mustard oil, another cleansing and antiseptic natural chemical; its sharpness offsets the sweetness of the elderflower and the rosehip syrup. Combined with the spiciness of ginger, one of the best of all digestive cleansers, and the delicate flavour of the lavender flowers, it makes a fabulous cooling, cleansing drink on a hot summer's day.

**nasturtium flowers** 6
**crushed ice**
**fresh root ginger** 2.5cm (1in) piece, peeled and grated
**pure rosehip syrup** 1 tbsp
**sparkling elderflower pressé** 700ml (1¼ pints), organic
**lavender flowers** 5g (⅛oz), rubbed off the stalk

**1** Put the nasturtium flowers into an ice-cube tray, fill with water and freeze. If you grow your own, make up a supply; they'll keep for at least 3 months.

**2** Fill a large glass tumbler a third full with crushed ice, add the ginger and rosehip syrup and stir well.

**3** Pour in the elderflower pressé and float the nasturtium ice cubes on the top. Sprinkle with the lavender flowers.

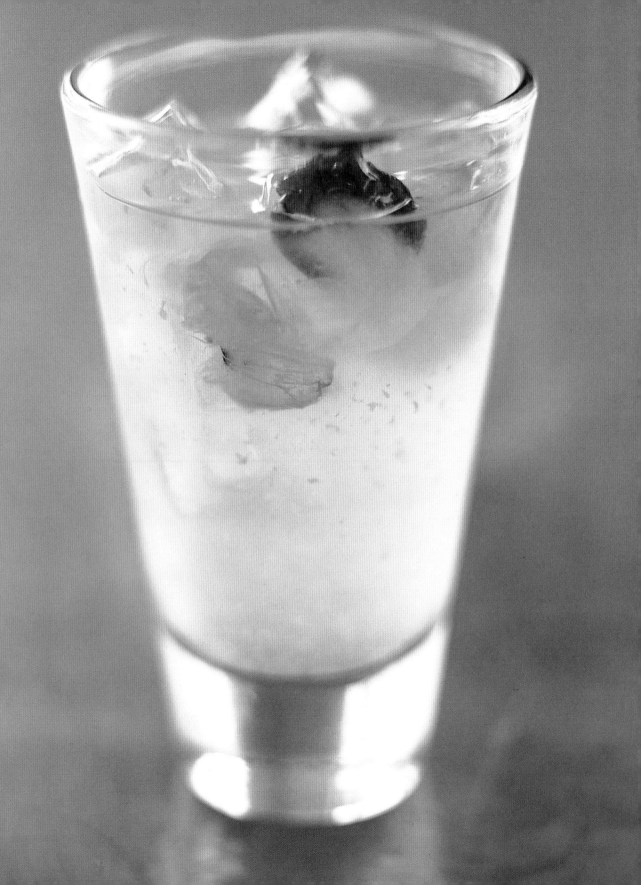

## vital statistics

This juice is rich in vitamins A, C and E. It contains folic acid, magnesium and potassium. It is particularly suitable for physically active men who enjoy regular sport (of course, women can take it, too). The mineral content will also replace losses experienced through sweating. As a regular cleansing juice taken once or twice weekly, it ensures a substantial intake of cancer-fighting nutrients thanks to the watercress and broccoli.

# the activator

Naturopaths regard melon as a cooling cleanser, and in Indian Ayurvedic medicine it's used as an effective diuretic. It is also cooling to the body and soothing to the digestion. The addition of watercress, broccoli and the tart cooking apple make this 'green juice' a perfect cleanser for men, because it has a testosterone-enhancing effect. It's gently laxative and a powerful immunity booster.

**cooking apple** 1, unpeeled, uncored and quartered

**green melon** ½, peeled and deseeded

**broccoli florets** 85g (3oz), without thick stalks

**watercress** 1 handful

**1** Put all the ingredients through a juicer.

## vital statistics

This drink is super-rich in vitamins A, C, E and folic acid, and is also rich in potassium and magnesium. As well as its strong diuretic effect, it will benefit the skin and is ideal for anyone with high blood pressure or heart disease, since it is very low in sodium.

# waterfall

Another powerful diuretic juice, Waterfall combines celery and parsley to help ease even the most stubborn fluid retention. Although English curly parsley is fine for this recipe, the European flat-leaf variety has a richer, fuller and slightly smoother flavour and is, if anything, an even better diuretic.

**carrots** 3, trimmed and peeled unless organic
**apples** 2, unpeeled, uncored and quartered
**celery** 2 sticks, with leaves
**parsley** 1 handful, with stalks

**1** Put all the ingredients through a juicer.

The cleansing plant chemicals in cowslips, dandelions and marjoram give this drink its real boost, though the very high vitamin-C content is a major cleansing factor, too. The lemon peel is rich in bioflavonoids, which are also cleansing and protective.

# granny's lemon barley water

Lemon barley water has been a traditional cleansing formula of herbalists for hundreds of years. It's particularly effective for all forms of urinary problem and is a great cleansing aid for most skin conditions, particularly those associated with oily skins and recurrent spots. The three herbs enhance the cleansing abilities of this drink, and the high fibre content of the barley means that one glass can provide up to a third of your daily fibre needs, making this an excellent bowel cleanser as well. Most importantly, it tastes delicious.

**pot barley** 125g (4½oz)

**demerara sugar** 55g (2oz)

**unwaxed lemons** 2

**cold water** 1.2 litres (2 pints)

**cowslip flowers, dandelion leaves or marjoram** 1 handful, well washed

**ice cubes**

**1** Wash the barley and put it into a large heatproof jug.

**2** Put the sugar into a bowl. Scrub the lemons with warm water and grate the rind into the sugar; mix together and add to the barley.

**3** Bring the water to the boil, pour over the barley, sugar and lemon rind, stir vigorously and leave to cool.

**4** Squeeze the juice from the lemons, add to the barley, stir again and strain through a fine sieve. If you have access to cowslip flowers or dandelion leaves, they make an unusual addition; if not, you can buy marjoram in the supermarket or grow your own.

**5** Serve over lots of ice cubes for a taste of the 'real thing' – far removed from the oversweetened, artificial bottled stuff that's commercially available.

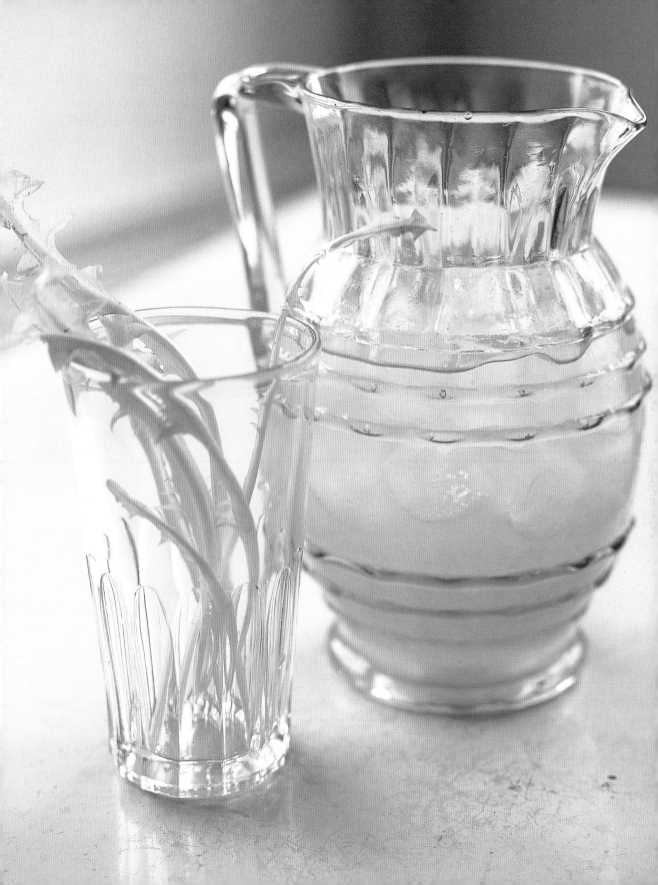

# lady windermere's fan club

This recipe was given to us by my wife Sally's oldest friend, Diana. She's a keen golfer and a Mancunian, and she spends a lot of her spare time travelling around the major golf tournaments, helping provide hospitality for the world's top players. According to Diana, this drink is a favourite with lady golfers and all the female golf fans in the north of England. It's the ginger and the lemons that have the cleansing effect – and of course, it tastes even better made with traditional ginger beer.

**ginger beer** 300ml (½ pint), chilled
**lemonade** 300ml (½ pint), chilled
**angostura bitters** 2 shots

1 Mix the ingredients together thoroughly and serve.

## vital statistics

This juice is super-rich in vitamin C. It contains potassium, calcium, folic acid and bioflavonoids. Oranges boost overall resistance and are good for the heart and circulatory system. They are also considered beneficial to the intestines, since they make it difficult for unwanted bacteria to survive. They also help with constipation and wind. Like most citrus fruits, oranges stimulate the flow of saliva.

# minty morning

This is a variation on what has to be the most popular breakfast juice of all. By combining the health-giving properties of oranges with the natural oils present in mint (the best digestive of all the herb family), this juice makes a powerful digestive aid and cleanser that gets to work right from the start.

**oranges** 4 large
**mint** 1 large sprig

**1** If using a citrus-fruit juicer, just halve the oranges. If using a regular juicer, peel the oranges, removing most of the white pith.

**2** Put the oranges through the citrus-fruit juicer. Chop the mint finely and stir into the juice. Alternatively, feed a few mint leaves into the regular juicer between each 2 or 3 pieces of orange.

## vital statistics

Saffron contains the natural ingredients saffronal, cinelle and crocins, and has anti-depressant and mood-enhancing properties. Its main cleansing attribute helps induce menstruation, thus preventing the build-up of waste products. The phyto-oestrogens in soya milk have a weak hormonal effect that is especially beneficial to women. Like all nuts, almonds are a rich source of vitamin E, essential fatty acids and minerals.

# soya with saffron

Here's a smoothie that's simply bursting with nutritional value. Lots of protein, minerals, plant hormones and all the digestive protection of honey are present in this mixture. The saffron adds a wonderful colour, but it is also a mood-enhancer and helps improve digestion. Throughout Asia, most women have a daily intake of some form of soya protein, and it is this component of their diets that is believed to protect them against heart disease, osteoporosis, hot flushes and the other unpleasant symptoms of the menopause in later life.

**soya milk** 450ml (16fl oz)
**runny honey** 2 heaped tbsp
**saffron threads** 1 large pinch
**ground almonds** 1 tbsp
**flaked almonds** 1 tsp

1 Put the soya milk, honey, saffron and ground almonds into a blender or food processor.

2 Whizz until smooth.

3 Serve with the flaked almonds floating on top.

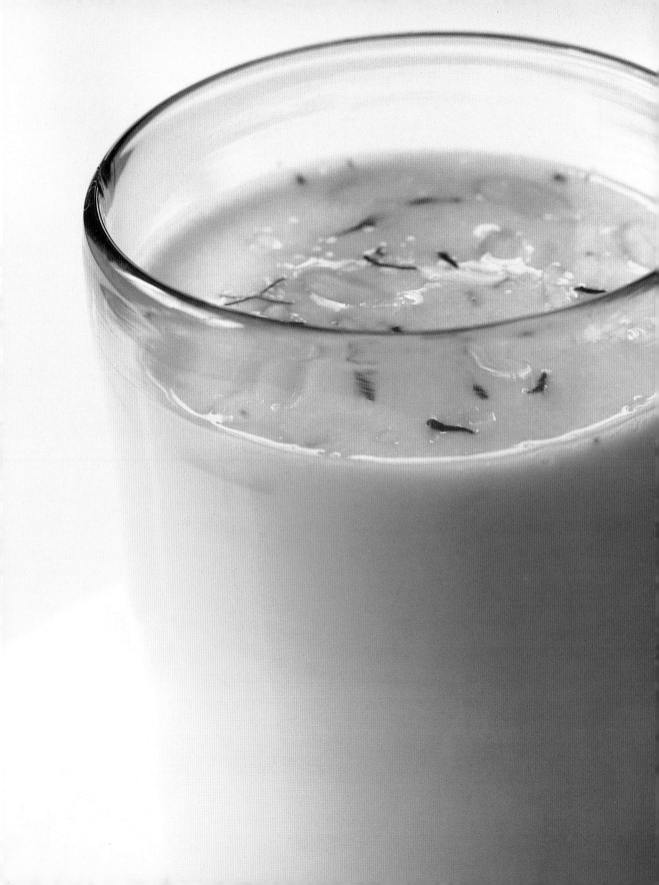

Prune juice is rich in betacarotene, iron, B vitamins and potassium. The fresh apricots provide soluble fibre, some iron and lots more betacarotene. It's the way these two ingredients stimulate bowel function and improve digestion that produces the cleansing benefits of this delicious smoothie.

# prune and apricot smoothie

Jokingly known as 'nature's little black-coated workers', prunes are an immensely effective cleanser due to their laxative effect. But they are much more than that since, weight for weight, they are the most powerful protective food of all. Regular consumption of prunes really does protect you against premature ageing, heart disease, many forms of cancer and even wrinkles. Add the nutrients and fibre from apricots and you have a double whammy of a cleanser.

**apricots** 6, stoned
**prune juice** 250ml (9fl oz)

**1** Put the apricots into a blender or food processor with the prune juice and whizz until smooth.

This juice is super-rich in vitamin C and rich in vitamin A. It contains useful amounts of potassium and calcium. The acidity of all these citrus-fruit juices helps remove unwanted bacteria from the digestive tract and encourages the growth of beneficial probiotic bacteria. This digestive aid should be drunk for two or three days after a course of antibiotics to get your system back in good running order as soon as possible.

# rainbow cocktail

This mixture of orange-, pink-, green- and yellow-skinned citrus fruits is a cleanser for both the liver and intestines. Its clean, tangy, wide-awake taste also makes it a favourite anytime drink. Use the Rainbow Cocktail as an excellent start to the detox cleansing day. And if you are unfortunate enough to wake up with a hangover, then this works better than the hair of any dog!

**oranges** 2, peeled but leaving white pith in place

**lemon** 1, unpeeled if thin-skinned

**lime** 1, peeled (unless key lime)

**pink grapefruit*** 1, peeled but leaving white pith in place

\* If taking prescribed medicines, consult your doctor before drinking large amounts of grapefruit juice.

**1** Put all the ingredients through a juicer.

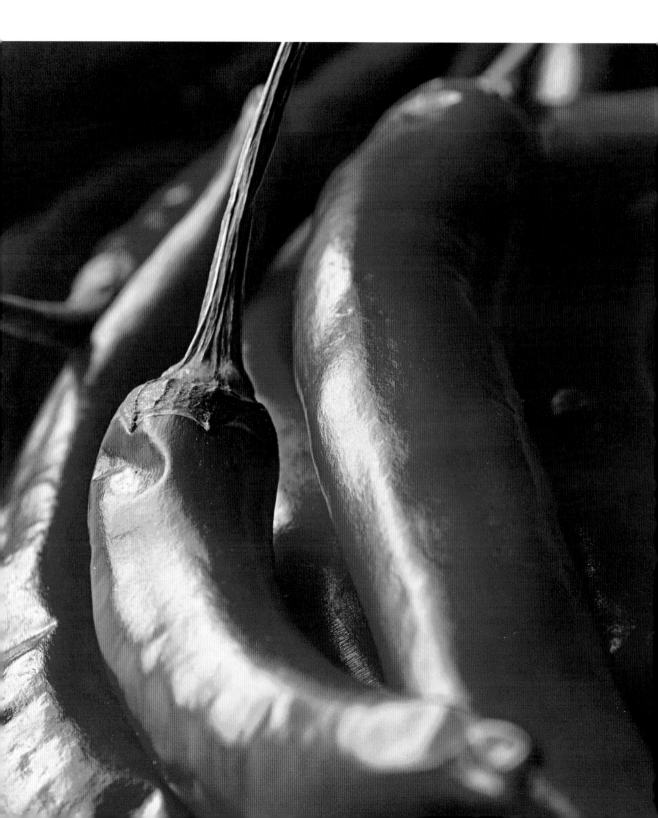

circulation

**A**lmost more than any other medical condition, circulatory problems are easier to prevent than to cure. Don't become a couch potato, don't put on too much weight and don't let your diet fall victim to burger chains, pizza parlours and convenience-food manufacturers. There's nothing wrong with an occasional treat, but as a staple diet they spell disaster.

One such circulatory disaster is high blood pressure. High blood pressure, or hypertension, is one of the most important factors in the cause of heart disease, which kills prematurely more people in the Western world than any other illness. It has no symptoms until the first stroke, kidney failure or heart attack. The good news is that you can reduce the chances of anyone in your family getting it. You can even do things to reduce blood pressure if it's already a problem by making simple changes.

Throughout daily life, the blood pressure varies considerably, depending on what is needed. Your brain must get a regular supply of 750cc of blood each minute, and this is regardless of what the rest of your body is doing. If your arteries are narrowed, due to hardening, silting up with cholesterol or if they are constricted by nicotine, caffeine and excess alcohol, then the heart has to pump harder to push the blood around the system, and up goes the blood pressure.

It is at this point that self-help is the first and most important step. Treating high blood pressure with drugs is not a cure for the condition – it's merely a way of controlling the symptom. This may be a vital step when the pressure is much too high, but you can do things to help, even when medication is unavoidable. Many of my patients have been able to reduce the amount of medicine that they need to take, or even cut it out completely. (Never change your drug regime without your doctor's advice, however.) If you follow some simple suggestions for helping to reduce your blood pressure, your own GP will soon see when the readings start to fall, and he will want to reduce your drug intake. The three steps to reducing blood pressure are to change your diet, take regular exercise and learn some form of relaxation.

Other circulatory problems include coronary heart disease, angina, strokes, visual disturbances, senile memory loss, Raynaud's disease, intermittent claudication, chilblains and complications of diabetes. Whatever the specific problem or symptoms, however, the general food advice remains the same.

## Eating for good circulation

Herbs and spices have a part to play in treating most circulatory problems. Horseradish, ginger, cinnamon, cayenne, paprika and chillies are all circulatory stimulants and should feature prominently in your diet. But no matter how well you're eating, a healthy circulation needs regular exercise in order to stimulate the entire cardiovascular system. You don't have to become a fitness freak, a marathon runner or an aerobics addict; just half an hour's brisk walk three or four times a week, ten minutes of vigorous housework or gardening two or three times a day, playing your favourite sport, going for a swim or bicycling are all fine. Exercise becomes even more vital for the elderly, the incapacitated and the disabled. Arm and hand movements, foot and ankle rotation, knee exercise, hip, thigh and even abdominal muscles can be exercised sitting in a chair or lying in bed. No matter how little you think you can do, the more you do, the more you'll be able to do.

## Circulation-boosting foods

The recipes in this section are full of stimulating spices like ginger. You'll also find oatmeal to improve digestive function, prevent constipation and protect the heart and blood vessels; nuts for vitamin E; dates for fibre and extra iron; citrus fruits for bioflavonoids; and oily fish like salmon to protect the heart and blood vessels from inflammatory changes and help maintain the elasticity of the larger arteries.

    This is a cookbook, not a medical textbook, but you will find references to some of the specific circulatory problems in the introductions to the recipes that follow.

# circulation checklist

- Eat more garlic, onions, oats, apples and pears for their cholesterol-lowering benefits; cabbage, carrots, broccoli and sweet peppers for betacarotene; blackcurrants, cherries and citrus fruits for vitamin C and bioflavonoids; buckwheat for its rutin; oily fish for omega-3 fatty acids; nuts, seeds, avocados and extra-virgin olive oil for vitamin E.
- Eat fewer saturated fats found in all meat and meat products – burgers, sausages, salamis, pâtés, pies – and fewer bakery goods such as Swiss rolls, Danish pastries, or cakes. Avoid all artificially hardened and hydrogenated fat, all trans fats and excess alcohol, and consume less caffeine, sugar and salt. Finally, of course, avoid smoking.

## vital statistics

This dish is a light but effective blood builder. Oranges are rich in protective vitamin C and bioflavonoids, and chives have many benefits for the heart and circulation.

# beetroot and orange with chives

Throughout Eastern Europe, beetroot has been a traditional remedy for blood and circulatory disorders for centuries; in fact, the juice is given to anyone suffering from leukaemia. Combining it with slices of fresh orange and chives, makes for a light, delicious and appealing dish.

**salad dressing** 3 tbsp (*see* below)
**cooked beetroot** 3 large, cooled
**oranges** 2 large
**chives** 1 bunch, plus 6 chive flowers (optional)

**Salad dressing**
**extra-virgin olive oil** 400ml (14fl oz)
**cider vinegar** 200ml (⅓ pint)
**runny honey & mustard** 1 tbsp each
**spring onions** 2, finely chopped
**garlic** 1 clove, finely chopped
**black pepper** freshly ground, to taste
**rosemary** 1 sprig
**bay leaves** 2

**1** For the salad dressing, whisk all the ingredients, except the rosemary and bay leaves, together in a jug and pour into a bottle with a tight-fitting stopper.

**2** Peel the beetroot and cut into thickish slices.

**3** Peel the oranges and remove as much white pith as you can. Slice into thin rounds.

**4** Arrange alternate slices of beetroot and orange on a large platter or 4 individual plates.

**5** Scatter the whole chives over the top.

**6** Decorate with the chive flowers, if desired; they are edible and taste delicious.

**7** Add the rosemary and bay leaves to the dressing, shake well and drizzle over the salad.

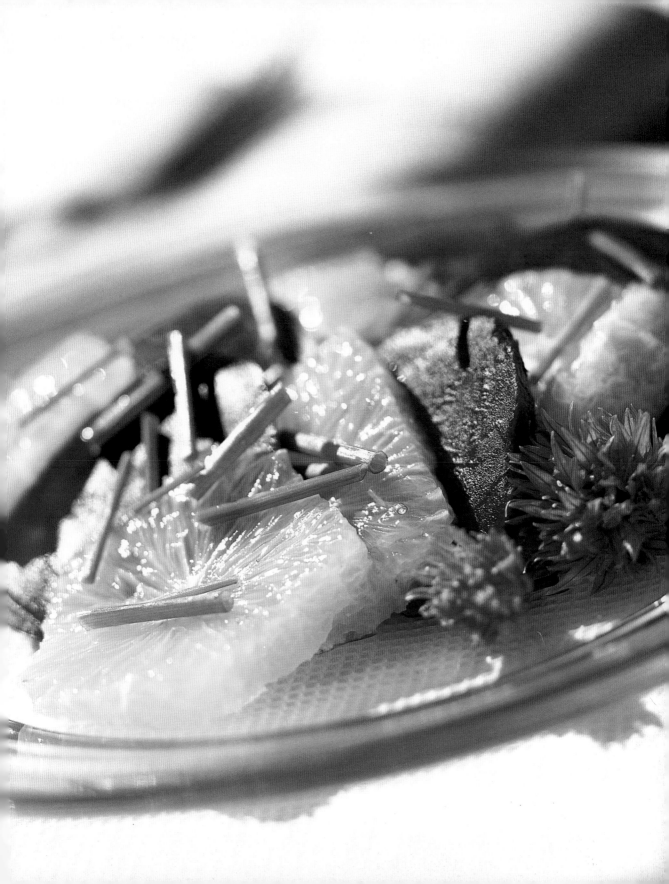

# fennel, rocket and radish salad

The familiar flavour of fennel used as a herb is found in many fish dishes, but this salad uses the large white bulb of the Florence fennel. Here, its crunchy texture and unusual flavour of mild liquorice is beautifully complemented by the sharp bite of rocket and radishes. Bringing together with the circulatory stimulus of the essential mustard oils in radishes, and the tannins and other volatile oils in the rocket, this dish will give a quick boost to even the most sluggish of circulations.

**fennel** 1 large bulb
**rocket** 1 generous bunch
**radishes** 12, quartered
**salad dressing** 3 tbsp (*see* page 182)

**1** Slice the fennel into rounds, reserving some of the green fronds, if there are any.

**2** Put all the ingredients, except the fennel fronds, into a salad bowl.

**3** Add the dressing and toss lightly.

**4** Sprinkle any fennel fronds over the top.

## vital statistics

This salad kick-starts the heart and circulation; it is also bursting with antioxidants. The betacarotene in the red, yellow and orange peppers protects the linings of your arteries and promotes a healthy heart and circulation.

# warming pepper salad

If you can, try to avoid the perfectly shaped, supermarket-packaged peppers, most of which are grown hydroponically – that means in artificially fertilized water. Instead, look for the long, pointed, misshapen peppers that are likely to have higher levels of essential nutrients.

**peppers** 1 each red, yellow and orange, cored, deseeded and diced

**garlic** 1 clove, finely chopped

**chilli oil** 1 tbsp

**extra-virgin olive oil** 2 tbsp

**balsamic vinegar** 1 tbsp

**cayenne pepper** ½ tsp

**mixed herbs** parsley, sage, thyme, marjoram, oregano and chives, 1 tbsp chopped

**1** Put the peppers into a salad bowl. Add the garlic and mix thoroughly with the peppers.

**2** Combine the oils and vinegar and whisk in the cayenne pepper. Pour over the peppers.

**3** Mix the herbs thoroughly with the peppers.

**4** Leave the salad to marinate for at least 3 minutes before serving.

This salad is a great circulatory stimulant, because figs contain the natural enzyme ficin, which improves the digestive absorption of the fruit's other constituents, especially iron, vital for healthy blood and circulation.

# citrus fig salad

Since the time of ancient Greece, figs have been renowned for their restorative and energy-building properties. They were so highly prized that the earliest Olympic athletes were fed pounds of them to improve their performance – with good reason, since figs are full of blood-building nutrients.

**lamb's lettuce** 1 generous bunch

**tarragon leaves** 2 tbsp coarsely chopped

**lemon** juice of 1

**extra-virgin olive oil** 1 tbsp

**fresh figs** 8 ripe, quartered

**1** Put the lamb's lettuce into a serving bowl with the chopped tarragon.

**2** Thoroughly mix the lemon juice with the oil. Add to the bowl and toss thoroughly to coat all the surfaces.

**3** Arrange the fig quarters over the top.

## vital statistics

Bean sprouts are rich in vitamin E, essential for a healthy heart and circulation; dates are an excellent source of iron, the blood-building mineral; and grapes contain many circulation-friendly antioxidants.

# nutty dates and grapes

An unusual mixture of bean sprouts from the culinary traditions of the Far East, almonds and dates from the Middle East and grapes from southern Europe makes this a super circulation booster.

**bean sprouts** 1 bag
**black and white seedless grapes** 20, halved
**fresh dates** 12, halved and stoned
**walnut oil** 1 tbsp
**sesame oil** 1 tsp
**balsamic vinegar** 1 tsp
**light soy sauce** 1 tsp
**almond halves** 2 tbsp, blanched
**black pepper** freshly ground, to taste

**1** Thoroughly wash and dry the bean sprouts – even if they're 'ready-washed'.

**2** Arrange the salad in 4 serving bowls, putting the bean sprouts in the bottom and sprinkling the grapes and dates on top.

**3** Whisk the oils, vinegar and soy sauce together.

**4** Drizzle each bowl with a little of the dressing – but don't toss.

**5** Scatter over the almonds and season to taste with black pepper.

## vital statistics

This dish provides good winter protection with a bite of chilli and warming spices.

# tiger, tiger

This is a bit of a luxury – but why not? It will really cheer you up in the depths of winter – or at any time of year, actually. There's lots of immunity-boosting zinc from the prawns, the warming spiciness of chilli and ginger, more winter protection from the spring onions and lots of artery-protecting lycopene from the tomatoes. This salad makes a wonderful light lunch or a really showy starter.

**cucumber** ½ large, peeled, halved, deseeded and chopped into small pieces

**tomatoes** 4 large firm, chopped into small pieces

**groundnut oil** 2 tbsp

**sesame oil** 3 tsp

**green pepper** 1, cored, deseeded and chopped into small pieces

**fresh red chilli** 1, deseeded and chopped into small pieces

**fresh root ginger** 6 thin slices, peeled

**garlic** 2 cloves, flattened with the blade of a large knife

**tiger prawns** 12 large in their shells, cooked or uncooked

**light soy sauce** 1 tsp

**spring onions** 6, thinly sliced lengthways

**1** Mix the cucumber and tomatoes together and put into a large serving bowl.

**2** Heat the oils in a large wok or deep frying pan over a high heat, add the green pepper, chilli, ginger and garlic and stir briskly.

**3** Add the prawns: if they're already cooked, they'll only take 2 minutes at maximum heat; if they're uncooked, they'll take 4 minutes at most; you'll know they're done when they turn from grey to pink all over. Shake vigorously while cooking to make sure that they're well coated with the oil and spices. When almost done, add the soy sauce.

**4** Arrange the prawns on top of the salad.

**5** Remove the garlic and pour the remaining oil on top. Garnish with the spring onions.

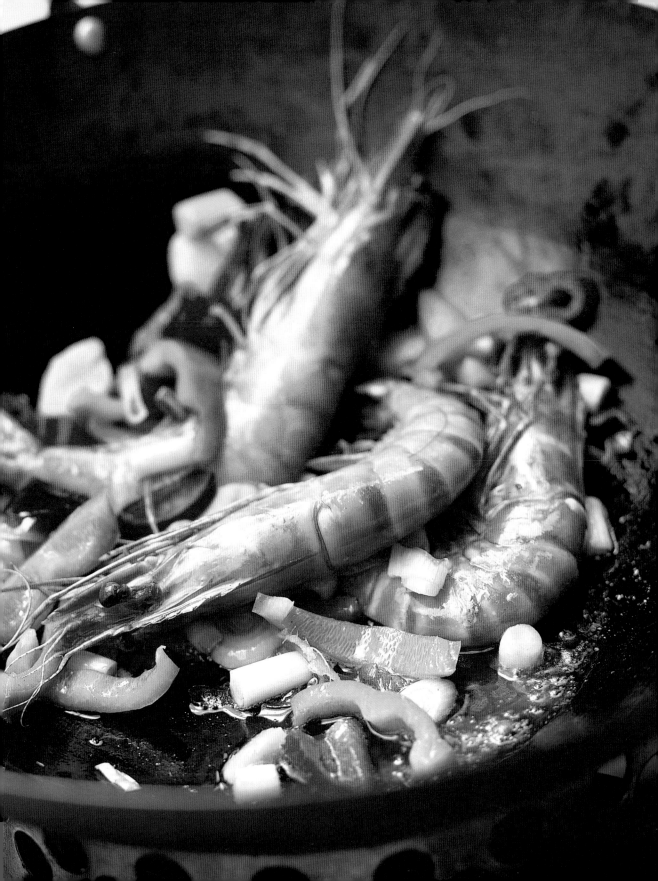

# shades of salmon red

All oily fish is good for the circulation, and salmon is one of the best. Although it is more expensive, it's really worth choosing wild salmon, since it not only tastes better, but it will not contain the chemicals added to the feed of farmed fish. The omega-3 fatty acids in the fish protect both the heart and arteries, and help prevent the build-up of plaque inside the blood vessels. With a slice of good, crusty wholemeal bread, this salad makes a meal for four. To use as a starter, reduce the quantities accordingly.

**fresh wild salmon** 675g (1lb 8oz)

**bay leaves** 2

**peppercorns** 6

**dill** 1 sprig

**red pepper** 1 large, cored, deseeded and chopped into small cubes

**fresh green chilli** 1 small, deseeded and very thinly sliced

**garlic** 1 clove, chopped

**cucumber** 7.5cm (3in) chunk, peeled and chopped

**natural low-fat live bio-yogurt** 1 small carton (about 125ml/4fl oz)

**radicchio** 1 head

**1** Put the salmon into a large saucepan of cold water with the bay leaves, peppercorns and dill. Bring slowly to the boil, then turn off the heat and leave to cool.

**2** Remove the salmon and flake the flesh.

**3** Stir the red pepper, chilli, garlic and cucumber into the yogurt, pour over the flaked salmon and stir gently to combine.

**4** Separate the radicchio leaves. Arrange the salmon on top and serve.

This spicy salad stimulates blood flow and is packed with wintertime nutrients.

# curried bean and egg salad

Commercially produced curry powder is almost never used by real Indian cooks, since nearly every family makes its own. However, it is still a wonderful winter warmer. The spices in this salad stimulate increased blood flow, and turmeric – an essential part of any curry powder or paste – is a particularly powerful antioxidant that protects against many forms of cancer. The beans provide natural plant hormones, while the eggs are a rich source of body-building protein and winter-resistance nutrients.

**free-range eggs** 4, hard-boiled

**curry powder** 2 tsp

**mayonnaise** 6 tbsp

**green flageolet beans** 300g can, drained and rinsed

**borlotti beans** 300g can, rinsed

**red onion** 1, thinly sliced

**fresh coriander leaves** 2 tbsp chopped

**1** Shell and slice the eggs into rounds.

**2** Whisk the curry powder into the mayonnaise and stir into the beans, mixing thoroughly.

**3** Add the onion to the bean mixture.

**4** Arrange the egg slices on top and sprinkle with the chopped coriander.

# b-warm salad

This delicious combination of ingredients is a real winter blood builder – and good blood is the key to keeping warm in the winter. Chicken livers take minutes to cook and are an amazingly good source of protein, easily absorbed iron and vitamin B12, high levels of which are essential for the oxygen-carrying ability of blood.

**unsalted butter** 55g (2oz)

**extra-virgin olive oil** 4 tbsp

**garlic** 2 cloves, flattened with the blade of a large knife

**chicken livers** 500g (1lb 2oz), washed and dried, white membranes removed

**cos lettuce** 1 head, torn into small pieces

**black seedless grapes** 20, halved

**parsley** 1 generous bunch, coarsely chopped

**black pepper** freshly ground, to taste

**1** Put the butter, oil and garlic into a large frying pan and heat gently. When hot, remove the garlic and add the chicken livers.

**2** Turn the heat up and fry the livers for 3 minutes, shaking the pan frequently to make sure that they're all coated with the oil. Don't overcook – they should be slightly pink in the middle.

**3** Put the lettuce into the bottom of a shallow dish. Add the livers, pouring over any remaining fat from the pan.

**4** Scatter the grapes on top. Sprinkle with parsley and black pepper, and serve while still warm.

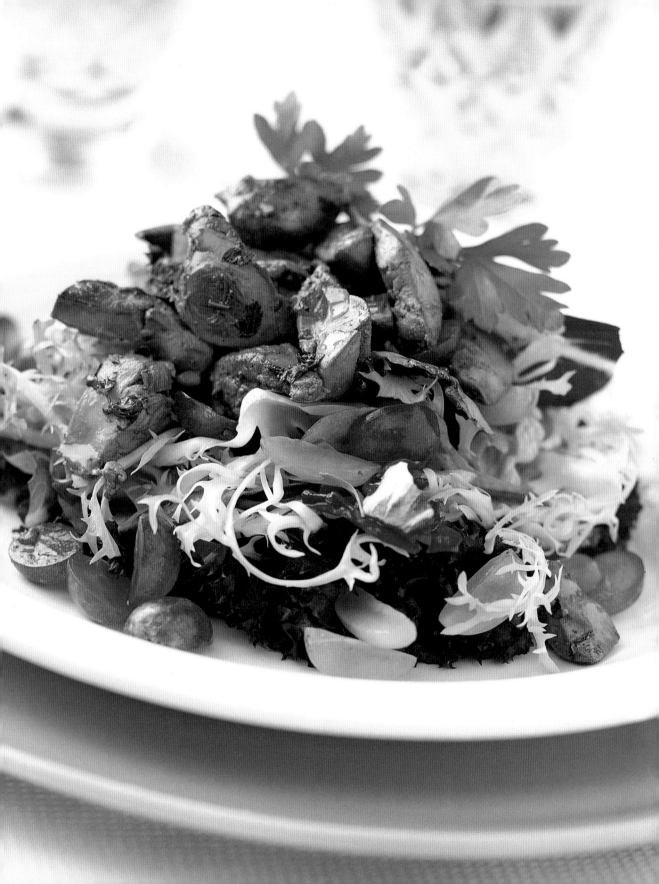

This hot and healthy treat will thaw you out even on the coldest winter's day. The tomatoes in the passata are full of artery-protecting lycopene, while the chillies are a great source of vitamin C, carotenoids and capsaicin, and they will help promote good circulation and prevent chilblains.

# devil's pasta

This salad is based on a traditional Italian dish, known as *pasta arrabbiata* or *diavolo* – 'devil's sauce'. Make it as hot as you like – the more chilli it has, the more warming it is. This is an ideal dish for the freezing months of winter.

**parsley** 2 sprigs
**dried oregano** 1 tsp
**chilli powder** 1 tsp
**cayenne pepper** 1 pinch
**garlic** 2 cloves
**red wine vinegar** 2 tsp
**extra-virgin olive oil** 1 tbsp
**passata** 25g (1oz)
**penne** 400g (14oz)
**mangetout** 100g (3½oz), cut into short pieces
**courgettes** 2, coarsely grated
**chestnut mushrooms** 6, thinly sliced
**baby sweetcorn** 200g (7oz)
**parmesan cheese** 3 tbsp freshly grated

**1** Put the parsley, oregano, chilli, cayenne pepper, garlic, vinegar and oil into a food processor or blender and whizz together.

**2** Add the passata and whizz again briefly.

**3** Put the penne into a large saucepan of salted boiling water and cook according to the packet instructions until al dente.

**4** Drain and shake off the surplus water. Return to the saucepan, add the sauce and stir over a low heat until the pasta is well coated and the sauce is hot.

**5** Add all the vegetables, turn into a large bowl and eat while still warm, sprinkled with the Parmesan.

## vital statistics

This risotto is a great detoxifier, because it stimulates digestive functions, as well as relieving varicose veins, high blood pressure and hardening of the arteries.

# complete eastern risotto

Here's a complete meal in under half an hour. This dish is given a very different texture and flavour by using bulgur wheat, and it offers all the heart and circulatory benefits of onions and garlic into the bargain. Serve it in the traditional Middle Eastern way, with yogurt, onions and a green salad.

**unsalted butter** 60g (2¼oz)

**onion** 1 large, finely chopped

**garlic** 2 cloves, chopped

**bulgur wheat** 250g (9oz)

**chicken or vegetable stock**
450ml (16fl oz) – *see* page 396 or use a good stock cube or bouillon powder

**sea salt** 1 pinch

**To garnish**

**groundnut or rapeseed oil** 1 tbsp

**onion** 1 large, sliced into rings

**natural live bio-yogurt** 1 small carton
(about 125ml/4fl oz)

**1** Melt the butter in a large, heavy-based saucepan over a low heat and sauté the chopped onion and garlic gently until they start changing colour.

**2** Add the bulgur wheat and stir well until coated with the butter.

**3** Add enough stock to cover the mixture and the salt and bring to the boil. Cover and simmer gently for 10 minutes or until the liquid is absorbed. (Add more stock if it seems to be drying out too quickly.)

**4** While the bulgur wheat is cooking, heat the oil in a frying pan and fry the onion rings until they begin to crisp. Serve the bulgur wheat garnished with the fried onion rings and yogurt.

# spiced lentil soup

In this soup, spices come into their own, working together to get your circulation buzzing. Add B vitamins and good fibre from the lentils, and calcium, phosphorus and magnesium from the coconut milk, and you have an effective, delicious and satisfying dish for circulatory health.

**extra-virgin olive oil** 3 tbsp

**onion** 1, thinly sliced

**garlic** 1 clove, finely chopped

**fresh root ginger** 2.5cm (1in) piece, peeled and finely grated

**coriander seeds** 1 tbsp, crushed

**ground allspice** 1 tbsp

**chilli powder** 1 tsp

**vegetable stock** 700ml (1¼ pints) – *see* page 396 or use a good stock cube or bouillon powder

**coconut milk** 400ml can

**green lentils** 150g (5½oz)

**1** Heat the oil in a large saucepan and sweat the onion gently for 5 minutes.

**2** Add the garlic and ginger and continue sweating for 4 minutes.

**3** Stir in the coriander, allspice and chilli powder and cook, stirring continuously, for 3 minutes.

**4** Stir in the stock and the coconut milk and bring to a simmer.

**5** Stir in the lentils and continue to simmer for about 30 minutes.

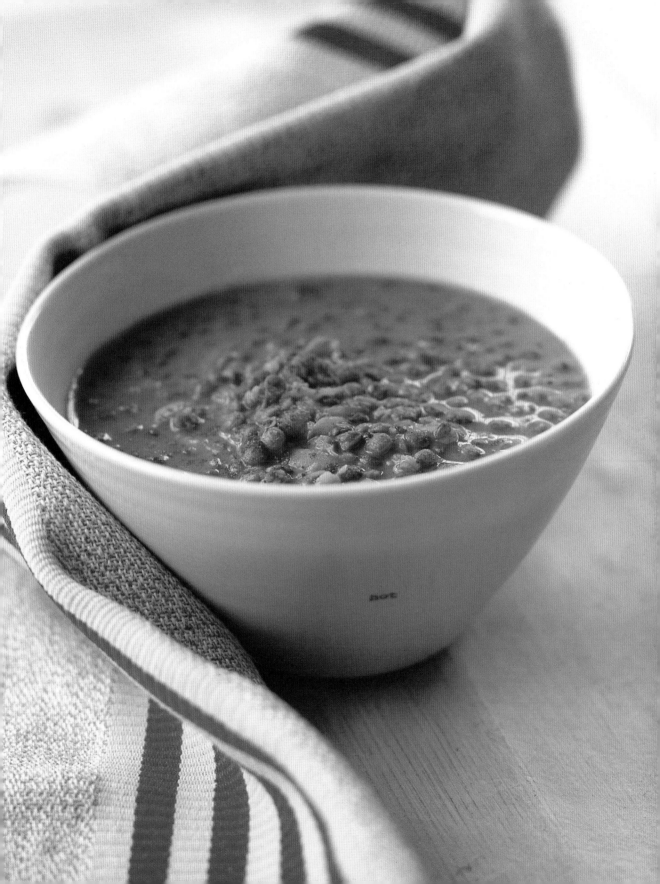

## vital statistics

This fragrant soup will help keep your blood flowing freely. Parsnips are rich in minerals and fibre, while beans and peas supply beneficial plant hormones.

# curried parsnip and vegetable soup

Putting parsnips together with stimulating spices such as curry produces a soup that is seriously good for your circulation. Adding beans and peas increases the fibre content and supplies beneficial protein, while the crème fraîche gives it a wonderfully creamy texture and supplies calcium, too.

**extra-virgin olive oil** 4 tbsp

**onion** 1 large, finely chopped

**curry powder** 1 heaped tbsp

**plain flour** 2 tbsp

**parsnips** 2, about 500g (1lb 2oz), peeled and diced

**vegetable stock** 1.2 litres (2 pints) – *see* page 396 or use a good stock cube or bouillon powder

**crème fraîche** 200ml (⅓ pint)

**french beans** 100g (3½oz), cut into 2.5cm (1in) lengths

**peas** 100g (3½oz), fresh or frozen

**1** Heat the oil in a saucepan and sweat the onion gently for 10 minutes.

**2** Remove from the heat and stir in the curry powder and flour.

**3** Return to the heat and cook, stirring continuously, for 3 minutes.

**4** Add the parsnips and cook, stirring, for 2 minutes.

**5** Pour in the stock and bring to the boil.

**6** Turn the heat down and simmer for 20 minutes or until the parsnips are tender.

**7** Whizz the mixture in a food processor or blender – or use a hand blender – until smooth, return to the pan and bring back to a simmer.

**8** Stir in the crème fraîche.

**9** Add the beans and peas and simmer the soup for another 7 minutes.

## vital statistics

This soup is great for reducing blood pressure, since leeks contain phytochemicals that help lower cholesterol.

# ginger, leek and carrot soup

The leek is a member of the *Allium* genus of plants and, just like its onion and garlic relatives, it is a rich source of natural sulphur-based chemicals that improve the circulation. This recipe provides a triple boost from all three. As an extra circulatory bonus, there's plenty of ginger as well.

**extra-virgin olive oil** 3 tbsp

**red onion** 1 large, thinly sliced

**garlic** 3 plump cloves, finely chopped

**leeks** 3 large, finely chopped

**fresh root ginger** 2.5cm (1in) piece, peeled and grated

**carrots** 1kg (2lb 4oz), trimmed and peeled unless organic, finely diced

**vegetable stock** 1.2 litres (2 pints) – *see* page 396 or use a good stock cube or bouillon powder

**1** Heat the oil in a large saucepan and sweat the onion, garlic, leeks and ginger gently for 10 minutes.

**2** Add the diced carrots and stir until coated with the oil mixture.

**3** Pour in the stock and bring to the boil.

**4** Turn the heat down and simmer until the carrots are tender – about 20 minutes.

**5** Whizz in a food processor or blender – or use a hand blender – until puréed.

**6** Pour through a fine sieve, being careful to remove any unpuréed ginger.

## vital statistics

Lentils provide energy, fibre, folic acid and iron. Feel-good essential oils come from thyme and bay leaves, while onions and garlic offer winter protection.

# lovely lentils

This soup is the embodiment of that wonderful image we all have of a great pot of warming peasant soup bubbling on the stove. Yes, there is bacon, which means salt and fat, but it's a very small percentage of the total, and there's no other animal fat in the recipe. Lentils may be small, but nutritionally they're mightily powerful. Some studies have indicated that a diet rich in legumes such as lentils can significantly reduce your risk of dying from heart disease. This is a comforting soup, with slow-release energy that also controls blood sugar and helps get rid of bad cholesterol.

**olive oil** 3 tbsp

**bacon** 115g (4oz), cut into thin strips crossways (or the same quantity of tofu, cubed)

**onions** 2 small, finely chopped

**celery** 2 sticks, sliced

**garlic** 6 cloves, crushed

**puy lentils** 175g (6oz)

**tomatoes** 400g can, crushed

**vegetable stock** 600ml (1 pint) – *see* page 396 or use a good stock cube or bouillon powder

**thyme** 3 sprigs

**bay leaves** 2

**1** Heat the oil in a large saucepan and cook the bacon, onions and celery until the vegetables are soft – about 10 minutes.

**2** Add the garlic and cook, stirring, for about 1 minute until soft.

**3** Add the lentils and stir until coated with the oil and bacon fat.

**4** Add the tomatoes, stock, thyme and bay leaves and bring to the boil. Turn the heat down and simmer for about 35 minutes or until the lentils are tender.

**5** Remove the thyme and bay leaves before serving.

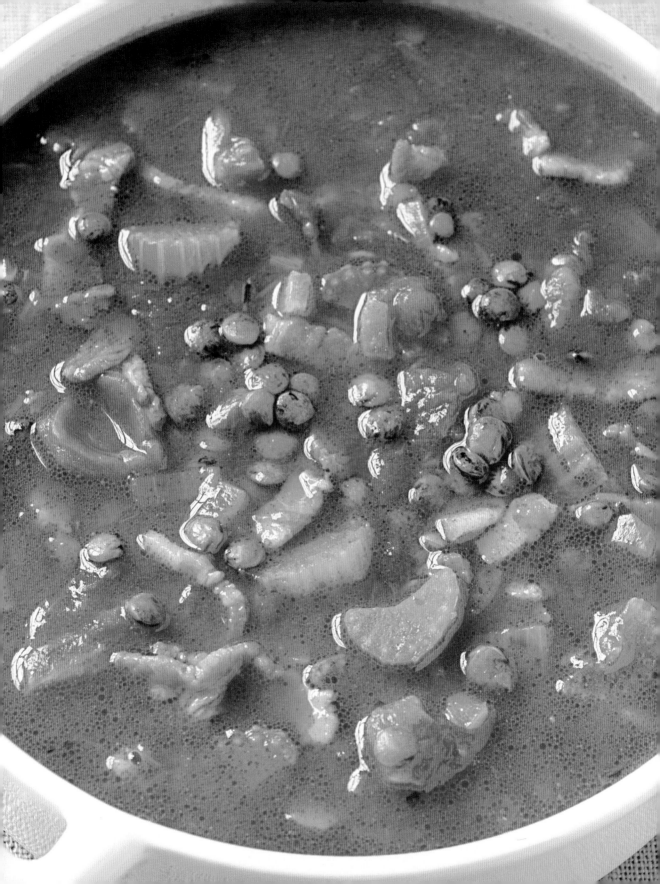

## vital statistics

This is a great soup for protecting the heart. Oats are rich in B vitamins and soluble fibre, while broccoli supplies vitamin C and betacarotene, which protect the heart and help prevent cancer.

# oatmeal and broccoli soup

As well as being a healthy breakfast food in the form of porridge, oats are a versatile ingredient and can be used to delicious advantage in many other ways. In this unusual soup, they're combined with broccoli to make a surprisingly light and delicate dish that offers huge health benefits.

**extra-virgin olive oil** 2 tbsp

**spring onions** 6, finely chopped

**broccoli florets** 600g (1lb 5oz), halved if very large

**oatmeal** 75g (2³/₄oz)

**semi-skimmed milk** 700ml (1¼ pints)

**vegetable stock** 750ml (1¼ pints) – *see* page 396 or use a good stock cube or bouillon powder

**sea salt and black pepper** freshly ground, to taste

**natural live bio-yogurt** 4 tbsp

**chives** 1 generous bunch, finely snipped, or Herb Croûtons (*see* page 95), to serve

**1** Heat the oil in a large saucepan and sweat the springs onions gently for about 5 minutes until soft.

**2** Add the broccoli and cook gently, stirring continuously, for 3 minutes.

**3** Mix in the oatmeal and continue cooking for 4 minutes, still stirring.

**4** Pour in the milk and stock, cover and simmer for 10 minutes. Season to taste with salt and black pepper.

**5** Serve with a spoonful of yogurt in each bowl.

**6** Scatter with the chives or the herb croûtons.

## vital statistics

This soup supplies heart-friendly olive oil with monounsaturated fat. Garlic and onion contain protective chemicals; courgettes provide betacarotene; and natural Greek yogurt delivers calcium, protein and friendly bacteria.

# greek cold courgette soup

It's no coincidence that Greek men live the longest in Europe and that Cretan men have the live longest in Greece. This is all down to their traditional diet, which is based on fish, olive oil, fruit, vegetables, nuts and seeds. Thanks to these foods, Greeks have the lowest level of heart and circulatory disease. This soup is a typical Cretan recipe, full of heart-friendly ingredients and containing nothing to interfere with good health.

**olive oil** 2 tbsp

**onion** 1, finely chopped

**garlic** 1 clove, flattened with the blade of a large knife and finely chopped

**ground ginger** 1 tbsp

**courgettes** 2 large, cut into large cubes

**unwaxed lemon** juice and finely grated rind of 1 large

**vegetable stock** 1.2 litres (2 pints) – see page 396 or use a good stock cube or bouillon powder

**natural greek yogurt** 4 tbsp

**1** Heat the oil in a large saucepan and add the onion, garlic and ground ginger. Mix well and cook gently until the onion and garlic are soft – about 5 minutes.

**2** Add the courgettes and lemon juice and rind, and pour in the stock.

**3** Bring to the boil, then turn the heat down and simmer gently until the courgettes are tender – about 20 minutes.

**4** Whizz in a food processor or blender – or use a hand blender – until smooth and return to the pan.

**5** Add the yogurt, mix well and leave to cool.

**6** Chill in the refrigerator until really cold.

# beetroot soup

Throughout Eastern Europe, beetroot is renowned for its blood- and circulation-boosting properties. Served as soup or juice, this vegetable has been used in the treatment of anaemia, poor circulation and even leukaemia. In this recipe, it is combined with carrots and lemon juice to provide a refreshing, nourishing soup for healthy blood.

**raw beetroot** 1kg (2lb 4oz), unpeeled

**carrots** 2 large, trimmed and peeled unless organic

**white onion** 1, peeled

**garlic** 1 clove, peeled

**extra-virgin olive oil** 5 tbsp

**vegetable stock** 1.4 litres (2½ pints) – see page 396 or use a good stock cube or bouillon powder

**lemon** juice of 1

**natural live bio-yogurt** 400ml (14fl oz)

**croûtons or white seedless grapes** to serve (optional)

**1** Grate the beetroot, carrots, onion and garlic, or chop them in a food processor.

**2** Heat the oil in a large saucepan and sweat the vegetables gently for 10 minutes.

**3** Add the stock and simmer, covered, for 40 minutes.

**4** Strain the soup into a clean saucepan and bring back to a simmer.

**5** Stir the lemon juice into the yogurt.

**6** Serve the soup with a swirl of the flavoured yogurt on top, along with croûtons, if desired. Alternatively, serve the soup cold, substituting white seedless grapes for the yogurt.

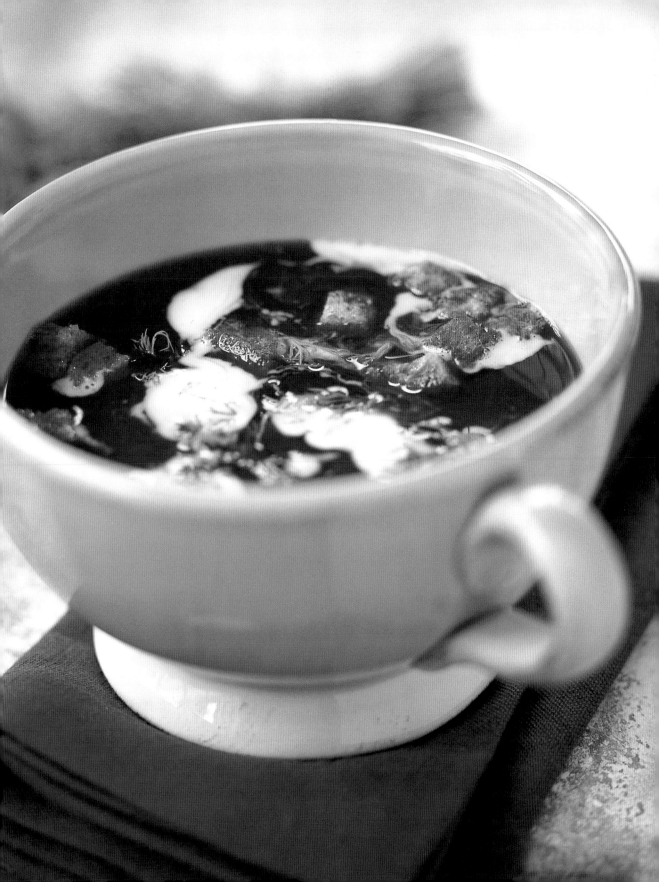

Cooking the rice in good stock means the grains absorb all the nutrients from the vegetables. The stimulating oils from the chillies boost the circulation, and the spicy curry powder adds more tropical heat to this strange but delicious soup.

# hot, sweet and spicy soup

Egg yolk, curry, cocoa and chilli in the same soup sounds disgusting. Thankfully, I had no idea of the ingredients when I first tasted this. I'd been travelling for three days: London, Frankfurt, Rio de Janeiro, São Paulo and finally Manaus, the capital of Amazonas, Brazil. I ate this soup in a street-side café a stone's throw away from the Rio Negro: little more than a tin shack with a sheet of sacking between the diners and the kitchen. It was a meeting place of South American cultures: the rainforest Indians, the Spanish, the Portuguese and, of course, the French. Raw eggs are not suitable for young children and the elderly.

**unsalted butter** 25g (1oz)

**onion** 1, finely chopped

**chillies** 2, deseeded and very finely chopped

**long-grain rice** 60g (2¼oz)

**vegetable stock** 1 litre (1¾ pints) – see page 396 or use a good stock cube or bouillon powder

**crème fraîche** 200ml (⅓ pint)

**cocoa powder** 1 tbsp

**curry powder** 1 tbsp

**free-range egg yolk** 1

**1** Melt half the butter in a large frying pan and sauté the onion and chillies until the onion is soft and golden. Set aside.

**2** Cook the rice in the stock in a large saucepan according to the packet instructions under just tender – normally about 10 minutes.

**3** Add the onion and chillies and whizz the mixture in a food processor or blender – or use a hand blender.

**4** Soften the rest of the butter slightly and mix with the crème fraîche, cocoa powder, curry powder and the egg yolk.

**5** Add to the rice mixture and mix well.

## vital statistics

Peanuts contain artery-protecting monounsaturated fats. Chilli, paprika and ginger are rich sources of plant chemicals that stimulate blood flow, while sweet potato offers abundant supplies of skin- and immunity-protecting betacarotene.

# sweet potato and peanut soup

Why on earth do so many people think peanuts are unhealthy? The truth is just the opposite: they help reduce cholesterol and prevent type 2 diabetes, both of which spell disaster for the circulation. The spices give your circulation a short, sharp boost, and the rich supply of phytochemicals from the tomatoes and sweet potato all add to the heart and circulatory benefits of this African treasure.

**groundnut oil** 2 tbsp

**onion** 1 large, finely chopped

**garlic** 2 cloves, finely chopped

**mushrooms** 4 large, finely chopped

**dried chilli flakes** 1 tsp

**paprika** ½ tsp

**fresh root ginger** 1cm (½in) piece, grated

**vegetable stock** 850ml (1½ pints) – *see* page 396 or use a good stock cube or bouillon powder

**canned tomatoes** 275g (9¾oz), with juice

**sweet potato** 2 large: 1 peeled and cubed, 1 peeled, cooked and mashed

**smooth peanut butter** 4 heaped tbsp

**1** Heat the oil in a large saucepan and sauté the onion, garlic and the mushrooms gently until the onion is soft and golden.

**2** Tip in the chilli flakes, paprika and ginger. Mix well and cook gently for 2 minutes.

**3** Pour in the stock, tomatoes and raw sweet potato cubes and simmer until the sweet potato is tender – about 15 minutes.

**4** Whizz in a food processor or blender – or a hand blender – until smooth.

**5** Add the mashed sweet potato and the peanut butter and blend again.

**6** Reheat, if necessary, to serve.

## vital statistics

You'll get a massive circulatory boost from the ginger, a blood-flow bonus from the hot harissa paste and lots of beneficial oils from the coriander. Lycopene, one of the most protective of all carotenoids, is more abundant in canned and puréed tomatoes than fresh.

# hot harissa

For at least 5000 years, herbs and spices have been used in food and as medicine to stimulate the circulation. Harissa is a prime example. Chillies, caraway, cumin, hot peppers and paprika are all used in this fabulous North African condiment. Ginger and fresh coriander leaves give an extra circulatory boost to this very different tomato soup. Be warned: one of the '57 varieties' it isn't!

**unsalted butter** 25g (1oz)

**onion** 1, finely chopped

**garlic** 2 cloves, finely chopped

**ground cumin** 1 tsp

**fresh root ginger** 2.5cm (1in) piece, grated

**tomato purée** 2 tsp

**harissa** 1 tsp

**tomatoes** 400g can, crushed

**vegetable stock** 1 litre (1¾ pints) – *see* page 396 or use a good stock cube or bouillon powder

**fresh coriander leaves** 1 handful

**crème fraîche** about 300ml (½ pint)

**1** Melt the butter in a large saucepan and sauté the onion and garlic gently until soft and golden.

**2** Add the cumin and ginger and cook for 2 minutes, stirring well.

**3** Add the tomato purée and harissa, stir well and cook for 2 minutes.

**4** Pour in the tomatoes and stock. Bring to the boil, then turn the heat down and simmer for 20 minutes.

**5** Tip the mixture into a food processor or blender – or use a hand blender – and whizz until smooth.

**6** Chop most of the coriander finely, reserving a few leaves, and whip with the crème fraîche.

**7** Serve the soup with the crème fraîche on top, garnished with the reserved coriander leaves.

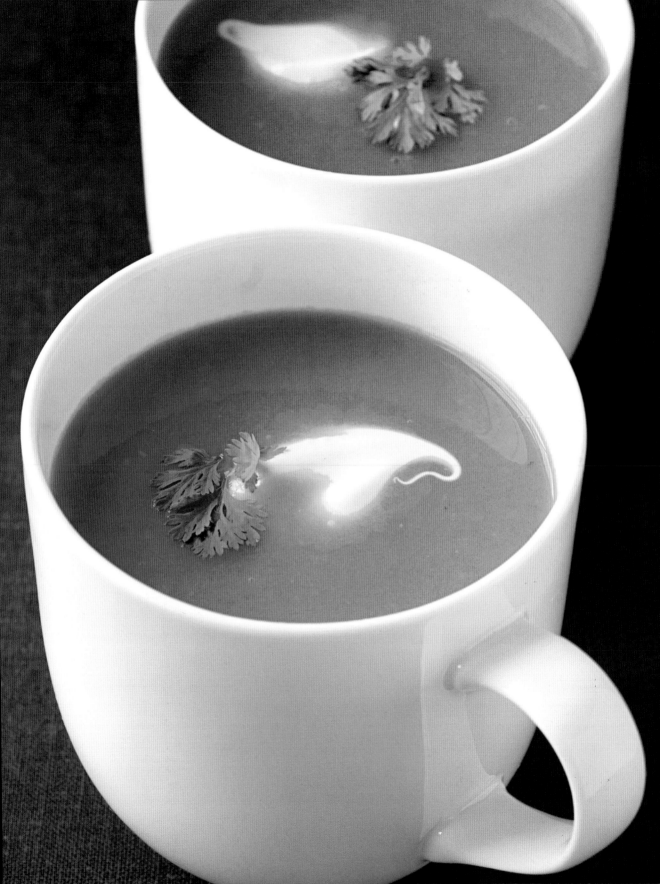

# oxtail soup

## vital statistics

This soup will revitalize the circulatory system. Oxtail bursts with B vitamins and iron for healthy blood, while turnips, swede and carrot provide betacarotene and minerals for good circulation.

I can't recommend this robust, hearty soup strongly enough. Make sure that you buy organic oxtail. Add the stimulating spices in Worcestershire or Tabasco sauce, and this soup is sure to warm the very cockles of your heart.

**oxtail** about 8 x 2.5cm (1in) chunks

**plain flour** 1 large cupful, seasoned with plenty of freshly ground black pepper and a little sea salt

**extra-virgin olive oil** 5 tbsp, plus a little extra for searing the oxtail

**onion** 1 large, coarsely chopped

**garlic** 2 cloves, finely chopped

**carrot** 1 large, trimmed and peeled unless organic, very finely diced

**turnip** 1, peeled and finely diced

**swede** ½ large, peeled and finely diced

**beef stock** 1.4 litres (2½ pints) – *see* page 397 or use a good stock cube or bouillon powder

**tomato purée** 3 tbsp

**worcestershire or tabasco sauce** 2 tsp

**bay leaves** 2

**parsley** 1 generous handful, finely chopped

**1** Trim as much fat as possible off the oxtail.

**2** Coat the meat in the seasoned flour and set aside.

**3** Heat the oil in a large saucepan and sweat the vegetables gently for 10 minutes, stirring continuously.

**4** In another pan, sear the seasoned oxtail in a little extra oil.

**5** Add the meat to the vegetables.

**6** Pour in the stock and add the tomato purée, Worcestershire or Tabasco sauce and bay leaves.

**7** Simmer gently for 50 minutes or until the meat is tender.

**8** Remove the bay leaves.

**9** Serve scattered with the parsley, either with the oxtail still intact or with the bone removed.

## vital statistics

Smoked salmon and avocado are excellent sources of fatty acids. Vitamin C from the lemon juice helps to reduce the risk of blood clots. Tabasco, like the other chilli derivatives, stimulates blood flow.

# avocado smokie

I'm no longer surprised by women who refuse to eat avocados in the false belief that they're unhealthy and fattening. Combined here with lemon juice, soured cream, Tabasco sauce and smoked salmon, they produce a soup that not only tastes great and would grace the most elegant dining table, but is also a cornucopia of health-giving and circulation-stimulating nutrients.

**avocados** 3 ripe, peeled and stoned

**lemons** juice from 2 large

**soured cream** about 300ml (½ pint)

**vegetable stock** about 1.2 litres (2 pints) – *see* page 396 or use a good stock cube or bouillon powder

**tabasco sauce** 3 good dashes

**smoked salmon** 200g (7oz) best-quality

**1** Put the avocado flesh into a food processor or blender with the lemon juice, soured cream, half the stock and the Tabasco sauce and whizz until smooth.

**2** Add more of the stock to give you the texture you want.

**3** Cover and transfer to the refrigerator to chill for an hour – no longer, otherwise it will discolour.

**4** Chop the smoked salmon finely.

**5** Stir half into the soup and serve the rest scattered on top.

## vital statistics

The ginger and chillies in this dish provide circulation-boosting phytochemicals. Protein and zinc are abundant in the prawns, as are fat-free nutrients in the fish stock and mushrooms.

# my thai

First it was Italian, then Indian, followed by Chinese; now all the ingredients for Thai cooking can be found in your local supermarket. As well as improving circulation, this is an all-round healthy soup that tastes fabulous and is very easy to make. Here again, ginger and chillies are the obvious ingredients to improve blood flow, but the absence of any animal fat makes this a double bonus for anyone with heart or circulatory problems.

**fish stock** 700ml (1¼ pints) – *see* page 396 or use a good stock cube or bouillon powder

**mushrooms** 100g (3½oz), finely chopped

**lemon grass** 1 small stalk, very finely chopped

**fresh root ginger** 2.5cm (1in) piece, peeled and finely grated

**soy sauce** 2 tsp

**red chillies** 3 small, deseeded and very finely chopped

**coconut milk** about 300ml (½ pint)

**prawns** 4 large in their shells, cooked

**fresh coriander leaves** 1 handful, chopped

**1** Put the stock into a large saucepan and bring to the boil.

**2** Add the mushrooms, lemon grass, ginger, soy sauce and chillies and boil for 5 minutes.

**3** Add the coconut milk and prawns and leave to stand off the heat for 5 minutes.

**4** Serve with the coriander sprinkled on top.

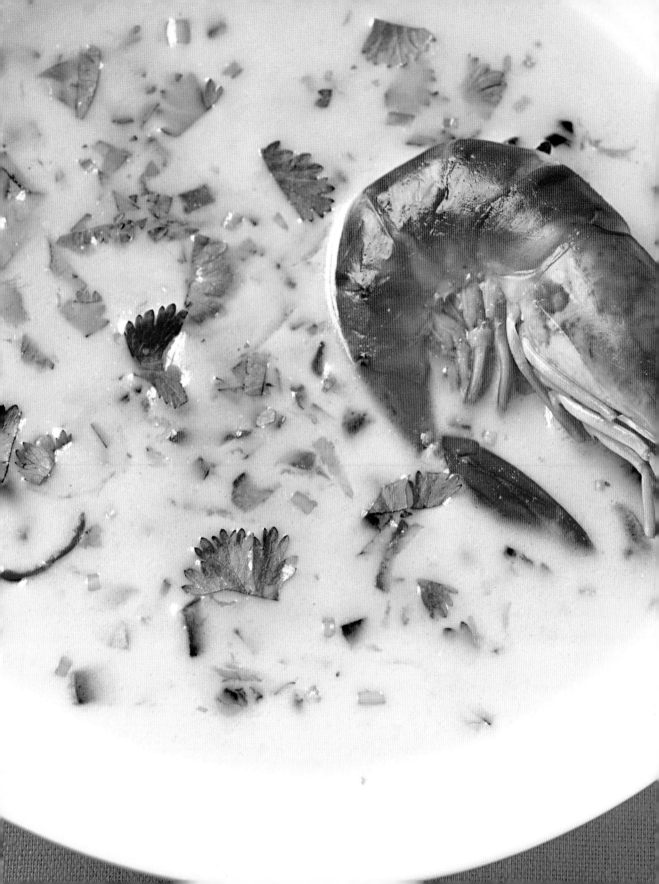

## vital statistics

Pectin, the natural fibre in apples, helps reduce cholesterol, while pumpkins provide betacarotene for good skin and a strong immune system. Onions contain circulation-boosting phytochemicals.

# apple and squash

If an apple a day keeps the doctor away, a bowl of this soup should keep you out of the clutches of medicine for a month. Spoon by spoon, you'll boost your immunity to all sorts of infections and help your body get rid of artery-clogging cholesterol. With heart- and circulation-protecting nutrients, this is a very simple and quick health-giving soup.

**unsalted butter** 25g (1oz)

**onion** 1, thinly sliced

**acorn squash** 1, peeled, deseeded and cubed

**apple juice** 350ml (12fl oz)

**vegetable stock** 350ml (12fl oz) – see page 396 or use a good stock cube or bouillon powder

**dessert apple** 1 Granny Smith, unpeeled, cored and diced

**crème fraîche** about 300ml (½ pint)

**1** Melt the butter in a large saucepan and sauté the onion and squash gently until the onion is golden – about 5 minutes.

**2** Pour in the apple juice and stock, bring to a simmer and add the apple pieces.

**3** Continue simmering until the vegetables are tender.

**4** Whizz in a food processor or blender – or use a hand blender – until smooth.

**5** Serve with a spoonful of crème fraîche in each bowl.

# papaya soup

Like most tropical fruits, papayas are both wonderfully tasty and incredibly healthy. They're a rich source of the protective antioxidants, minerals and vitamins that help promote a healthy heart and circulation. They also contain a digestive enzyme called papain. Eaten on their own, papayas are a powerful prescription for a healthy heart and circulation. The coriander gives an added dimension, since it's not only a traditional anti-inflammatory remedy in India, but has recently been shown to have cholesterol-lowering benefits, too.

**papayas** 3 large ripe, peeled, deseeded and cut into small chunks

**coconut milk** 250ml (9fl oz)

**semi-skimmed milk** 250ml (9fl oz)

**runny honey** 4 tbsp

**ground coriander** 1 tsp

**1** Put the papaya flesh into a large saucepan, add the coconut milk and milk and cook gently for 20 minutes.

**2** Add the honey and whizz in a food processor or blender – or use a hand blender – until smooth.

**3** Serve warm with the ground coriander sprinkled on top.

This fruity soup gives a great circulatory boost, because cherries are rich in bioflavonoids and vitamin C, both of which support healthy blood.

# sweet cherry soup

It's easy to think of cherries as simply one of those delicious summer treats, but they're much more than that. Ripe, plump cherries are a storehouse of circulation-boosting nutrients. Here, they are combined with an extra dose of vitamin C from the cranberry juice, ensuring that this soup will benefit anyone's circulatory system.

**cherries** 1kg (2lb 4oz) (stoned weight)

**cranberry juice** 250ml (9fl oz)

**cold water** 500ml (18fl oz), plus 2 tablespoons

**sweet white wine** 1 glass, such as Muscat de Beaumes-de-Venise or the less expensive Monbazillac

**arrowroot** 1 tbsp

**mint** 4 sprigs

**1** Purée the cherries in a food processor or blender and sieve to remove the skins.

**2** Put the pulp into a large saucepan with the cranberry juice, the large quantity of water and wine and bring slowly to the boil, stirring well.

**3** Stir the arrowroot into the 2 tablespoons of water and mix thoroughly.

**4** Pour the arrowroot mixture into the fruit stock and cook, stirring continuously, until slightly thickened.

**5** Serve garnished with the sprigs of mint.

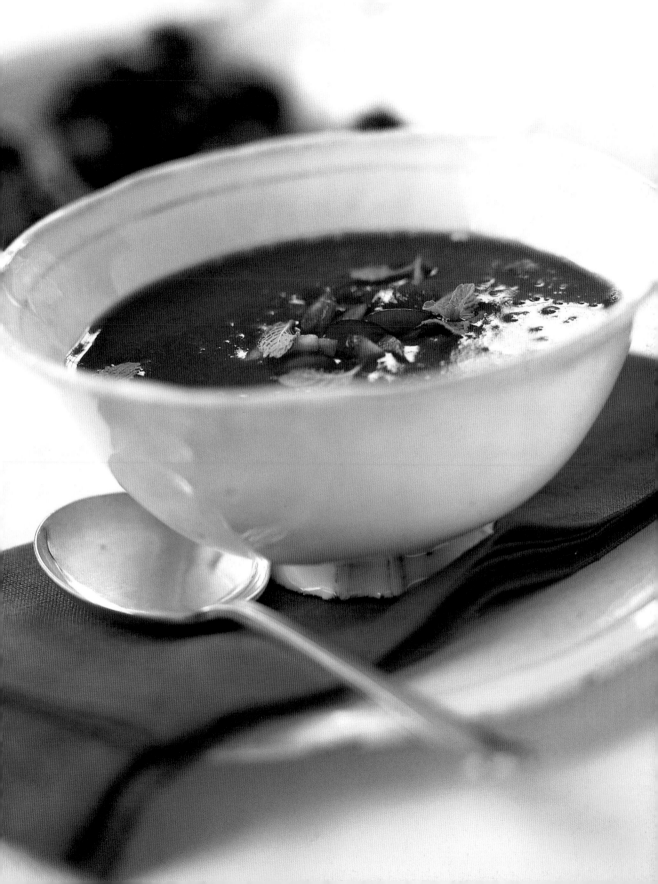

Beetroot was considered to be food of the gods by the ancient Greeks, and it was equally valued by the true European Romanies for its circulatory benefits. Horseradish is one of the great circulatory stimulants, containing a chemical called sinigrin, which speeds up the circulation and when crushed is converted into a powerful antibacterial called allylisothiocyanate.

# beetroot bopper

Throughout Eastern Europe, beetroot has been used for centuries as a blood tonic, and even as a treatment for leukaemia. It is reputed to improve the oxygen-carrying capacity of the blood, making circulation more efficient. Surprisingly, the combination of beetroot and horseradish is widely used as a pickle-type condiment in Eastern Europe, and the flavours are just brilliant together.

**fresh horseradish** 1 tsp freshly grated (or use a strong commercial variety)

**beetroot juice** 500ml (18fl oz)

**1** Whizz the horseradish in a blender or food processor with 125ml (4fl oz) of the beetroot juice until blended.

**2** Put the rest of the juice into a saucepan.

**3** Add the blended horseradish mixture and stir until well combined.

**4** Heat gently until just boiling.

**5** Pour into mugs and serve.

## vital statistics

Mango contains masses of vitamins A, C and E, together with potassium and iron, making it a super-protector of the heart and circulatory system. The hot South American chillies contain the circulatory stimulant capsaicin. Within moments of enjoying this drink, the tiny blood vessels dilate, your skin flushes and you're suffused with a warm and comforting glow.

# hot chilli mango

Now we're really getting down to the nitty-gritty of circulation boosters. The hot chilli sauce will get the blood fairly whizzing round your circulatory system, but the taste of this drink is less fiery than you'd expect, thanks to the soothing sweetness of the mango. This is the perfect drink when you come in from a brisk winter's walk, a frosty afternoon's leaf-sweeping or a cold morning on the edge of a sports field while the kids compete; if you've got any sense, you'll take a flask with you.

**mango juice** 500ml (18fl oz) home-pressed (or a good commercial variety)

**hot chilli sauce** 2 tsp

1  Put both ingredients into a saucepan.

2  Heat until just boiling.

3  Serve immediately in mugs or heatproof glasses.

## vital statistics

Apart from being an immunity booster, vitamin C has many valuable properties. Most importantly, it's one of the most powerful antioxidants, helping to protect individual cells from damage and vital for the protection of the entire circulatory system. The bioflavonoids in the rind and pith of citrus fruits improve your absorption of vitamin C and have their own strengthening effect on the walls of blood vessels.

# oranges and lemons

All citrus-fruit juices protect and improve the circulation, thanks to their exceptionally high vitamin C content. Adding some rind helps to protect the integrity and strength of the walls of both arteries and veins. There is also an additional benefit in the enormous increase in natural immune resistance, which is necessary to fight off everyday infections such as coughs, colds and flu.

**unwaxed oranges** 4
**unwaxed lemon** 1 large
**orange-blossom water** 2 tbsp

**1** Juice the oranges and lemon, then take 2 curls of both orange and lemon rind, including the white pith.

**2** Mix the juices together and heat gently in a saucepan until just simmering.

**3** Pour into 2 heatproof glasses.

**4** Divide the orange-blossom water and rind curls between the glasses to serve.

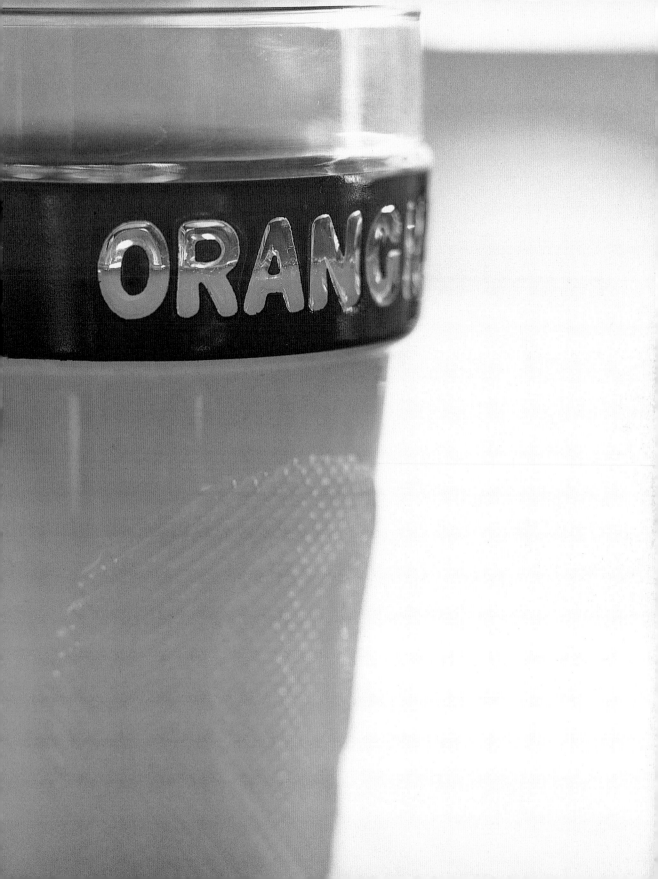

Sorrel is believed by herbalists to both improve and cleanse the circulating blood. Its natural phytochemicals, including flavonoids and anthraquinones, are the active ingredients.

# sorrel tea

This tea is one of the favourite tonics of the herbalist. Roman soldiers used to eat such wild sorrel when they were marching, because it was said to stop them feeling thirsty, and the earliest Roman physicians knew that it helped the body get rid of surplus fluid. In the time of Henry VIII, sorrel was a highly prized vegetable, which the king adored, and his doctors used it as one of the earliest spring blood tonics.

**sorrel leaves** 1 large handful
**boiling water** 250ml (9fl oz)
**runny honey** to taste

1 Tear the sorrel leaves roughly.

2 Put in a mug or infuser and cover with the water.

3 Cover and leave to stand for 10 minutes.

4 Strain and sweeten to taste with honey.

## vital statistics

Essential oils such as saffronal and crocins from the saffron, myristicin from nutmeg, cinnamaldehyde from cinnamon and eugenol from the cloves are all circulation stimulants, and the antioxidants in green tea make this drink powerfully protective. Apart from these chemical actions, the mellow, spicy flavours are warming on their own.

# slemp

A favourite from Holland, where this is drunk by everyone who has managed (or can still manage) to get their skates on and go for a stimulating winter race along frozen canals between the dykes. They return with cheeks aglow, healthily out of puff and ready for this drink to get them warm and add to the circulation boost of a few hours' exercise in the fresh air. The spices are the biggest stimulant.

**cinnamon stick** 4cm (1½in) piece

**saffron threads** 2

**cloves** 3

**nutmeg** 1, halved

**dried green tea** 1 tbsp

**milk** 850ml (1½ pints)

**unwaxed lemon** grated rind of 1

**sea salt** ¼ tsp

**sugar** preferably golden caster sugar, to taste

1  Tie the spices and tea into a piece of kitchen muslin.

2  Put the milk into a saucepan and add the muslin bag.

3  Add the lemon rind and salt to the pan.

4  Simmer gently for 1 hour.

5  Remove the spice bag.

6  Pour into mugs and let everyone sweeten to taste.

## vital statistics

Bananas are rich in potassium, which is important for normal heart function and for the prevention of high blood pressure, making them a circulatory superfood. Thanks to their high content of vitamin B6 and their ability to prevent fluid retention, they also help reduce the distressing and uncomfortable symptoms of PMS. Add the theobromine in the cocoa and volatile oils from the cinnamon, and you'll soon be glowing.

# hot banana smoothie

There's something very comforting about this combination of bananas, milk and cocoa, which gets its hidden punch and flavour from the added cinnamon. This drink not only helps improve circulation, it also protects against heart disease and high blood pressure, and will even relieve the distress of PMS.

**bananas** 2 small, peeled

**milk** 300ml (½ pint)

**natural live bio-yogurt** 1 small carton (about 125ml/4fl oz)

**mixed cocoa powder and ground cinnamon** 1 heaped tsp

**1** Put the bananas, milk and yogurt into a blender or food processor – or use a hand blender – and whizz until very smooth.

**2** Pour the mixture into a saucepan and heat gently until just simmering.

**3** Use a cappuccino wand or whisk to stir up a froth.

**4** Pour into 2 mugs or heatproof glasses and serve with the cocoa powder and cinnamon scattered on top.

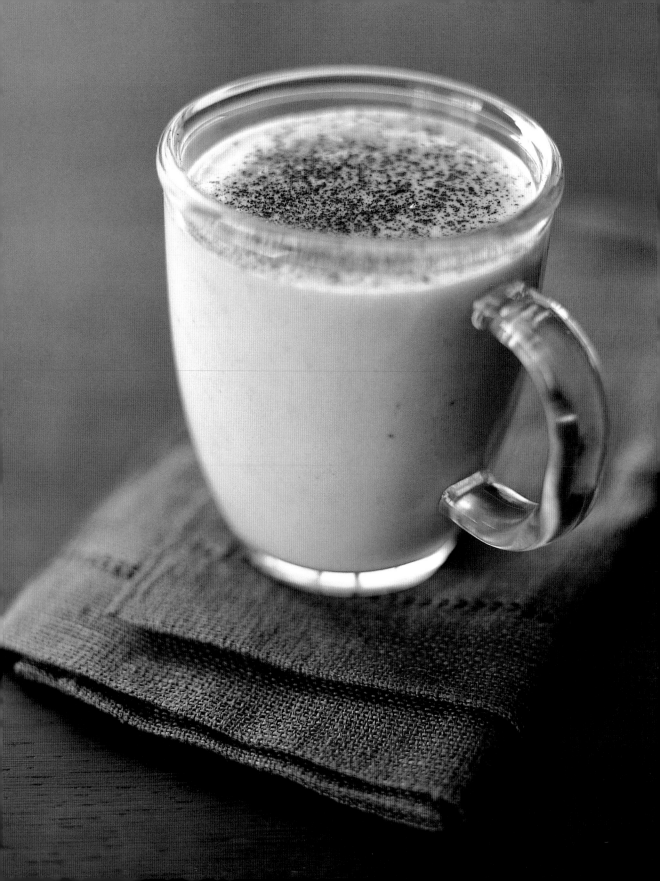

## vital statistics

This punch overflows with vitamin C, carotenoids and an abundance of cancer-fighting phytochemicals. The natural pigments that give the berries their deep red, blue and purple skins are some of the most powerful of all cancer-protective substances, which is why blueberries, blackberries, strawberries, raspberries and blackcurrants feature so widely in all healthy cookery.

# winter berry punch

Fruit is one of the healthiest and most life-supporting of all food groups, but berries come top of the class in the health-promotion tables. They're the richest sources of the protective antioxidants that guard every cell in the body, warding off damage and disease, especially cancer. Adding ginger and cinnamon gives a boost to the circulation, as well as a lift to the spirits.

**mixed berries** 350g (12oz), fresh or frozen
**cold water** about 600ml (1 pint)
**fresh root ginger** 2.5cm (1in) piece
**cinnamon sticks** 4

**1** Put the berries into a saucepan and add the water.

**2** Peel and bruise the ginger, but leave it in one piece, and add to the pan.

**3** Bring slowly to a simmer and continue simmering for 10 minutes.

**4** Remove the ginger and strain the liquid through a sieve, pressing the fruit to extract all the juices.

**5** Warm through if necessary.

**6** Serve with cinnamon sticks as stirrers.

The powerful antioxidants in red grape juice help protect every cell in your body, but most notably they have anti-cancer and heart-protective properties. The mixed berries not only deliver a huge dose of vitamin C, but they, too, are bursting with antioxidants, which also do a great job at protecting the skin from ageing.

# fruity mulled wine

The brandy in this drink is optional, and without it this is a perfect winter warmer for children. For all its festive feel, it also makes a great everyday drink, especially when those first frosts bring a nip to the air. It is also a valuable protective mixture that helps boost natural immunity and is particularly good for the heart and circulation.

**red grape juice** 75cl bottle

**apple juice** 850ml (1½ pints)

**caster sugar** 60g (2¼oz)

**cinnamon stick** ½

**mixed berries** 85g (3oz), fresh or frozen, not dried

**brandy** 1 tbsp (optional)

**1** Put the fruit juices, sugar and cinnamon stick into a large saucepan.

**2** Heat gently until the sugar has dissolved.

**3** Remove the pan from the heat and leave the mixture to stand for 10 minutes.

**4** Add the berries and heat gently for 5 minutes.

**5** If using frozen fruit, heat for a further 5 minutes.

**6** Stir in the brandy, if using, and serve.

For 7000 years, Chinese herbalists used ginger as an important medicine, as well as a flavouring. The pungent shogaols and the stimulating gingerols and zingiberene have a dramatic effect on blood circulation, making this root a great remedy for poor circulation, chilblains and Raynaud's disease. The bioflavonoids in lemon help by strengthening the blood-vessel walls.

# ginger and lemon zizz

In terms of real physics, a cup of a hot drink when you're freezing has about the same effect on your body temperature as adding a pint of boiling water to an ice-cold bath. But there's no doubting the psychological comfort of clutching a warm mug between your hands, sipping its contents and inhaling the heady vapours. The difference here is that this drink really does 'ginger you up' and gets those blood corpuscles fairly whizzing round your veins and arteries.

**fresh root ginger** 2.5cm (1in) piece, peeled and grated

**boiling water** 200ml (⅓ pint)

**lemon** ½

1 Put the ginger into an infuser or mug and add the boiling water.

2 Cover and leave to stand for 10 minutes.

3 Juice the lemon half, reserving 2 slices.

4 Strain the ginger tea into a mug and add the lemon juice.

5 Serve with the lemon slices on top.

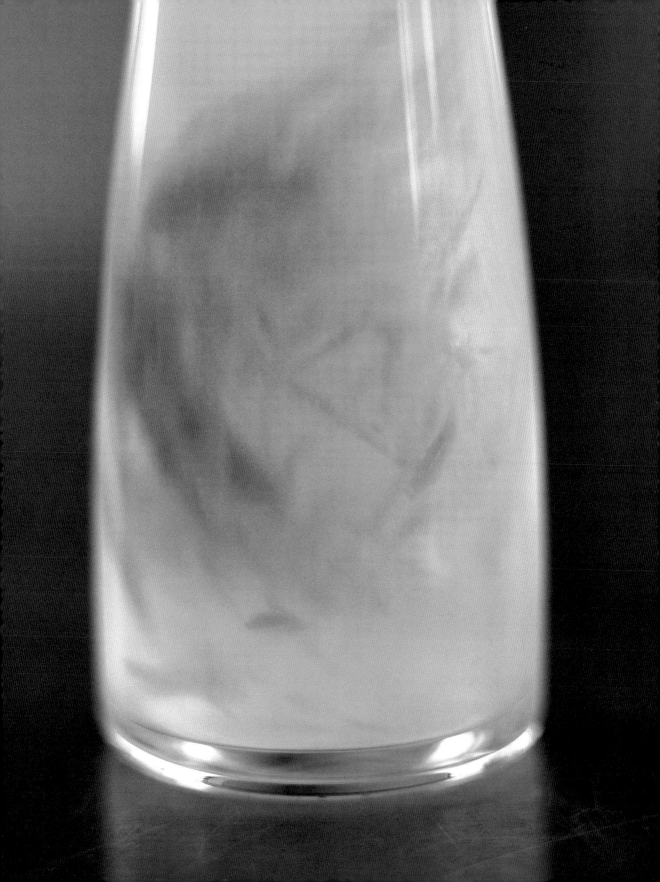

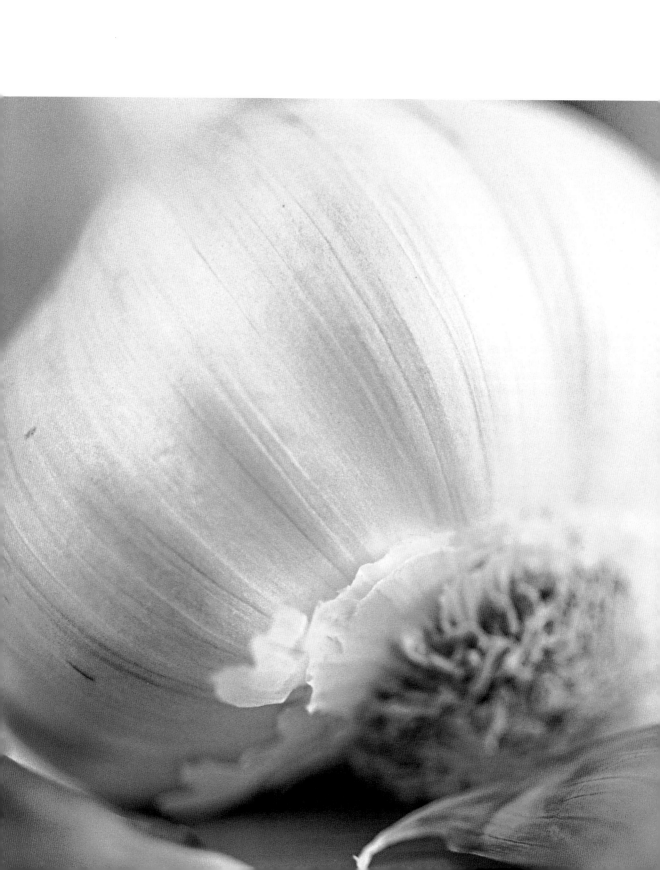

# positive thinking

When Granny said, 'Eat your fish, it will make you brainy', she wasn't far off the mark. All oily fish contains essential fatty acids, which makes it a vital food for any woman planning to have a baby or who's pregnant or breast-feeding. Fatty acids form a major part of a developing baby's brain tissue, and there's now substantial evidence that women whose diets are very low in fish oils have children who tend to be slower at mental development.

It's not just oily fish that makes good brain food; the protein in all fish provides slow-release energy that helps keep a constant supply of blood sugar flowing to the brain, helping it to function consistently. Poultry, game and lean free-range beef are ideal too, especially if you remove all visible fat and avoid eating the skin on chicken, duck or turkey. While all forms of protein are good brain nourishment, you should avoid animal protein that contains large amounts of saturated fat. Saturated fat can lead to raised cholesterol, which consists of fatty deposits in the arteries and narrowing of the blood vessels that supply the brain. This is often the first step towards declining brain function.

## Cerebral eating plan

Wholegrain cereals, beans, garlic, leeks and onions should be regular ingredients in your cerebral eating plan. These help the body to get rid of cholesterol and so work towards keeping the levels of this damaging deposit healthily low, ensuring the maintenance of an adequate and continuous blood supply that carries essential nutrients to brain cells.

Modest amounts of alcohol are good for your brain, too. The high levels of antioxidants that prevent brain-cell damage are a major component of red wines, so a couple of glasses a day are a great ally in the maintenance of good mental function and the power of positive thought. Alcohol itself is also valuable, whether it comes from white wine, beer, spirits or liqueurs; in small amounts, it has the effect of opening up the tiniest blood vessels at the end of the circulatory system and improving blood flow to the brain.

That's the good news, and istrue for two or three glasses of wine, two or three pub measures of spirits or up to two pints of beer a day. However, once you start to exceed this, alcohol has the opposite effect, making these minute vessels contract, depriving the brain of blood and leading to rapid deterioration in mental ability and decision-making. Thoughts become negative. Depression is a hallmark of those abusing alcohol.

## The role of herbs and spices

Herbs and spices have a vital role as brain foods. Some, like basil, nutmeg, lemon balm and coriander, have an effect on mood and emotion. Others have a more direct impact on mental function; the two most powerful of these are sage, synonymous with wisdom, and rosemary, which has been linked with improved memory since the times of the ancient Greeks.

The most important of the spices is chilli, which has an almost immediate effect on the circulation, opening up the tiniest blood vessels and leading to an almost instant rush of blood to the head. This accounts for the beads of sweat on the forehead within seconds of your first mouthful of a strong chilli con carne. Ginger comes a pretty close second and will also provide really quick brain stimulation, whether taken as tea, a sprinkle of ground ginger on your melon or fresh in a stir-fry.

Since we live in an age of an ever-older population, the maintenance of good brain function assumes even greater significance. By accentuating all the positive aspects of diet and eliminating the negatives, you dramatically increase your chances of maintaining the ability to think positively, as well as mental agility, well into old age. But food alone isn't enough. The brain is like any muscular part of the body: if you don't use it, you lose it. Keep it active by reading, engaging in conversation, doing crossword puzzles, learning a few lines of poetry and playing memory games. Most important of all is the process of calculation; following these recipes and working out the quantities is a start. So, for your brain's sake, get cooking!

# positive-thinking checklist

- Eat more oily fish, white fish, poultry, game, lean free-range beef for protein and the iron needed to carry oxygen in the blood to the brain. Avoid narrowing of the brain's blood vessels by eating wholegrain cereals, beans, garlic, leeks and onions. Modest quantities of alcohol, sage and chilli are excellent brain boosters and a top aid to positive thinking.
- Eat less saturated fat in manufactured meat products; and avoid excessive quantities of alcohol and foods with a high refined-sugar content, which can lead to fluctuating blood-sugar levels and an inability to concentrate and focus mental energy.

The benefits of this wonderful treatment come from a combination of touch and smell. This mood-boosting salad assaults your olfactory senses with the pungency of onion and the heavy, sweet scent of basil. You'll hardly have to eat it to feel better.

# aromatherapy salad

This salad provides a calming combination of ingredients that benefits the senses. After all, aromatherapy doesn't just mean a special type of massage...

**tomatoes** 6 ripe organic, the freshest and best you can buy, thinly sliced

**red onion** 1 large, thinly sliced

**extra-virgin olive oil** 4 tbsp

**basil** 1 generous bunch

**black pepper** freshly ground, to taste

**crusty wholemeal bread** cut into chunks, to serve

**1** Layer the tomatoes and onion in a fairly large, shallow dish.

**2** Pour on the oil.

**3** Tear the basil into small pieces and sprinkle over the top of the salad.

**4** Season to taste with black pepper.

**5** Serve with the bread, making sure that you have a chunk left over to mop up the succulent mixture of oil and tomato juices.

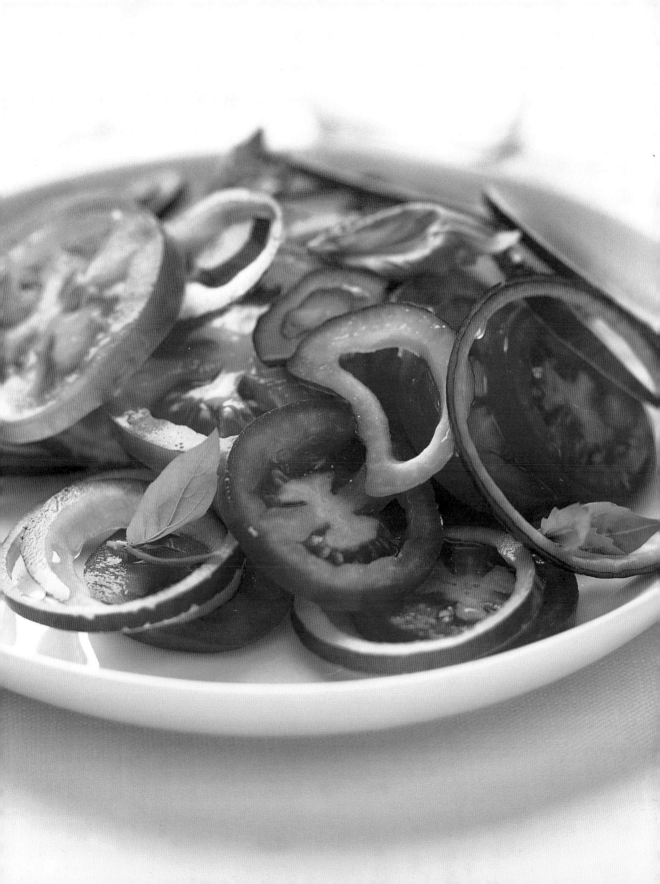

The calming power of basil, the soothing effects of all types of lettuce and the mind-clearing power of mint, combined with the memory-boosting benefits of sage, make this beautifully light salad a mental marvel.

# good-mood green salad

This soothing salad gently lifts the spirits and clears the mind. With parsley, sage, and thyme, this may sound like a song from the past, but our ancient forebears knew a thing or two about the mood-boosting benefits of these extraordinary herbs. They weren't used for flavour alone but for their medicinal properties as well. Don't forget that all medicine started in the kitchen.

**basil, chives, parsley, mint, sage and thyme** 1 handful each
**extra-virgin olive oil** 2 tbsp
**lemon** juice of ½
**mixed green leaves** a good selection

1 Tear the basil into small pieces.

2 Snip the chives with scissors.

3 Chop the parsley, mint and sage.

4 Mix the thyme leaves with all the other herbs.

5 Mix the oil and lemon juice together.

6 Add the herbs to the leaves and combine thoroughly.

7 Add the dressing and toss very lightly – just enough to coat the leaves.

Lemon balm is a traditional anti-depressant and heart tonic, and the phytochemicals in tarragon are calming and sleep-inducing. The blood-building benefits of beetroot and probiotic bacteria from the yogurt imbue this recipe with health-giving properties.

# upbeet herbal salad

An unusual salad, with mood-enhancing properties, this creamy, pink mixture brings a blaze of colour as an unusual starter, a light lunch dish served with wholemeal bread, or a side dish with cold meat or fish, or an accompaniment to a barbecue. It has the added piquancy of horseradish – a popular combination in Eastern Europe.

**cooked beetroot** preferably baby bulbs, about 700g (1lb 9oz)

**unwaxed lemon** juice and grated rind of ½

**fresh horseradish** 1 tsp freshly grated (or 2 tsp ready-made sauce)

**chives** 1 heaped tbsp finely snipped

**tarragon** 1 tsp finely chopped

**lemon balm** 1 tsp finely chopped

**natural live bio-yogurt** 250ml carton

1 Cut the beetroot into chunks – or slice if large.

2 Sprinkle with the lemon juice and stir in the rind.

3 Stir the horseradish and herbs into the yogurt and pour over the beetroot.

4 Leave for 1 hour to allow the flavours to combine.

# traditional tabbouleh

Keep blood-sugar levels on course for a calm, assured day. This staple salad comes from Lebanon, but it's popular throughout North Africa and the Middle East. You can vary this recipe to suit your personal tastes. The basic ingredient is bulgur wheat, sometimes known as burghul or cracked wheat.

**bulgur wheat** 150g (5½oz)
**garlic** 2 cloves, finely chopped
**extra-virgin olive oil** 6 tbsp
**lemon** juice of 1
**plum tomatoes** 2 ripe
**cucumber** ½
**spring onions** 4
**flat-leaf parsley** 4 tbsp chopped
**mint** 4 tbsp chopped
**black pepper** freshly ground

**1** Leave the bulgur wheat to soak in a bowl of cold water for 30 minutes.

**2** Mix the garlic with the oil and lemon juice, and leave to infuse while you prepare the rest of the salad.

**3** Coarsely chop the tomatoes.

**4** Peel, deseed and chop the cucumber.

**5** Finely chop the spring onions.

**6** Drain the bulgur wheat, getting it as dry as possible, then put into a serving bowl. Add the tomatoes, cucumber, spring onions, parsley and mint.

**7** Add the garlic dressing and stir thoroughly. Season with plenty of black pepper.

**8** Cover tightly with clingfilm. It will taste good in 1–2 hours but fantastic if you leave it until the next day.

## vital statistics

Cottage cheese is rich in protein – important for brain function – and easily digested. Add it to the walnuts for more protein, minerals and essential fats, and the celery for its cleansing action, and you couldn't find a quicker or easier mood booster.

# protein plus

This delicious, quick-and-easy salad boosts brain function with plenty of good protein and vital essential minerals.

**cottage cheese** 300g (10½oz) full-fat, preferably organic

**black pepper** freshly ground, to taste

**celery** 1 large stick, preferably with leaves, thinly sliced and any leaves chopped

**radishes** 10, quartered

**green pepper** ½, cored, deseeded and cubed

**walnuts** 100g (3½oz) chopped

**1** Put the cottage cheese into a large bowl and season to taste with black pepper.

**2** Mix the celery, radishes and green pepper with the cottage cheese, then sprinkle the walnuts on top.

## vital statistics

This is the perfect combination of brain-activating protein, slow-release energy for extended concentration and gently calming phytochemicals from the lettuce.

# fruity duck salad

This salad looks terrific, tastes great and is packed with protein and energy for good concentration. In fact, it's the perfect lunch to prepare for an afternoon of mental exertion. It is substantial enough to be a meal, and the bit of extra work involved in making it is honestly worth the effort.

**duck breasts** 4, preferably organic, skinned

**chinese noodles** 300g (10½oz)

**mixed salad leaves** 1 bag

**groundnut, rapeseed or safflower oil** 3 tbsp

**rice vinegar** 1 tbsp

**light soy sauce** 1 tsp

**papaya** 1 large ripe, deseeded and sliced

**kiwi fruit** 2 ripe, peeled and sliced

**1** Put a large saucepan of water on to boil and preheat the grill to high.

**2** Bash the duck breasts gently to flatten them.

**3** Cook the duck breasts under the grill for about 3 minutes on each side or until they're just pink in the middle.

**4** Meanwhile, add the noodles to the boiling water.

**5** Wash and dry the salad leaves – even if they're 'ready-washed'. Cover a serving plate with them.

**6** Drain the noodles and toss with the oil, vinegar and soy sauce.

**7** Pile the noodles on top of the leaves, then arrange the duck breasts on top of the noodles. Arrange the fruit around the plate, and enjoy!

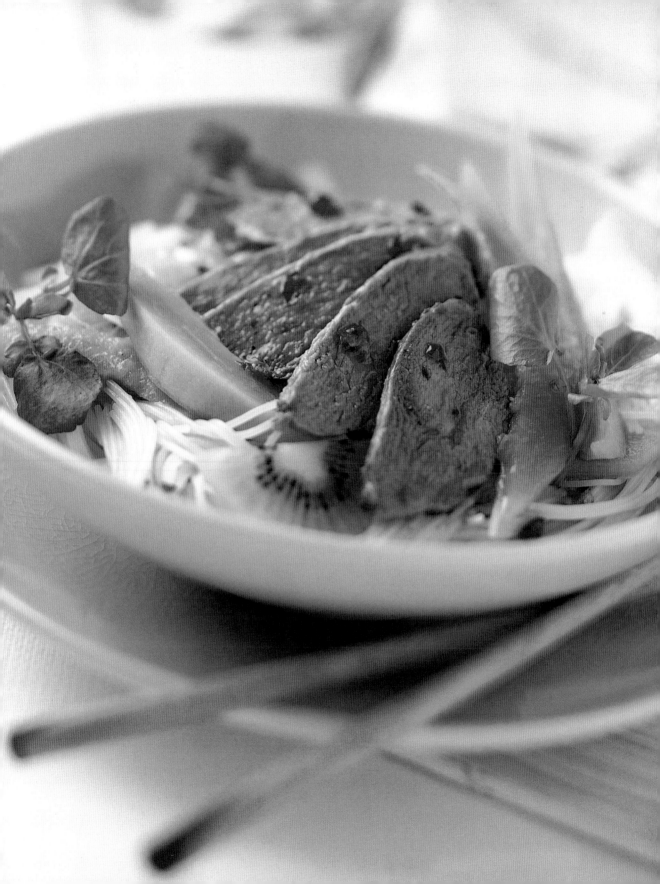

## vital statistics

High in protein and low in fat, duck breasts are a good source of iron and B vitamins. Rosemary's volatile oils enhance memory, anise has aphrodisiac properties and saffron contains substances that lift the spirits.

# canard aux herbes

This is a dish of unsurpassed mood food. The unusual combination of saffron and anise is a perfect complement to the rich meatiness of the duck – which tastes even better if it's wild. The memory-enhancing benefits of rosemary, the increased libido generated by anise and the general mood-improving properties of saffron make this the perfect meal to mend those lovers' quarrels.

**duck breasts** 4, preferably organic, skinned
**extra-virgin olive oil** 150ml (¼ pint)
**white wine or sherry vinegar** 4 tbsp
**oregano** 4 large sprigs
**rosemary** 2 large sprigs
**anise seeds** 4, crushed
**saffron threads** 1 pinch

**To serve**
**mashed potatoes**
**french beans** lightly cooked
**parsley** chopped

1 Remove any tendons from the duck breasts.

2 Mix the rest of the ingredients together and pour over the duck breasts. Cover and leave to marinate in the refrigerator for at least 2 hours.

3 Preheat the grill to high.

4 Cook the duck breasts under the grill for 7 minutes on each side, basting frequently with the marinade.

5 Serve with mashed potatoes and French beans, sprinkled with chopped parsley.

## vital statistics

Rich in protein and B vitamins and a good source of iron, this recipe combines all the protective benefits of onions and garlic with the mood-enhancing essential oils of oregano and mint's mind-stimulating properties.

# minty lamb meatballs

Just to smell these meatballs cooking will transport you back to a Greek taverna in an unspoilt village – or make you yearn to visit this magical country if you haven't been there before. The traditional Greek way of cooking with lamb, herbs and spices creates an amalgam of wonderful flavours as well as a unique and mind-altering aroma.

**lamb** 700g (1lb 9oz) lean, minced

**onion** 1 large, very finely chopped

**garlic** 2 cloves, very finely chopped

**sea salt and black pepper** freshly ground, to taste

**dried oregano** 1 tsp

**mint** 3 tbsp finely torn leaves

**flat-leaf parsley** 3 tbsp chopped

**ground cumin** 1 tsp

**free-range eggs** 2 small

**1** Combine the lamb, onion and garlic in a large bowl until thoroughly mixed. Season to taste with salt and black pepper.

**2** Combine the oregano, mint, parsley and cumin and blend into the lamb mixture.

**3** Beat the eggs and mix into the meat and herbs.

**4** Form the mixture into walnut-sized balls (makes approximately 20), cover and refrigerate for 1 hour.

**5** Preheat the oven to 180°C/350°F/gas mark 4.

**6** Transfer the meatballs to a greased baking dish. Cover with foil and cook in the oven for 45 minutes.

**7** Remove the foil. Turn the heat up and cook for another 10 minutes, shaking the dish frequently, until the meatballs are slightly crisp.

## vital statistics

The volatile oils in the rosemary act specifically on the brain, clearing muddled or tired heads. This recipe is also ideal for anyone with arthritis, gout or rheumatism, because it's rich in the essential fatty acids that have natural anti-inflammatory properties and are beneficial to the central nervous system. It is an excellent source of protein too.

# rosemary salmon

The traditional belief that fish is 'brain food' is well founded – especially when it's combined with the aromatic properties of rosemary. The essential fatty acids in oily fish are vital for human brain development, and since the time of ancient Greece, rosemary has been used as an all-round mental tonic. Besides aiding memory, it also helps lift depressive moods. Food for thought, indeed!

**salmon** 4 steaks
**rosemary oil** 2 tbsp (*see* below)
**lemon** 8 thin slices
**dried rosemary** 4 large sprigs
**onion** 1, thinly sliced
**dry white wine** 2 tbsp

**Rosemary oil**
**fresh rosemary leaves** 1 tbsp
**extra-virgin olive oil** 150ml (¼ pint)

**To serve**
**minted boiled potatoes**
**green vegetables**

1 For the rosemary oil, put the leaves into a mortar with a little oil and crush with the pestle. Add to the rest of the oil and pour into a tight-fitting screw-top jar. Leave on a sunny windowsill for 3 weeks, shaking gently every day or so. Strain through a muslin and pour into a dark-coloured bottle with a tight-fitting stopper. Store in a cool place (but not the refrigerator) out of sunlight.

2 Preheat the oven to 190°C/375°F/gas mark 5.

3 Rub both sides of the fish with the rosemary oil. Lay on a baking sheet lined with a piece of foil large enough to fold over the top of the fish.

4 Put 2 slices of lemon and a sprig of rosemary on each steak. Drizzle with a little more oil, surround the fish with the onion slices and sprinkle with the wine.

5 Seal the parcel loosely. Bake for 20 minutes. Serve with minted boiled potatoes and green vegetables.

Bay has been used as a mood improver since ancient times; its volatile oil, laurenolide, is a powerful mood lifter. The fenchone present in fennel helps regulate women's hormone levels, thus preventing mood swings. The combination of herbs with the essential fatty acids in the herring makes this a perfect dish for affairs of the heart – emotional or physical.

# hearty herring

The traditional combination of herring with lemon, olive oil and fennel leaves is given a new and interesting twist in this recipe by the addition of curry-plant and bay leaves. Due to its spirit-lifting effects, this makes a perfect meal if you're feeling a bit blue, but its nutritional value makes it equally good during pregnancy – and it's a four-star superfood if you're breast-feeding.

**extra-virgin olive oil** 6 tbsp
**white wine vinegar** 3 tbsp
**lemon** 1, sliced
**fennel fronds** 1 bunch
**curry-plant leaves** 6
**bay leaves** 2
**herrings** 4, filleted
**sea salt and black pepper**
freshly ground, to taste
**olive oil** for shallow-frying
**tarragon-flavoured herb mustard** 2 tsp

**1** Mix the extra-virgin olive oil, vinegar, lemon slices, fennel fronds and curry-plant and bay leaves together.

**2** Season the fish fillets to taste with salt and black pepper, then pour on the oil mixture.

**3** Cover and leave to marinate in the refrigerator for at least 3 hours.

**4** Drain the fish, reserving the marinade, wipe dry and shallow-fry in olive oil for about 4 minutes on each side.

**5** Strain the marinade and heat through. Add the mustard to the marinade and pour over the fish.

## vital statistics

The aromatic oils in apples contain volatile substances that, when inhaled, act directly on the brain. Just smelling an apple can relieve migraines and lower blood pressure, so this combination is the ideal dessert to elevate your mood at the end of a meal. Used by the ancient Persians, advised by Hippocrates and mentioned in the Bible, hyssop is a naturally calming herb.

# aromatic apples

The Bramley cooking apple is unique to the British Isles, and its tart acidity mixes well with the Mediterranean flavours of hyssop and scented geranium and the sweet smoothness of mascarpone cheese. This recipe makes a great breakfast dish, as well as being an ideal source of easily digestible nutrients for anyone recovering from illness.

**cold water** 100ml (3½fl oz)

**caster sugar** 60g (2¼oz)

**hyssop** 1 sprig

**cooking apples** 900g (2lb) Bramleys, peeled, cored and sliced

**mascarpone cheese** 500g (1lb 2oz)

**scented geranium leaves** 2 tsp chopped (optional)

**orange rind** finely pared strips, to decorate

**1** Pour the water into a saucepan. Add the sugar and hyssop and boil gently until the sugar has dissolved.

**2** Remove the hyssop. Add the apples to the sugar mixture, cooking very gently over a low heat. When cooked to a smooth purée, fold in the mascarpone.

**3** Transfer the mixture to individual dishes, sprinkle with the geranium leaves, if using, and leave in the refrigerator to chill before serving.

**4** Serve decorated with strips of orange rind.

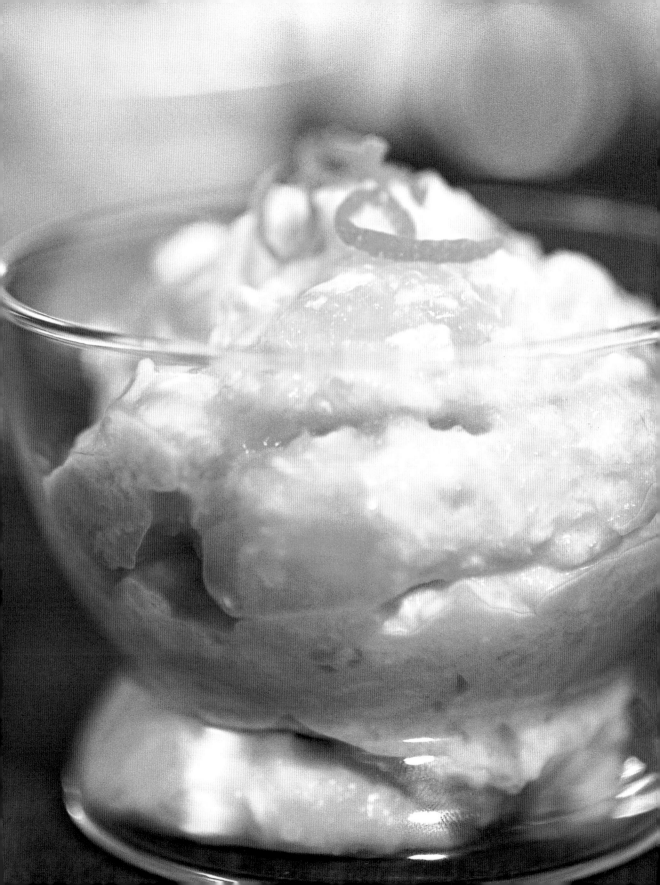

## vital statistics

The protein, vitamins and fibre in the flour and the tremendous calming effects of lavender make these biscuits a far better (and more enjoyable) alternative to sleeping pills or tranquillizers. Lavender oil is also a traditional remedy for the relief of headaches.

# lavender biscuits

Most people associate its sweet aroma with the garden, but lavender is a great herb to use for flavouring food. Its ability to calm the nervous, relax the stressed and grant sleep to long-suffering insomniacs is legendary. Once you've tried these, you'll never want to eat shop-bought biscuits again!

**butter** 115g (4oz)

**caster sugar** 55g (2oz)

**75% wholemeal self-raising flour** 175g (6oz)

**lavender leaves** 2 tbsp freshly chopped

**lavender flowers** 1 tsp, rubbed off the stalk

1 Preheat the oven to 230°C/450°F/gas mark 8.

2 Beat the butter and sugar together in a bowl until pale and fluffy. Mix in the flour and lavender leaves and knead into a dough.

3 Roll the dough out on a floured board, sprinkle with the lavender flowers and press them into the dough with the rolling pin.

4 Cut into shapes and bake on a greased baking sheet for about 10 minutes.

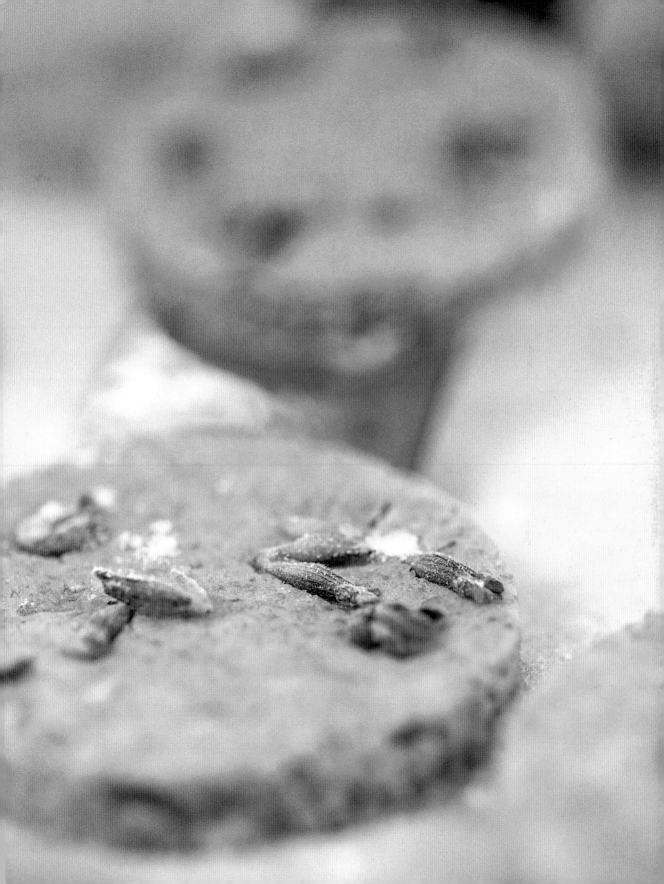

## vital statistics

Chestnuts aren't rich in protein, but they do provide vitamins B1, B2 and the PMS-relieving B6. They're also a good source of potassium. The pancetta provides some protein and salt, so don't add extra salt.

# chestnut soup

Chestnuts are underused and seriously underrated, often seen only as stuffing for the Christmas turkey or for roasting by the fire. Unlike most nuts, they're virtually fat-free and have only 170 calories per 100g (3½oz). They make great gluten-free flour and also purée – as used in this recipe. Their delicious taste disguises their nerve-nourishing vitamin B content. With a little butter, a dollop of crème fraîche and a splash of cognac, of course this soup will make you feel good.

**unsalted butter** 10g (¼oz)

**onion** 1, very finely chopped

**garlic** 1 clove, flattened with the blade of a large knife and very finely chopped

**chestnut purée** 500g (1lb 2oz)

**beef stock** 1.4 litres (2½pints) – *see* page 397 or use a good stock cube or bouillon powder

**crème fraîche** 100ml (3½fl oz)

**cognac** 3 tbsp

**pancetta** 200g (7oz), grilled until crisp

**1** Melt the butter in a large saucepan and sauté the onion and garlic gently until softened.

**2** Tip in the chestnut purée and stock and stir well.

**3** Add the crème fraîche and cognac, stir and bring to a simmer.

**4** Serve with the pancetta crumbled on top.

## vital statistics

All the alliums provide phytochemicals that help reduce cholesterol, lower blood pressure, lessen the risk of blood clots and boost natural resistance to bacterial and fungal infections. Lemon balm (*Melissa*), a member of the mint family, contains mood-enhancing essential oils.

# alli-um-yum

Thirty years ago, garlic was thought of as something only 'foreigners' ate – so much so that, because I recommended it so often, I was nicknamed 'Dr Garlic' by a leading UK political broadcaster at the station where I began my radio career. Today, I'm sure that most of my readers know about the heart-protective and cholesterol- and infection-fighting properties of this amazing bulb. What may be a surprise is the idea that garlic and its relatives from the allium family, combined with lemon balm, make this a great mood-enhancing recipe.

**onions** 2, finely chopped

**leeks** 2, thinly sliced

**spring onions** 3 large, thinly sliced

**garlic** 2 cloves, flattened with the blade of a large knife and finely chopped

**fresh root ginger** 2.5cm (1in) piece, peeled and grated

**vegetable stock** 1.2 litres (2 pints) – *see* page 396 or use a good stock cube or bouillon powder

**soy sauce** 5 tbsp

**lemon balm** 1 tbsp finely chopped

**1** Put the onions, leeks, spring onions, garlic and ginger into a large saucepan.

**2** Just cover with water and simmer for 5 minutes.

**3** Add the stock and soy sauce and simmer for 45 minutes, adding extra water if necessary.

**4** Whizz in a food processor or blender – or use a hand blender – until smooth.

**5** Sprinkle with the lemon balm to serve.

## vital statistics

This soup provides a little iron and vitamin C and very few calories. Lentinan, which fights cancer cells, and eritadenine, which helps lower cholesterol, are both present in mushrooms. Calcium is provided by the cheese and crème fraîche.

# very different mushroom soup

An old Spanish proverb says: 'Between soup and love, the first is better.' That's certainly true of this mood-enhancing mushroom mixture. All mushrooms are healthy, since they're fat-free, low in calories and a good source of nutrients. In Chinese and Japanese medicine, mushrooms are revered as medicinal treatments: shiitake for immunity, reishi for the liver and asthma, maitake for blood pressure and liver disease. The combination of mushrooms with cheese is a certain mood-booster.

**unsalted butter** 25g (1oz)

**onion** 1, finely chopped

**shiitake mushrooms** 600g (1lb 5oz), finely chopped, plus extra whole fried mushrooms to garnish (optional)

**plain flour** 1 heaped tbsp

**vegetable stock** 1 litre (1¾ pints) – *see* page 396 or use a good stock cube or bouillon powder

**manchego cheese** about 150g (5½oz), grated

**half-fat crème fraîche** 200ml (⅓ pint)

**1** Melt the butter in a large saucepan and sauté the onion and mushrooms gently, stirring continuously, until the onion is soft and golden.

**2** Sprinkle on the flour, mix well and continue cooking, stirring continuously, for 2 minutes.

**3** Pour in the stock, stir and simmer for 20 minutes.

**4** Add the cheese and the crème fraîche. Stir well and continue cooking for 2 more minutes, until the cheese has softened.

**5** Whizz in a food processor or blender – or use a hand blender – until smooth. Serve garnished with extra whole fried mushrooms, if desired.

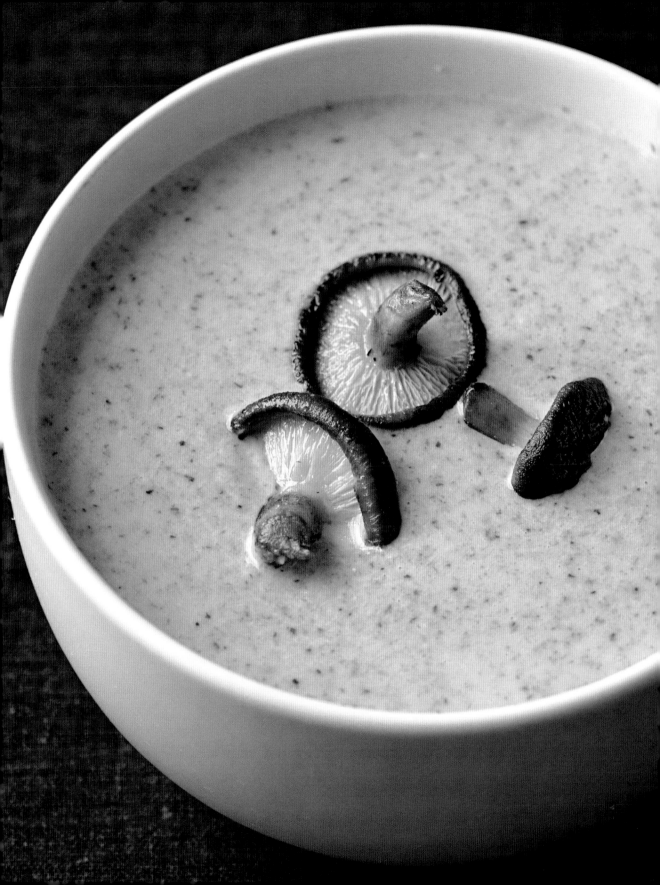

## vital statistics

This is a wonderful soup to soothe and alleviate stressed nerves. Sorrel is an excellent source of mood-enhancing phytochemicals, and the yogurt supplies brain-soothing tryptophan.

# sorrel soup

Sorrel isn't used nearly as much as it deserves to be. In addition to its mood-enhancing qualities, this delicious herb also works as an effective detoxifier. This recipe is particularly helpful for those suffering from anxiety, especially when it is associated with insomnia – another common cause of mood swings.

**sorrel leaves** 2 large handfuls, stripped from the stalks

**unsalted butter** 55g (2oz)

**shallots** 4, thinly sliced

**potatoes** 200g (7oz), peeled and cubed

**vegetable stock** 1.2 litres (2 pints) – *see* page 396 or use a good stock cube or bouillon powder

**natural set greek yogurt** 400ml (14fl oz)

**1** Reserve 8 of the sorrel leaves and whizz the rest briefly in the small bowl of a food processor or blender until puréed. (Alternatively, rub through a sieve.)

**2** Melt the butter in a small saucepan over a low heat – don't allow it to smoke or burn.

**3** Mix the puréed sorrel into the melted butter, cover and refrigerate.

**4** Simmer the shallots and potatoes in the stock until tender – about 15 minutes.

**5** Whizz in a food processor or blender – or use a hand blender – until smooth.

**6** Just before serving, stir in the sorrel and butter mixture and the yogurt. Heat gently.

Cherries are a rich source of potassium, with almost no sodium, making them a perfect fruit for anyone with high blood pressure or heart disease. They have significant amounts of protective bioflavonoids and ellagic acid, which adds to their anti-cancer properties.

# coriander and sweet-cherry soup

When it comes to feeling good, a drop of cherry brandy can't hurt, but the cherries themselves in this unusual Middle Eastern soup have extraordinary healing powers and are pretty near the top of the list of protective foods. They probably started life in Mesopotamia and were used medicinally by ancient Greek physicians. Anyone suffering from arthritis, rheumatism, gout or muscle pain will benefit from this soup.

**ground coriander** 1 heaped tsp
**runny honey** 2 tbsp
**cherries** 400g (14oz), stoned
**crème fraîche** 100ml (3½fl oz)
**milk** 600ml (1 pint)
**cherry brandy** 2 tbsp (optional)
**fresh coriander leaves** about 10, finely chopped

**1** Mix the ground coriander and honey together.

**2** Put into a food processor or blender, add the cherries, crème fraîche, milk and cherry brandy, if using, and whizz until smooth. (Alternatively, use a hand blender.)

**3** Cover and chill thoroughly in the refrigerator.

**4** Serve with the chopped coriander leaves on top.

## vital statistics

This soup is great for providing therapeutic energy. Parsnips, turnips and swedes are rich sources of slow-release energy, and garam masala supplies mood-elevating spices.

# spicy parsnip soup

The slow-release energy provided by the parsnips, turnips and swedes helps keep your blood-sugar level on an even keel and prevent mood swings. This soup also gives you a bonus in the form of the instant energy in the honey, making it the perfect soup to take to work for a hot, sustaining lunch.

**unsalted butter** 50g (1³/₄oz)

**onion** 1 large, thinly sliced

**mixed parsnips, turnips, celeriac, swede and potatoes** 600g (1lb 5oz), peeled and cubed

**runny honey** 3 tbsp

**vegetable stock** 1.4 litres (2½ pints) – *see* page 396 or use a good stock cube or bouillon powder

**natural live bio-yogurt** 150ml (¼ pint)

**garam masala** 2 tsp

To garnish

**flat-leaf parsley sprigs**

**mixed peppercorns** crushed

**1** Melt the butter in a large saucepan over a low heat and sweat the onion gently for 5 minutes.

**2** Add the mixed root vegetables and stir to coat well in the butter.

**3** Remove from the heat and drizzle in the honey, stirring to coat all the vegetables.

**4** Pour in the stock and bring to the boil.

**5** Turn the heat down and simmer until the vegetables are tender – about 20 minutes.

**6** Whizz in a food processor or blender – or use a hand blender – until smooth.

**7** Return to the heat. Stir in the yogurt and garam masala and heat through.

**8** Serve garnished with sprigs of flat-leaf parsley and crushed mixed peppercorns.

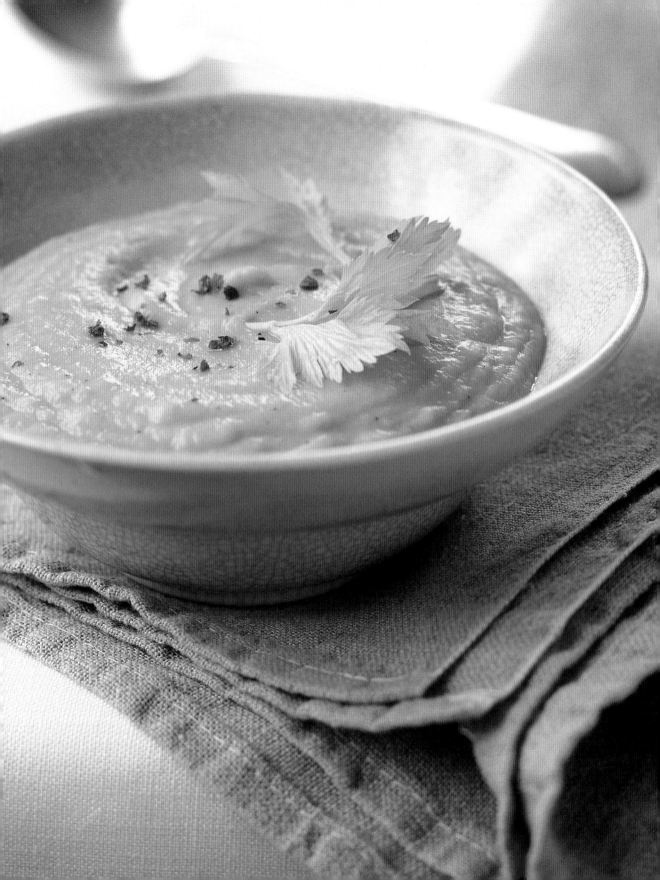

## vital statistics

Tomatoes are the richest of all sources of the nutrient lycopene. This member of the carotenoid family is one of the most protective of all the phytochemicals and will quickly boost your lowered vitality. Sago, made from the starchy pith of the sago-palm tree, is a quickly digested energy source, providing the healthiest form of carbohydrates. Minerals from the vegetable stock, and calcium and B vitamins from the milk, add to the energy-boosting value.

# hot tommy

Whether you've been laid low by a cold or flu, you're recovering from illness or an operation or you're just ground down by an extended period of work or stress, this is the drink you need. Packed with vitality, energy and valuable nutrients, this tomato-based, almost soup-like beverage is an instant shot in the arm. Easily digested and with a savoury tang to please even the most jaded of palates, it will soon be on your list of favourites.

**vegetable stock** 300ml (½ pint) – *see page* 396 or use a good stock cube or bouillon powder

**milk** 200ml (⅓ pint)

**tomatoes** 400g can, crushed

**onion** 1 large, finely grated

**sago** 20g (3/4oz)

1 Put all the ingredients into a large pot or saucepan.

2 Simmer for 2 hours.

3 Strain and serve in mugs.

## vital statistics

Enormously rich in betacarotenes, this dish is a valuable protector against heart and circulatory disease and some cancers. Its mood-enhancing properties come from the eugenol in the basil and the coriandrol from the fresh coriander.

# carrotiander soup

I defy anyone who claims to hate 'boring old carrots' not to be captivated by this variation on a traditional recipe. The combined flavours of basil and coriander and the calcium-rich smoothness provided by the crème fraîche give this easily digestible soup a completely new dimension. It's a calming and effective feel-good dish that tastes great.

**extra-virgin olive oil** 2 tbsp

**onion** 1, finely chopped

**carrots** 900g (2lb), finely cubed

**basil** ½ tsp dried, plus 10 large fresh leaves, roughly torn, to garnish

**coriander** ½ tsp dried, plus 5 fresh leaves, roughly torn, to garnish

**herb or vegetable stock** 1 litre (1¾ pints) – *see* page 396 or use a good stock cube or bouillon powder

**crème fraîche** 250ml carton

**1** Heat the oil in a large saucepan and sweat the onion gently for 5 minutes.

**2** Add the carrots and dried herbs, stir thoroughly and continue sweating for 15 minutes, stirring occasionally.

**3** Pour in the stock and bring back to the boil, then turn the heat down and simmer until the carrots are soft but not mushy.

**4** Purée using a mouli or blender, or cool slightly, put through a food processor and gently reheat.

**5** Serve with a dollop of crème fraîche and garnish with the fresh herbs.

Spinach is a rich source of folic acid, one of the essential B vitamins, making this the ideal soup to lift the spirits.

# spicy spinach soup

Here is a valuable, nutritious soup that also promotes a good mood. Spinach mixed with lots of chilli (a mood stimulant) and fresh coriander – the essential oils that have enhanced moods for centuries – turns this soup into a nutritional powerhouse, providing vitamins that help keep both mind and body healthy.

**extra-virgin olive oil** 6 tbsp

**red onions** 2, finely chopped

**garlic** 3 cloves, thinly sliced

**fresh chilli** 1 tsp chopped and deseeded

**parsley, mint and coriander leaves** ½ handful each, chopped

**spinach** 600g (1lb 5oz) (no need to remove stalks)

**vegetable stock** 1.4 litres (2½ pints) – *see* page 396 or use a good stock cube or bouillon powder

**crème fraîche** 200ml (⅓ pint)

**Emmental croûtons**

**stale wholemeal bread** 4 slices

**emmental cheese** 125g (4½oz), finely grated

**1** Heat 4 tablespoons of the oil in a large saucepan and sweat the onions for 2 minutes.

**2** Add the garlic and continue sweating for 2 minutes.

**3** Stir in the chilli, parsley, mint and coriander and heat for a further 2 minutes.

**4** Finely chop the spinach and add to the pan with about 3 tablespoons of the stock. Heat for 2 minutes, stirring continuously.

**5** Add the rest of the stock and simmer for 10 minutes.

**6** Meanwhile, for the Emmental croûtons, heat the remaining oil in a frying pan until slightly smoking. Remove the crusts from the bread and cut the slices into 1cm (½in) cubes. Roll the bread in the cheese, pressing it in firmly. Fry in the oil, turning continuously, until golden on all sides.

**7** Stir the crème fraîche into the soup and serve with the croûtons.

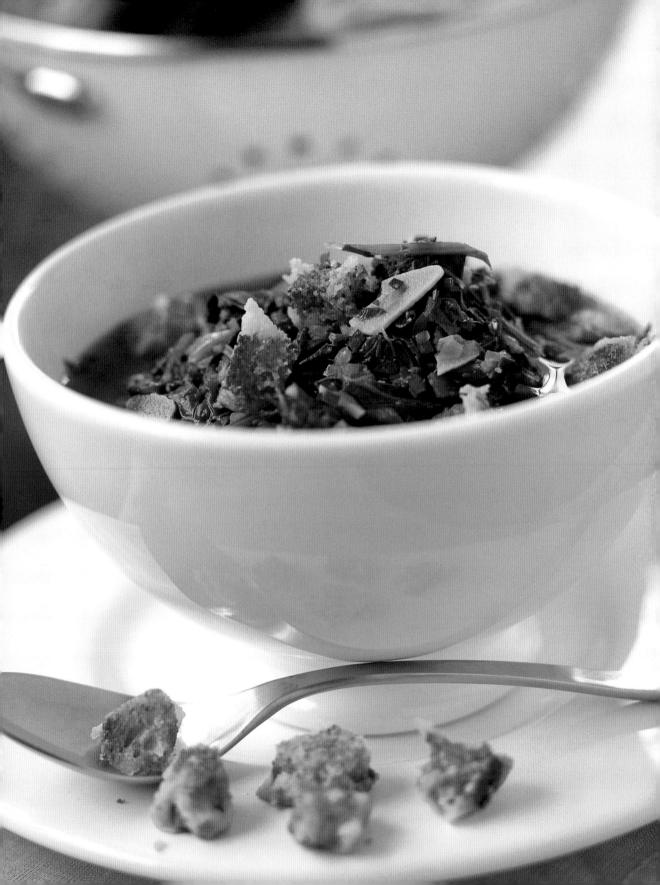

# spiced lettuce soup with goats' cheese

If insomnia is your problem, this soup is a better remedy than all but the most powerful of pills. What's more, it makes you feel good, it's highly protective and it helps keep bones strong and healthy. Although any lettuce will do, the darker the leaves, the higher the content of valuable nutrients – especially betacarotene – you'll get.

**unsalted butter** 25g (1oz)

**onion** 1, finely chopped

**garlic** 1 clove, flattened with the blade of a large knife and finely chopped

**ground cumin** 1 tsp

**green pepper** 1 small, cored, deseeded and very finely chopped

**lettuce** 1 large (any type), roughly shredded

**vegetable stock** 1.4 litres (2½ pints) – *see* page 396 or use a good stock cube or bouillon powder

**soft goats' cheese** 150g (5½oz), finely diced

**1** Melt the butter in a large saucepan and sauté the onion and garlic gently for 5 minutes.

**2** Sprinkle in the cumin, stir thoroughly and cook for 2 minutes.

**3** Add the green pepper, lettuce and stock and simmer for 5 minutes.

**4** Whizz in a food processor or blender – or use a hand blender – until smooth, then return to the saucepan to heat through.

**5** Serve hot with the diced cheese on top.

Jerusalem artichokes are a great source of inulin, a special type of fibre that ends up in the large bowel, where it feeds beneficial probiotic bacteria. Parsnip, pasta and artichokes contribute complex carbohydrates, supplying continuous slow-release energy.

# pasta, pear and blue cheese

At times of stress, carbohydrates can help stimulate the release of relaxing, feel-good brain chemicals. But they do need to be complex carbs – those with the lowest glycaemic index. This recipe has low-GI carbs in abundance from the pasta, artichokes and parsnips. Also featuring the mood-boosting effects of ginger, this is a stress-busting, feel-good soup.

**olive oil** 2 tbsp

**shallots** 2, finely chopped

**fresh root ginger** 2.5cm (1in) piece, peeled and grated

**parsnip** 1, peeled and finely cubed

**carrot** 1, trimmed and peeled unless organic, diced

**jerusalem artichokes** 5, finely cubed

**pears** 2 large, sliced

**chicken or vegetable stock** 1 litre (1¾ pints) – *see* page 396 or use a good stock cube or bouillon powder

**low-fat crème fraîche** 200ml (⅓ pint)

**blue cheese** 150g (5½oz), crumbled

**tiny pasta** such as farfalline, 150g (5½oz)

**1** Heat the oil in a large saucepan and sauté the shallots and ginger gently until the shallots are soft and golden.

**2** Add the vegetables, pears and stock and bring to the boil. Turn the heat down and simmer for 30 minutes.

**3** Add the crème fraîche and blue cheese and then whizz in a food processor or blender – or use a hand blender – until smooth.

**4** Pour back into the pan, add the pasta and leave off the heat until the pasta is al dente – about 10 minutes, depending on the type of pasta.

## vital statistics

Just 100g (3½oz) of cornmeal provides 30 per cent of a day's supply of B6, 38 per cent of fibre, 20 per cent of protein, 20 per cent of thiamine and around 25 per cent of iron, magnesium, zinc and manganese. Scallops boost the protein, zinc and iron content, and add omega-3 fatty acids.

# cornmeal with scallops

Cornmeal is a traditional food of Native Americans, both north and south. Not widely used in the UK and the rest of northern Europe, it's popularly known as polenta in Italy. It makes an excellent base for this good-mood soup, thanks to its B vitamins and tryptophan. Like all shellfish, scallops provide minerals and essential fatty acids – both important brain foods.

**milk** 1 litre (1¾ pints)

**yellow cornmeal** 450g (1lb)

**potato** 1, peeled and finely diced

**garlic** 2 cloves, flattened with the blade of a large knife and finely chopped

**sage** 1 large sprig

**potato flour** 1 tbsp

**unsalted butter** 25g (1oz)

**scallops** 4

**1** Put the milk into a large saucepan and add the cornmeal, potato, garlic and sage.

**2** Simmer for 20 minutes, stirring occasionally, until the potatoes are soft.

**3** Remove the sage.

**4** Purée using a hand blender, then sieve into a clean saucepan.

**5** Sprinkle on the potato flour and reheat, stirring.

**6** Melt the butter in a separate large saucepan.

**7** Cut the scallops into quarters (or 6 or 8 pieces if large) and cook in the butter until firm – about 45 seconds.

**8** Transfer the soup to individual serving bowls and place the scallop pieces on top.

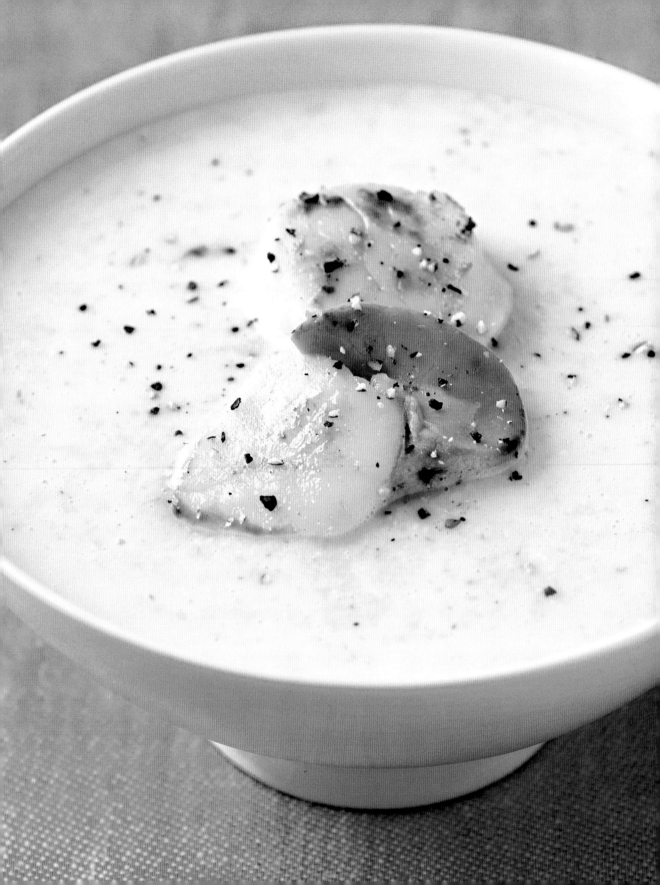

## vital statistics

Mackerel provides essential fatty acids, porridge oats are rich in B vitamins and soluble fibre, and olive oil provides vitamin E. – all in all it adds up to a great soup to boost energy and mood.

# smokie soup

This unusual combination of porridge and smoked mackerel gives a massive mood boost. In addition to the slow-release energy from the porridge oats and the protein content of the fish, the garlic, leeks and onion add flavour and protective phytochemicals.

**extra-virgin olive oil** 4 tbsp

**onions** 2 large, finely chopped

**leeks** 2, finely chopped

**garlic** 1 clove, finely chopped

**carrot** 1 large, trimmed and peeled unless organic, grated

**potato** 1 large, peeled and grated

**fish stock** 500ml (18fl oz) – *see* page 396 or use a good stock cube or bouillon powder

**water** 500ml (18fl oz)

**smoked mackerel fillets** 4 (not canned), skinned and boned

**unsalted butter** 55g (2oz)

**fine porridge oats** 100g (3½oz)

**double cream** 4 tbsp

**1** Heat the oil in a large saucepan and sweat the vegetables until soft – about 10–15 minutes.

**2** Add the stock and water and simmer for 15 minutes.

**3** Poach the mackerel fillets with the butter for about 6 minutes in just enough water to cover them.

**4** Pour the poaching liquid into the stock.

**5** Flake the fish, add to the soup and stir in the oats.

**6** Remove from the heat, cover and leave to stand for 10 minutes.

**7** Serve with a tablespoon of cream in each bowl.

## vital statistics

This soup will promote good general nutrition, especially because lentils are an excellent source of protein and complex carbohydrates.

# pancetta, onion and green lentil soup

Like all the legumes, lentils are rich in nutrients that fuel and maintain an even metabolism, which in turn promotes a sense of wellbeing. These components, together with exceptionally high levels of B vitamins and minerals from the other ingredients, make this a rich, filling and satisfying soup.

**extra-virgin olive oil** 4 tbsp

**onion** 1 large, very finely diced

**ham stock** 1.2 litres (2 pints) – *see* page 397 or use a good stock cube or bouillon powder

**green lentils** preferably Puy, 300g (10½oz)

**pancetta or unsmoked bacon** 250g (9oz), cut in one piece, rind removed, finely cubed

**1** Heat 3 tablespoons of the oil in a large saucepan and sweat the onion gently.

**2** Add the stock and bring to the boil.

**3** Add the lentils and simmer until tender – about 15–25 minutes, depending on the variety of lentils.

**4** About 5 minutes before the soup is ready, fry the pancetta or bacon in the remaining oil until crisp.

**5** Drain on kitchen paper.

**6** Serve the lentil soup scattered with the pancetta or bacon cubes.

## vital statistics

The aromatic esters from apples and the essential oils in basil are all calming and mood-enhancing. The cucumber and parsley have a gentle diuretic effect that helps with the fluid retention and swelling that some women get around their periods.

# the moody swinger

If the idea of strawberries, parsley and basil sounds a bit strange, wait till you try them with balsamic vinegar and black pepper – a truly stunning taste combination. Using the other fruit and yogurt to produce this smoothie creates a unique taste that will give you a lot of pleasure and help lift your mood if you're feeling down in the dumps.

**cucumber** 1, halved lengthways

**apples** 4, unpeeled, uncored and quartered.

**pineapple** 1 small, peeled and sliced

**flat-leaf parsley** 1 bunch

**basil** 3 large sprigs

**natural fat-free greek yogurt** 125ml (4fl oz)

**strawberries** 2, hulled and sliced

**1** Put the cucumber, apples, pineapple, parsley and 2 sprigs of basil through a juicer.

**2** Mix the yogurt with the juices.

**3** Serve with the strawberry slices and remaining basil on top.

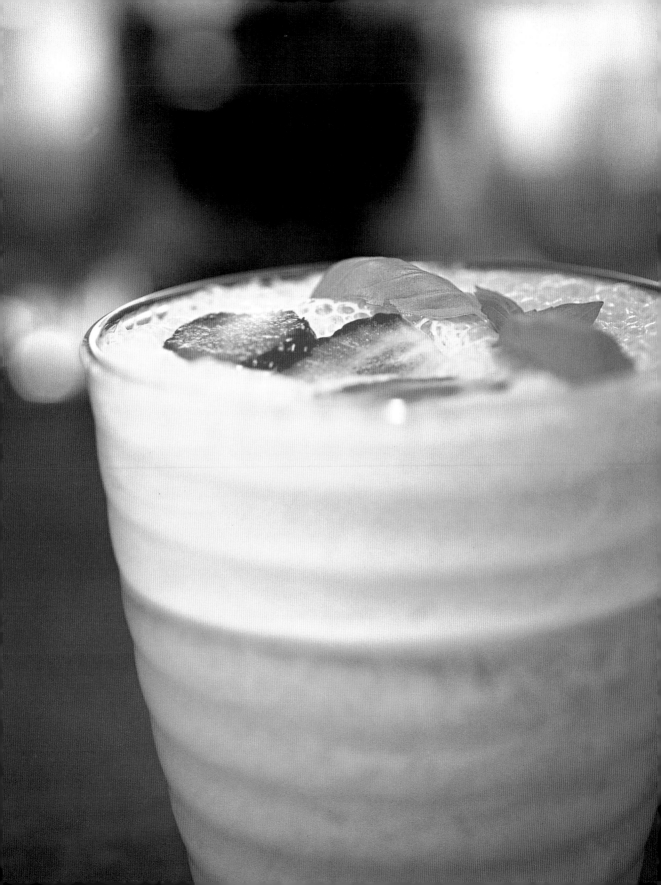

Super-rich in vitamin C and folic acid, and containing vitamin A, iron, calcium and masses of potassium, this superjuice is also a good source of protective flavonoids. Lettuce contains substances known as lactones and was used by the ancient Assyrians as a mild sedative. All of this makes the Life Saver an ideal calming and restorative juice for children recovering from illness.

# life saver

This is just the juice to revive that sinking feeling! Of all the lettuces, iceberg probably has the fewest nutrients – especially when compared with the dark-green and red-leafed varieties. However, it doesn't go slimy in your refrigerator after three days; in fact, it will keep well for two weeks if wrapped in clingfilm. It has a much sweeter flavour than other lettuce and contains the highest levels of natural calming substances. If you're tense, anxious and irritable, as well as run down, this is the cure.

**apples** 3, unpeeled, uncored and quartered
**oranges** 2, peeled but leaving white pith in place
**lemon** 1, unpeeled if thin-skinned
**iceberg lettuce** 2 handfuls

**1** Put all the ingredients through a juicer.

## vital statistics

Flaxseeds are the next best thing to fish oils in terms of omega-3 fatty acids, and they enhance mood and behaviour. Mint, surprisingly, is not only the best antacid of all but also contains essential oils that sharpen concentration and focus, while the green leaves in this juice provide betacarotenes and small but important amounts of iron.

# pear punch

Pears and celery normally go together with a strong piece of Cheddar, but not here, because this juice packs a real punch, thanks to the flaxseeds.

**conference pears** 2 large
**celery** 2 sticks, with leaves
**chard or sorrel leaves** 1 good handful
**mint** 2 large sprigs
**ground flaxseeds** 2 tsp

**1** Put all the ingredients except the seeds through a juicer.

**2** Stir in the flaxseeds.

## vital statistics

Lemons are a rich source of natural bioflavonoids, which help strengthen and protect the walls of your blood vessels. Add ginger's essential natural oils (gingerols and zingiberene), and you'll benefit from centuries of ancient wisdom, since it is one of the most effective stimulants in the ancient herbal repertoire.

# lemon and ginger tea

I'm not a great lover of the quick fix – especially since this usually means covering up the symptoms and sweeping the problem under the carpet. But when you're feeling a bit low, run down and one degree under, here's a quick fix that I really do recommend. Nothing works quite as well as this extremely simple but deliciously stimulating drink. The cleansing citrus flavour of the lemon is an ideal combination with the tropical heat of ginger. Together they provide an almost instant mood boost, raising energy and gingering up the circulation.

**fresh root ginger** 2.5cm (1in) piece, peeled and grated

**boiling water** 600ml (1 pint)

**lemon** 1, halved

1 Cover the ginger with the boiling water.

2 Add the juice from one lemon half and leave to cool.

3 Chill in the refrigerator.

4 Strain and serve with slices taken from the other lemon half.

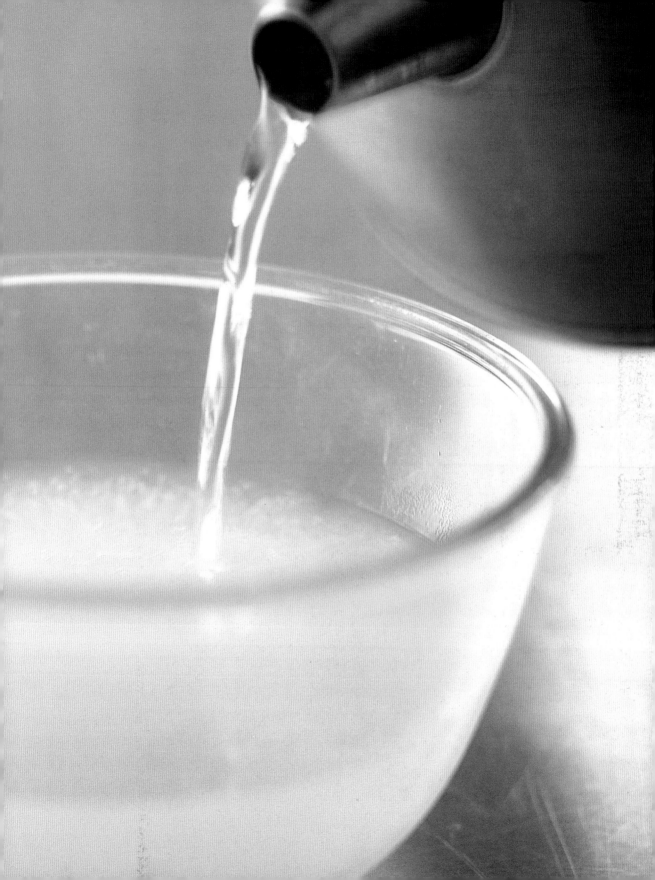

Nutmeg contains a mild hallucinogen that certainly makes you feel good, and the essential oils in basil make it one of the most mood-enhancing of all the herbs. Juiced together with calming celery, energizing apples and kiwi fruit, this is a real mood reviver at the end of a long, hard day.

# bounce back

The mood-enhancing properties of basil and nutmeg and the calming effect of celery in this drink will help you bounce back into a good mood.

**celery** 2 sticks, with leaves
**dessert apples** such as Russets, 3 good-sized, unpeeled, uncored and quartered
**kiwi fruit** 4, unpeeled
**basil leaves** 6 good-sized
**nutmeg** ½ tsp freshly grated

**1** Put all the ingredients except the nutmeg through a juicer.

**2** Stir in the nutmeg.

The natural enzymes and trace elements in the papaya and kiwi fruit help replace mood-sapping nutrient deficiencies. With the quick energy boost of the grapes as well as all their protective benefits, this is a great start to a lousy day.

# clever kiwis

Yes, they are clever, those New Zealanders. Once they found out they could grow the Chinese gooseberry so successfully, they renamed it kiwi fruit. Juiced together here with grapes and papayas, it makes for a simple, nourishing good-mood drink.

**red seedless grapes** 250g (9oz)
**papayas** 2, deseeded, flesh scooped out
**kiwi fruit** 3, unpeeled

**1** Put all the ingredients through a juicer.

## vital statistics

The essential oils of menthol and menthone are found in all varieties of mint, whether it's apple mint, ginger mint, Moroccan mint or any of the dozens of their relatives. Mint is most commonly thought of as a digestive remedy – which indeed it is – but the powerful peppermint is also mood-enhancing and protective against infections.

# pep up with peppermint

The sharp, almost astringent flavour of peppermint is a real eye-opener. There are, of course, many varieties of mint, probably the most popular of all culinary herbs. But peppermint has the most distinctive and unmistakable flavour. The bite of this mint tea, softened with the soothing flavour of honey, is a wonderful anytime mood booster.

**peppermint** 3 large sprigs
**boiling water** 250ml (9fl oz)
**runny honey** 1 tbsp

1 Put the mint into a heatproof jug.

2 Cover with the boiling water.

3 Leave to infuse for 10 minutes.

4 Strain the tea into a mug.

5 Add the honey and stir briskly until dissolved.

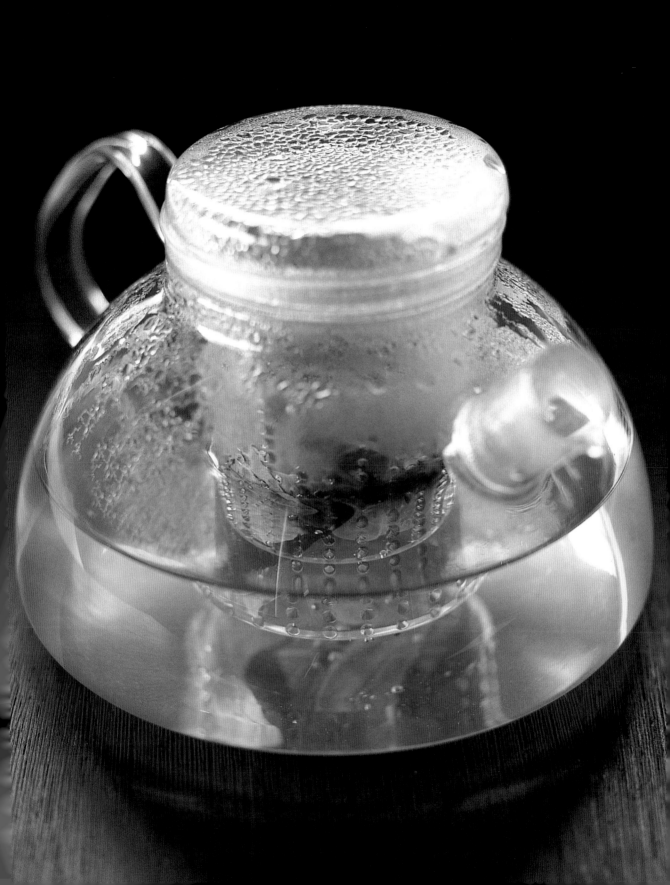

## vital statistics

The vitamin E and antioxidants from the pomegranates and the small quantities of essential oils from the orange-blossom water all help enhance your mood. The extra vitamin C from the apples and the lime will make sure you absorb sufficient iron from the food that follows this drink.

# middle eastern magic

The pomegranate, lime and orange-blossom water are certainly Middle Eastern, but the Granny Smith apples are not. However, that doesn't stop this delicious bit of magic helping you enjoy a good mood for the rest of the day.

**pomegranates** 2, seeds and flesh scooped out

**dessert apples** 4 Granny Smiths, unpeeled, uncored and quartered

**lime** 1, peeled (unless key lime)

**orange-blossom water** 1 dash

1 Put all the ingredients except the orange-blossom water through a juicer.

2 Stir in the orange-blossom water.

## vital statistics

With brain-nourishing omega-3 fats from the tahini, improved production of B vitamins in the gut through the friendly bugs, mood-enhancing phyto-oestrogens from the soya milk and all the protective nutrients in the berries and pomegranates, this has to be a double whammy of good mood and good health.

# ancient wisdom

This is a United Nations of a smoothie, starting with the ancient wisdom of the Greeks (who still make real yogurt full of beneficial bacteria) and tahini, which is like peanut butter but made from sesame seeds. Next come pomegranates, with an ancient history in the Middle East; raspberries and blackberries, traditionally gathered wild in the hills of Scotland and the hedgerows of England; and soya products, which come to us from the Far East. They all combine to make you feel happier.

**raspberries** 100g (3½oz)
**blackberries** 100g (3½oz)
**pomegranates** 2, seeds and flesh scooped out
**calcium-enriched soya milk** 300ml (½ pint)
**natural greek yogurt** 4 tbsp
**tahini** 3 tsp

**1** Put the fruit through a juicer.

**2** Add the rest of the ingredients to the juice and put into a blender or food processor – or use a hand blender. Whizz until blended.

## vital statistics

Rosemary is known as the herb of remembrance – and that's no coincidence. The natural chemicals it contains act as stimulants to the areas of the brain that control your memory, a fact well known to the ancient Greeks and Romans. The herb is also mood-enhancing, anti-inflammatory, antibacterial and stimulating.

# rosemary milk

Most people wouldn't automatically associate milk with rosemary. After all, they don't quite fit together in the same way as, say, fish and chips or bread and jam. But when you're feeling a bit low, getting over an illness or generally just under the weather, this drink will provide some comfort, calmness and a feeling of mental alertness.

**rosemary** 15cm (6in) stalk
**milk** 250ml (9fl oz)

1 Break the rosemary stalk into 4 pieces.

2 Put 3 of the pieces into a saucepan and add the milk.

3 Bring slowly to the boil, then turn the heat down and simmer for 5 minutes.

4 Press the rosemary against the side of the pan to extract the juices, then discard.

5 Serve with the reserved rosemary floating on top.

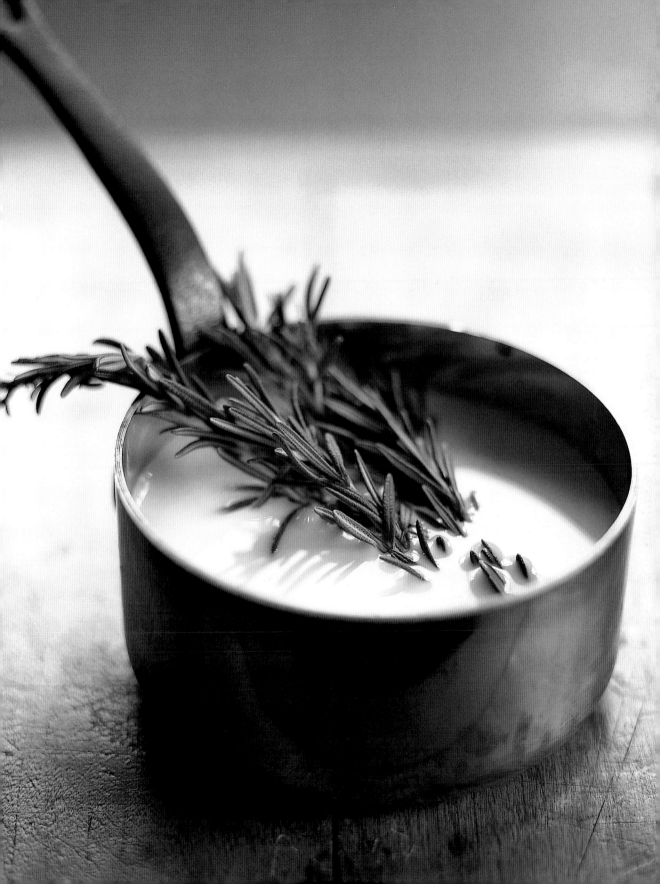

This juice has with enormous quantities of protective plant chemicals, B vitamins from the wheatgerm, potassium and B6 from banana, brain-essential fatty acids from the flaxseed oil and phyto-oestrogens from the soya milk. The latter will help even out any hormonal imbalances that might be dragging you down.

# perfect balance

To maintain emotional balance and good mood, enjoy this complex mixture of berries with wheatgerm and soya milk. Together, the ingredients provide a wide spread of good-mood nutrients that will also help build strong bones and provide a boost to your natural immunity.

**blueberries** 100g (3½oz)
**strawberries** 50g (1¾oz), hulled
**cranberries** 50g (1¾oz)
**wheat germ** 1 dessertspoon
**flaxseed oil** 1 tsp
**banana** 1 ripe, peeled
**soya milk** 300ml (½ pint)

**1** Put all the berries through a juicer.

**2** Put the juice with the rest of the ingredients into a blender or food processor – or use a hand blender – and whizz until smooth.

This juice offers amazing mood-lifting theobromines in the chocolate; mild, good-mood hallucinogenic action from the nutmeg; and a feel-good factor of instant energy from the honey. Finally, there's slower-release energy from the banana, together with its mood-enhancing vitamin B6.

# brainy bananas

You can't really get juice out of a banana, but they're so nutritious that, combined in this juice, they make a real restorative drink to help you sleep, have sweet dreams and ease any aching muscles if you've been boogieing the night away. Be sure to enjoy it while its still warm.

**hot chocolate** 3/4 mug, made from an organic 70 per cent cocoa solids mix

**banana** 1 ripe, peeled

**runny honey** 2 tsp

**ground cinnamon** 1 pinch

**nutmeg** 1 generous pinch freshly grated

**1** Put all the ingredients into a blender or food processor – or use a hand blender – and whizz until smooth.

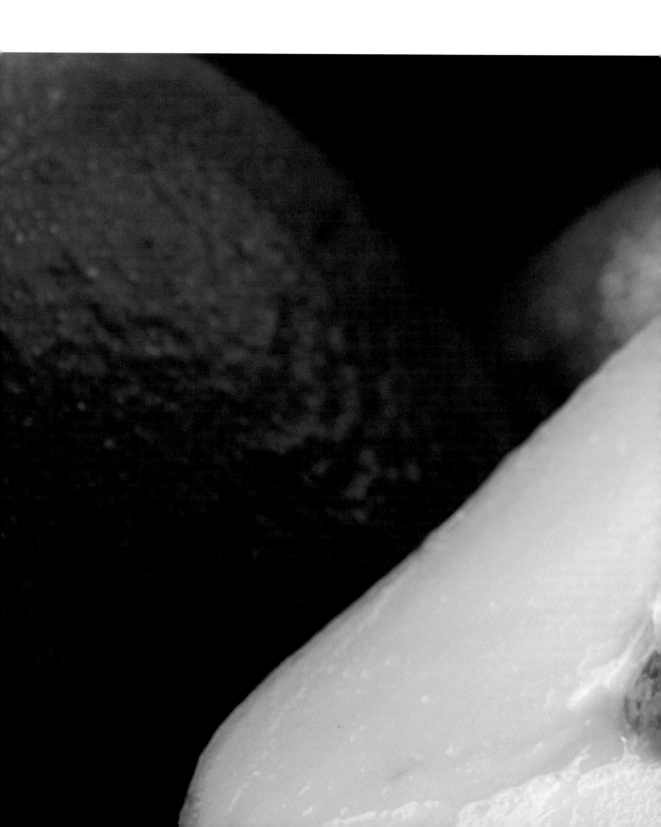

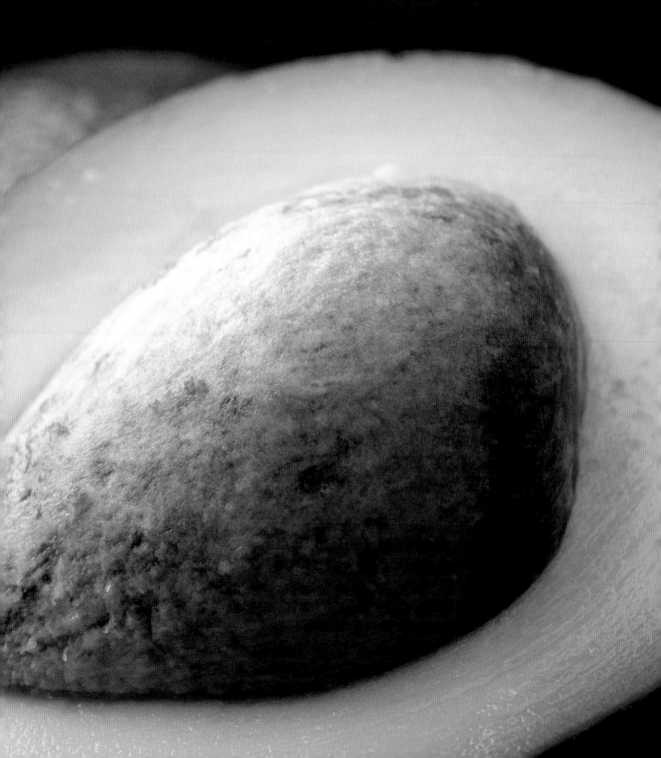

The human body has the most amazing ability to heal itself, yet it needs the right tools to do the job. Prevention is always better and easier than cure, and if your regular diet is rich in healing superfoods, then your chance of avoiding serious illness is greatly increased. This is particularly true in respect of the diseases of Western civilization: heart disease, high blood pressure, stroke, diabetes and many types of cancer, including lung, prostate and colon. In terms of healthy eating, it's what you do most of the time that really matters; the occasional treat, binge or gourmet holiday isn't going to do you any harm at all.

There's never a time when it's sensible to ignore the principles of following a diet made up predominantly of healing foods, because you never know when illness or accident might happen. A hospital bed is not the best place to get a wake-up call about your junk-food-eating habits. If your immune system is working well and you have a healthy level of the protective and healing foods in your system, then you are consuming a diet that increases your chances of a speedy recovery.

## Nutrition-aided healing

Convalescence used to be an integral part of all medical treatment. A period of time that allows recovery from illness or operation should still be considered an essential part of any cure. Nutritional needs depend on the type of illness, but the general principle is to include healing foods that are easily digestible, nutrient-rich, appetizing and easy to eat. Also essential for an effective convalescence are the antioxidant vitamins A, C and E, protective minerals like zinc and a high intake of iron to ensure good haemoglobin.

Hospital diets are notoriously poor. Virtually no fresh fruit, unappetizing, wilted salads and overcooked vegetables kept warm for hours result in a severe lack of vitamin C. This in turn makes the patient more liable to infection, causes slower wound healing and the development of bedsores. A study by Professor John Garrow published in the *British Medical Journal* shows that the poor quality of hospital food doubles the number of days spent in hospital by elderly patients recovering from hip fractures. Observations of well-nourished older patients demonstrate that the daily intake of a simple vitamin and mineral supplement shortens the time it takes for them to recover from illnesses.

Traditionally, all cookery books used to contain a section on convalescent and invalid cookery, with recipes that included healing foods. It saddens me that this is no longer the case. So, in case you don't have any old cookery books, here are some ideas.

**Food to aid recovery**

Breakfasts should include porridge, yogurt with honey and pine nuts, melon, soaked dried fruits with yogurt and cinnamon, wholemeal toast, and boiled, poached or scrambled eggs. Lunches: white fish, oily fish, broccoli, spinach, carrots, free-range chicken, rosemary, thyme, garlic and sage. Evening meals: light salads; soups made with root vegetables, barley and millet; fruit salads with almonds; low-fat cheeses and avocados. Extras: fresh fruit, especially grapes, dates, kiwi fruit, citrus fruits and berries; unsweetened fresh fruit juices; vegetable juices; dried fruit; fresh nuts and seeds.

This is also the place for the wonders of 'Jewish penicillin': chicken soup. That great antiviral, antibacterial, body-and-soul-healing recipe that's been passed from generation to generation really is a cure for colds, flu, chest infections and probably many other ailments. Made with real chicken, real vegetables, real herbs and, most of all, real love, it is a powerful healing food as confirmed by scientific studies.

# healing checklist

- Eat more blackcurrants, berries, citrus fruits and kiwi fruit – rich in vitamin C and bioflavonoids; cabbage and all its relatives for the antibacterial sulphur and cancer-protective phytochemicals they contain; apples for their ability to help the body eliminate cholesterol and toxic residues. Opt for live yogurt for the immunity-boosting benefits of probiotic bacteria; dates for iron and easily converted calories; oats for protein, B vitamins, calcium, potassium and magnesium; fish for easily digested protein and minerals. Choose root vegetables, broccoli and carrots for betacarotene; dried fruits for energy; and garlic, cinnamon, sage, rosemary and thyme for their antiseptic and circulation-stimulating properties.
- Consume fewer refined carbohydrates, less sugar and alcohol, and fewer high-bran foods, animal fats and red meat. Avoid convenience food, instant 'just-add-water' products and nutritionally poor takeaways.

As well as fibre, broad beans are rich in protein, offer loads of potassium, and they're a good source of selenium, zinc and iron. An added restorative boost comes from the mind-improving volatile oils in sage, and the lycopene from the sun-dried tomatoes.

# broad bean, tomato and sage

Throughout the Mediterranean, broad beans are known as fava beans, and many imaginative recipes use them fresh, raw, cooked or dried to provide a huge source of nature's nutrients. This dish provides a bundle of nutrients for a natural lift.

**broad beans** 400g (14oz), shelled fresh or frozen

**sun-dried tomatoes** 10, coarsely chopped

**purple sage leaves** 10, torn into small pieces

**sage flowers** 1 handful (optional)

**pumpkin seeds** 2 tbsp

**salad dressing** 3 tbsp (*see* page 182)

1 Cook the broad beans in a saucepan of unsalted boiling water until just tender. Plunge them into ice-cold water to cool and freshen.

2 Mix the sun-dried tomatoes, sage leaves and beans together in a shallow dish.

3 If you're lucky enough to grow your own sage, sprinkle the flowers on top.

4 Add the pumpkin seeds.

5 Add the dressing and leave to marinate for at least 1 hour before serving.

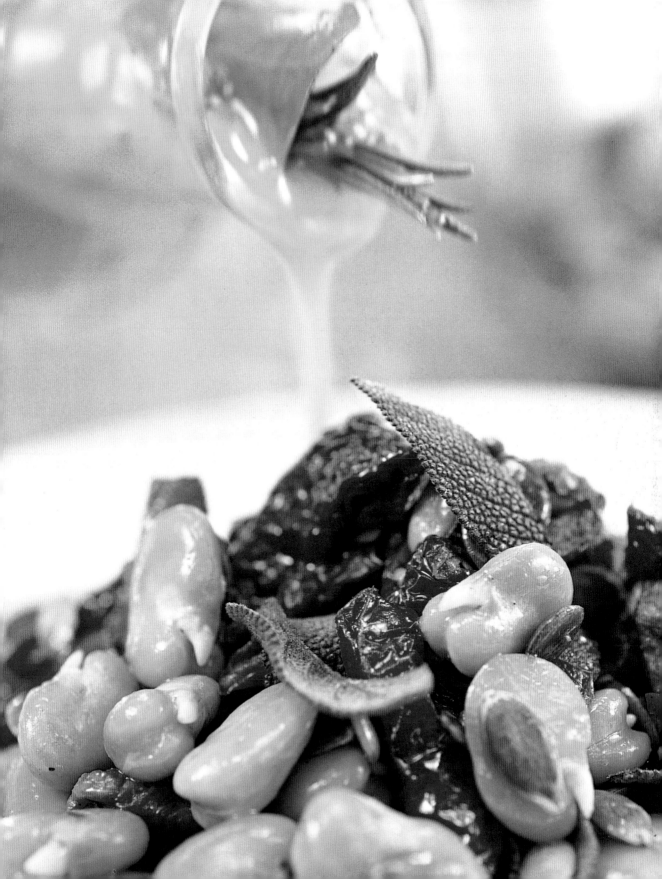

## vital statistics

This dish provides some protein, plenty of fibre and a good helping of vitamins A and E, potassium and phosphorus.

# byzantine broad beans

Ancient Greece was the cradle of bean cuisine. The international crossroads of exotic foodstuffs produced extraordinary combinations, of which this is a prime example. The unique properties of olive oil and dill make this piquant bean dish both delicious and digestible.

**extra-virgin olive oil** 2 dessertspoons
**broad beans** 450g (1lb), shelled fresh
**spring onions** 5, chopped
**black pepper** freshly ground, to taste
**dill** 3 tbsp chopped
**lemons** juice of 2

**1** Heat the oil in a saucepan over a medium heat and sauté the broad beans and spring onions, seasoned with black pepper to taste, for 5 minutes.

**2** Add enough water to cover the beans and simmer gently for 10 minutes.

**3** Add the dill and lemon juice, and simmer for another 10 minutes.

Seeds and sprouts contain enzymes, as well as other important nutrients. These help boost the activity of the body's own enzyme systems, which, in turn, enhances the body's absorption of essential substances. Adding walnuts increases the amount of B vitamins provided by this salad, as well as offering the extra benefits of essential fatty acids and protein.

# bean sprout booster

Sprouted beans and seeds of all types should be high on your list of favourites if you're in need of a quick burst of restoration. All sprouts are wonderful sources of vitamins and minerals – and they're cheap and easy to grow yourself if you fancy a bit of DIY therapy. All this makes this dish a good all-round source of vitamins and minerals.

**bean sprouts** 1 bag
**watercress** 1 bunch
**walnuts** 200g (7oz), coarsely chopped
**spring onions** 2, coarsely chopped
**avocado** ½ ripe
**walnut oil** 2 tbsp
**rice vinegar** 1 tbsp
**light soy sauce** 1 tsp
**black pepper** freshly ground, to taste

**1** Wash and dry the bean sprouts and watercress thoroughly – even if they're 'ready-washed'. Put them into a salad bowl.

**2** Add the walnuts and spring onions to the bowl.

**3** Peel, stone and mash the avocado together with the oil, vinegar and soy sauce. Add this dressing to the bowl.

**4** Toss well and season to taste with black pepper.

Not only is this salad full of vitamin C, but the natural substances that give strawberries and blueberries their colour are among the most powerful of the immunity-boosting antioxidants.

# strawberry fare

Restoring your immune system is the key to quick recovery after any period of excessive stress or illness – and this is just the salad to give you a kick-start.

**cottage cheese** 150g carton
**lime** juice of 1
**extra-virgin olive oil** 1 tbsp
**balsamic vinegar** 2 tsp
**cucumber** ½ large, peeled, deseeded and diced
**strawberries** 12 large ripe, hulled and quartered
**blueberries** 300g (10½oz)
**mint leaves** 6 (optional)

**1** Mix the cottage cheese, lime juice, oil and vinegar together in a bowl.

**2** Arrange the cucumber in a serving bowl. Scatter with the strawberries and blueberries. Add a large dollop of the cottage cheese dressing and mix lightly together.

**3** Sprinkle with mint leaves, if using, and serve.

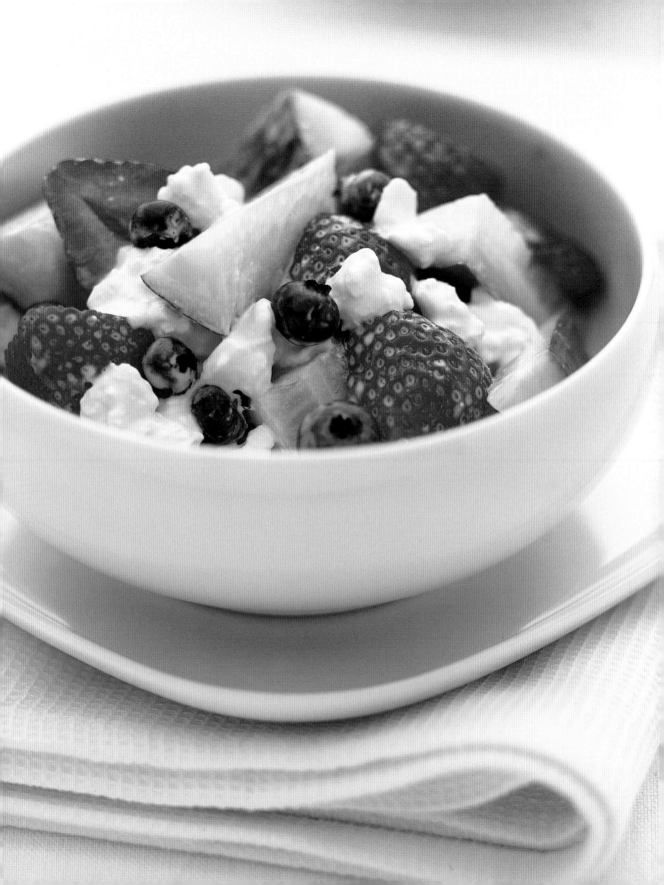

## vital statistics

Garlic's age-old tradition as an antibacterial and antifungal is now scientifically proven, while watercress is full of special mustard oils that guard against coughs and colds – it's specifically protective of lung tissue. The rich source of vitamin E found in sunflower seeds will help boost your overall resistance to infection.

# bitter green salad

If you're recovering from an illness, the last thing you need is to pick up another infection. In this salad you'll get multiple protection, since it helps prevent infection and increase natural resistance.

**watercress** 1 large bunch
**frisée lettuce** 1 head, leaves separated
**garlic** 2 cloves, finely chopped
**sunflower seeds** 2 tbsp
**salad dressing** 3 tbsp (*see* page 182)

**1** Thoroughly wash and dry the watercress – even if it's 'ready-washed'.

**2** Tear the lettuce into small pieces and put into a salad bowl. Add the watercress, garlic and sunflower seeds and mix well.

**3** Pour on the dressing and toss lightly.

The cabbage in this recipe provides vitamin C. Carrots give a huge boost of betacarotene, while the caraway seeds aid the digestion of sauerkraut and counteract its well-known flatulence factor.

# sauerkraut and caraway salad

It's a great shame that sauerkraut has never become as popular in Britain as it has in the rest of Europe, where most countries have a traditional recipe for this health-giving dish. Long before freezing, shredded cabbage was preserved with salt and fermentation to provide a valuable source of vitamin C during the winter months. The beneficial bacteria that live in the digestive system are encouraged by the lactic acid formed during fermentation, and this increases the amount of nutrients absorbed by the body. As a result, this salad restores digestive balance and increases nutritional uptake.

**caraway seeds** 2 tsp

**sauerkraut** 500g (1lb 2oz), drained

**carrots** 2 large old, peeled unless organic

**safflower oil** 2 tbsp

**cider vinegar** 1 tbsp

**parsley** 1 tbsp chopped

1 Mix the caraway seeds into the sauerkraut.

2 Grate the carrots finely.

3 Mix the oil and vinegar together and add to the grated carrots.

4 Put the grated carrots into the middle of a serving dish, arrange the sauerkraut around the outside and sprinkle with the parsley.

This delicious dish gives a gentle boost to the brain and nervous system, and helps the immune system.

# chicken and mango tango

This is a special dish for me. Our friend Caroline made it for us when my wife, Sally, and I got married. Sally now makes it frequently, and it's a particular favourite for friends who were at our wedding and are now so welcome in our home. Chicken is the perfect restorative food for the brain and nervous system, because it contains B vitamins as well as protein. Like most tropical fruits, mangoes are a terrific source of betacarotenes, which are not only protective antioxidants, but are also converted by the body into vitamin A, an essential nutrient for a healthy immune system.

**spring onions** 4 large

**mangoes** 1 large or 2 small ripe, peeled and stoned

**celery** 2 sticks, roughly chopped

**limes** juice of 2

**extra-virgin olive oil** 150ml (¼ pint)

**fresh coriander** 1 large bunch

**cooked chicken** 1 medium-sized (or use the leftovers from yesterday's roast)

**iceberg lettuce** about 4 large leaves

**cucumber** ½, peeled, halved, deseeded and diced

**1** Trim the spring onions, leaving any succulent green tips, and roughly chop.

**2** Put the onions into a food processor or blender with the mangoes, celery and lime juice, and whizz on a moderate speed.

**3** With the machine running, add the oil gradually.

**4** Roughly chop half the coriander and add to the dressing without whizzing any further.

**5** Remove all the white meat from the chicken (use the rest to make super-immunity-boosting chicken soup) and take off any skin and extra fat.

**6** Arrange the lettuce leaves on a plate and sprinkle over the cucumber pieces.

**7** Pile the chicken on top and pour on the dressing. Garnish with the rest of the coriander.

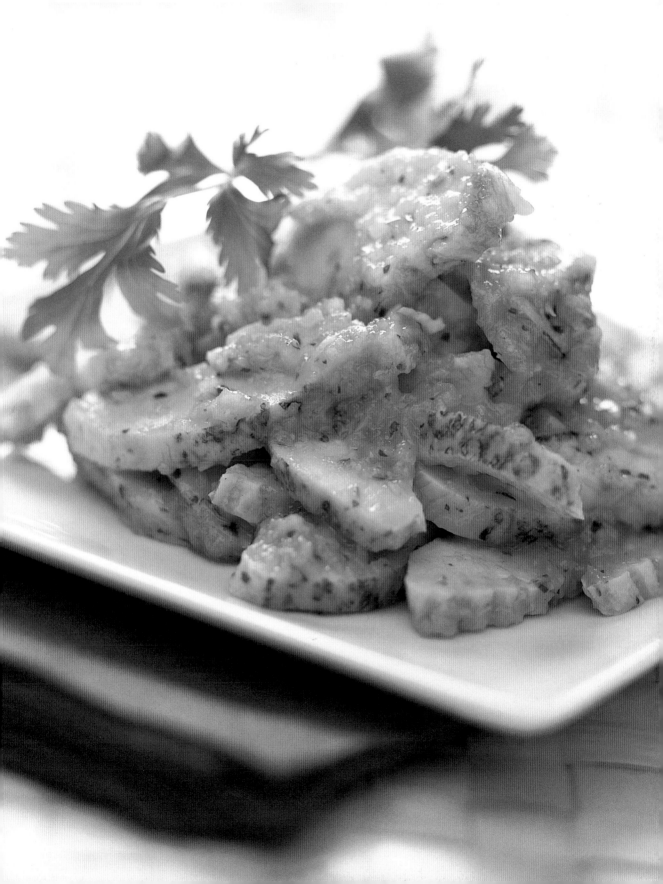

## vital statistics

Prebiotic fibre from the endive helps feed friendly bacteria. You'll get instant energy from the easily available gingerbread calories, plus stimulating spices.

# honey and spice and all things nice

Rapeseed oil has the very best balance between omega-3 and -6 fatty acids and a high smoking point, which means you can cook it at much higher temperatures. This results in faster cooking, less oil being absorbed by the food and much less risk of the dangerous by-products of overheated fats and oils. Two heads of chicory (endive or witloof) provide a scant 17 calories, a quarter of your daily fibre needs, lots of potassium and only 5mg of salt; consequently, this is a valuable restorative vegetable. With lots of protein and delicious calories from the gingerbread, this soup will stimulate the most jaded appetite.

**unsalted butter** 10g (¼oz)

**rapeseed oil** 2 tbsp

**smoked ham** 150g (5½oz), cut into small cubes

**chicory** 4 heads, roughly chopped

**full-fat milk** 600ml (1 pint)

**gingerbread** 200g (7oz), cubed

**crème fraîche** 300ml (½ pint)

**1** Melt the butter with the oil in a large frying pan and sauté the smoked ham until crisp.

**2** Remove from the pan with a slotted spoon and set aside to cool.

**3** Add the chicory to the pan and cook gently until softened, then tip into a food processor or blender.

**4** Pour in the milk, add the gingerbread and crème fraîche, and whizz until smooth.

**5** Pour into a saucepan and bring to the boil. Turn the heat down and simmer for 10 minutes.

**6** Leave to cool, then cover and chill in the refrigerator.

**7** Serve scattered with the smoked ham.

## vital statistics

You'll get a day's dose of vitamin C from one kiwi fruit, plus unique phytochemicals to protect DNA and enormous antioxidant properties from betacarotene and other nutrients. Kiwi fruit are essential for recovery from respiratory problems, particularly for children.

# cold and fizzy kiwi

Here's a restorative soup that's ready in minutes. It may sound like a smoothie, but I was served this as a cold soup before a meal of what my wife described as the best mussels she'd ever eaten. We were on the edge of Coromandel in New Zealand, where the best kiwi fruit and green-lipped mussels come from. Our hostess used local red apples, but the tang of a crisp Cox or Granny Smith gives a much better flavour.

**kiwi fruit** 6, peeled and roughly chopped

**dessert apples** 2, peeled, cored and roughly chopped

**crème fraîche** 300ml (½ pint)

**caster sugar** 100g (3½oz)

**fizzy lemonade** 150ml (¼ pint) good-quality, preferably homemade

**1** Put the fruit, crème fraîche and sugar into a food processor or blender and whizz until smooth.

**2** Cover and leave in the refrigerator to chill.

**3** Add the lemonade just before serving and mix well.

## vital statistics

This soup provides bioflavonoids to boost defences, carotenoids to protect the eyes and antibacterial essential oils from the thyme.

# pepper power

If you're just getting over a rotten cold, a bout of flu or a stay in hospital, this is the soup you need to restore your body and mind to tip-top performance. Sweet peppers are not only an enormous source of vitamin C – more than a day's dose from a mere 100g (3½oz) – they also supply considerable amounts of betacarotene, and this increases as they ripen from green to red. Protection against arthritis, heart and circulatory disease, some types of cancer and loss of vision all come from these simple and delicious fruits.

**rapeseed oil** 2 tbsp

**onion** 1, finely chopped

**paprika** 2 tsp

**plain flour** 1 tbsp

**peppers** 2 red, 1 yellow, cored, deseeded and finely chopped

**vegetable stock** 1 litre (1¾ pints) – *see* page 396 or use a good stock cube or bouillon powder

**thyme** 1 large sprig

**mascarpone cheese** 225g (8oz)

**black olives** 75g (2¾oz), pitted and roughly chopped, to serve

**1** Heat the oil in a large saucepan, add the onion and paprika and stir well. Sauté gently until the onion is soft.

**2** Sprinkle on the flour and mix in well.

**3** Add the peppers, stock and thyme, and stir. Bring to the boil, then turn the heat down and simmer until the peppers are soft.

**4** Whizz in a food processor or blender – or use a hand blender – until smooth and return to the pan.

**5** Bring back to a simmer and gradually add the mascarpone, mixing well.

**6** Serve with the olives scattered on top.

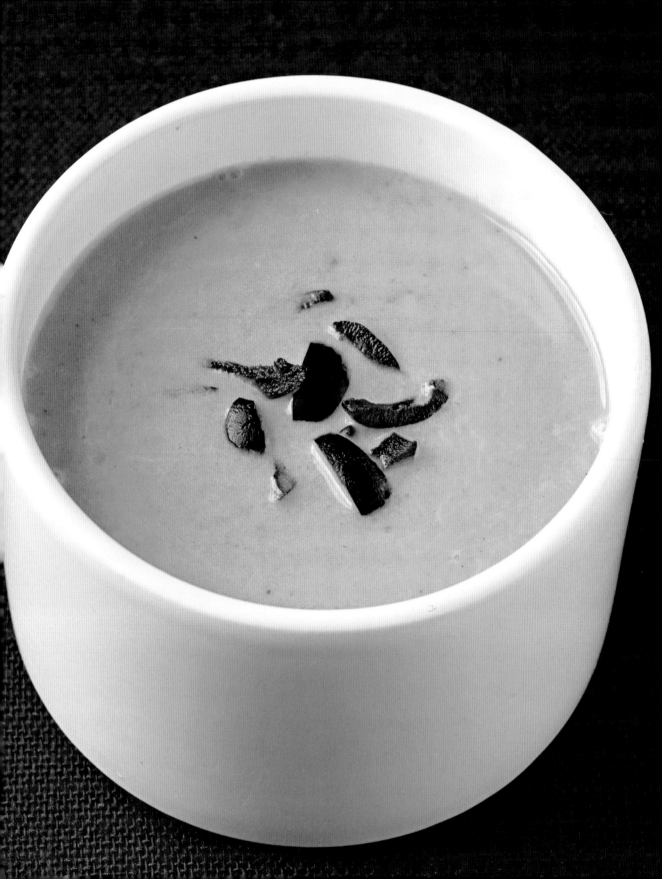

## vital statistics

The perfect soup for a speedy recovery from illness, this contains garlic, which is antibacterial and antifungal, and live yogurt, which provides probiotic bacteria that help restore the immune system.

# ajo bianco

This traditional garlic soup of southern Spain provides the extreme healing properties of garlic's sulphur compounds. Combined here with the instant energy derived from natural sugars in the grapes and the extra protein from the almonds, the result is a super-restorative bowl of strengthening nutrients.

**ground almonds** 175g (6oz)

**extra-virgin olive oil** 3 tbsp

**garlic** 4 cloves, very finely chopped

**white breadcrumbs** 100g (3½oz)

**cold water** 700ml (1¼ pints)

**grape juice** 250ml (9fl oz)

**natural live bio-yogurt** 100ml (3½fl oz)

**seedless white grapes** 400g (14oz), halved (and peeled if you can be bothered) to garnish

**1** Mix the almonds, oil and garlic together thoroughly.

**2** Put into a food processor or blender, add half the breadcrumbs, half the water and half the grape juice, and whizz until completely combined.

**3** Pour into a clean bowl.

**4** Put the rest of the breadcrumbs, water and grape juice into the food processor or blender – no need to rinse it out.

**5** Add the yogurt and pulse about 5 times until the ingredients are combined.

**6** Pour the yogurt mixture into the first breadcrumb mixture and stir thoroughly.

**7** Cover and chill in the refrigerator for about 1 hour.

**8** Serve garnished with the halved grapes.

## vital statistics

This is the ideal soup to heal throat and chest infections. Leeks contain antibacterial phytochemicals, and lentils supply easily digested protein and the essential trace minerals zinc and selenium.

# leek and lentil soup

Like all members of the *Allium* genus of plants, leeks have a long and effective history in the folklore of healing foods. They've been used as a medicinal food since the time of the ancient Romans, and they are valued just as much today. If you're recovering from a cold, flu or bronchitis, then this is the soup to choose.

**vegetable, ham or beef stock**
1.4 litres (2½pints) – *see* pages 396–7 or use a good stock cube or bouillon powder

**puy lentils** 200g (7oz)

**extra-virgin olive oil** 1 tbsp

**back bacon** 200g (7oz) organic, cut into thin shreds

**leeks** 3 large, very finely chopped

**garlic** 2 cloves, finely chopped

**matzo dumplings** (*see* page 316)

**1** Heat the stock in a large saucepan. Stir in the lentils.

**2** Leave them to cook for about 20 minutes.

**3** Meanwhile, heat the oil gently in a separate pan and sweat the bacon for 5 minutes.

**4** Stir in the leeks and garlic and cook very gently until softened.

**5** Once the lentils are tender, add the vegetables and bacon to the stock.

**6** Add the matzo dumplings to the soup and simmer for 15 minutes.

## vital statistics

Special flavonoids rutin and quercitin, combined with anethole, make fennel an unusually generous provider of phytochemicals. Lots of fibre, folic acid and potassium – again in the fennel – add to the benefits.

# fennel soup

American Dr James Duke is one of the world's leading ethno-botanists and an expert on the medicinal benefits of all plants. He is famously quoted as saying: 'An old-fashioned vegetable soup, without any enhancement, is a more powerful anti-carcinogen than any known medicine.' This is a great example. Eating can be a problem when you're getting over illness, and this soup is a brilliant solution. The Greeks, Romans, Anglo-Saxons and the American Puritans all understood the value of fennel as food and medicine. Fennel stimulates digestion and uniquely helps reduce inflammation and prevent some cancers. The gnocchi provide valuable energy for convalescence.

**rapeseed oil** 2 tbsp

**fennel** 3 bulbs, finely sliced

**onion** 1, very finely chopped

**garlic** 2 cloves, flattened with the blade of a large knife and very finely chopped

**plain flour** 2 tbsp

**vegetable stock** 1 litre (1³/₄ pints) – *see* page 396 or use a good stock cube or bouillon powder

**crème fraîche** 200ml (⅓ pint)

**gnocchi** 115g (4oz)

**1** Heat the oil in a large saucepan and sauté the fennel, onion and garlic gently until golden – about 5 minutes.

**2** Sprinkle on the flour and continue cooking for 2 minutes, stirring continuously.

**3** Pour in the stock and bring to the boil, stirring, then turn the heat down to a simmer.

**4** Add the crème fraîche and stir well.

**5** Cook the gnocchi in a separate saucepan according to the packet instructions.

**6** Serve the soup with the gnocchi floating on top.

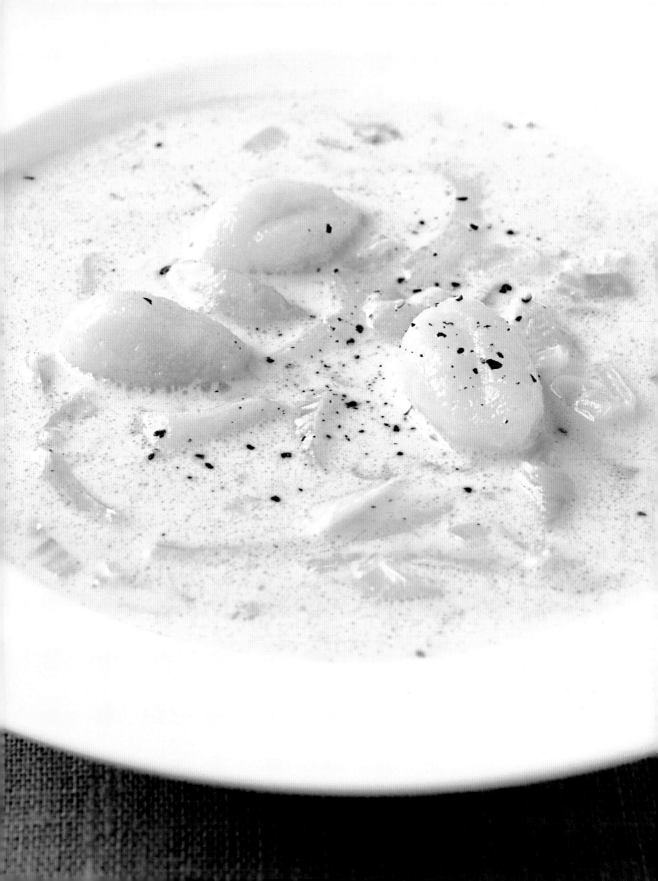

Cynarin in the artichoke hearts improves liver function, stimulates the gall bladder and encourages fat digestion and nutrient absorption. Milk and cheese are excellent sources of protein, calcium and calories. Sulphur-based chemicals in the onion help prevent infection.

# hearty help

Frequently, even minor illnesses can lead to unpleasant and lingering digestive problems. More serious conditions involving the liver or gall bladder can make the digestion of fats a serious problem. If this happens, the body's absorption of the fat-soluble vitamins A, D, E and K is soon compromised, resulting in delayed recovery. The artichoke in this soup improves fat digestion, encouraging quicker recovery.

**unsalted butter** 50g (1³/₄oz)

**onion** 1, finely chopped

**carrot** 1 large, trimmed and peeled unless organic, grated

**celery** 2 sticks, finely diced

**plain flour** 2 tbsp

**vegetable stock** 600ml (1 pint) – *see* page 396 or use a good stock cube or bouillon powder

**milk** 400ml (14fl oz)

**cheddar cheese** 225g (8oz), grated

**canned artichoke hearts** 400g (14oz) (drained weight), rinsed and quartered

**1** Melt the butter in a large saucepan and sauté the onion, carrot and celery, stirring continuously, until soft.

**2** Sprinkle in the flour, mix well and continue cooking for 2 minutes.

**3** Add the stock and milk, continue stirring and bring back to a simmer.

**4** Tip in the cheese and stir until melted.

**5** Add the artichoke hearts and continue simmering until warmed through – about 10 minutes.

## vital statistics

Lycopene in the tomatoes protects the eyes and the prostate. Protein and phyto-oestrogens from the beans rebuild tissues and help hormone problems. Natural cancer-fighting chemicals are abundant in the kale. Essential oils in the coriander stimulate appetite.

# five-a-day soup

I'd normally run a mile from any recipe calling for 15 ingredients. But this spicy soup tastes great and is easy to make. It's really worth the effort, as it actually tastes better by the second or third day. It's a blockbuster restorative soup, with virtually every protective nutrient you can think of – and a lot more besides.

**vegetable stock** 1 litre (1³/₄ pints) – *see* page 396 or use a good stock cube or bouillon powder

**onion** 1, very finely chopped

**garlic** 3 cloves, finely chopped

**green pepper** 1, cored, deseeded and diced

**green chillies** 6 small, deseeded and finely chopped

**chilli powder** 1 tsp

**courgette** 1, diced

**kale** 2 handfuls, roughly torn

**canned tomatoes** 225g (8oz), crushed

**canned kidney beans** 225g (8oz), rinsed

**canned sweetcorn** 225g (8oz), rinsed

**dried oregano and ground cumin** 1 tsp each

**sesame seeds** 2 tbsp, toasted

**fresh coriander** 3 heaped tbsp chopped

**1** Heat 1 tablespoon of the stock in a large saucepan.

**2** Add the onion, garlic, green pepper and chillies and simmer, stirring continuously, for 5 minutes.

**3** Add the chilli powder and continue cooking, again stirring continuously, for 1 minute.

**4** Pour in the rest of the stock and add the courgette, kale, tomatoes, beans, sweetcorn, oregano and cumin.

**5** Bring to the boil, then turn the heat down and simmer for 20 minutes.

**6** Add the sesame seeds and fresh coriander just before serving.

## vital statistics

Any form of extended stress, anxiety or depression drains the body's vitamin B stores. Fresh or frozen peas are an excellent source of vitamin B1 and folic acid. They also provide useful quantities of vitamins A and C, and fatigue-fighting minerals zinc and iron. Antibacterial and antiviral compounds in the onions help fight infection, making this an extra-valuable remedy for depressing infections like flu.

# peas please

This is a sort of instant pea soup – and just what's needed for anyone feeling a bit under the weather, miserable, depressed, anxious or suffering from seasonal affective disorder (SAD). Frozen peas are ideal for this delicious tonic, because they're quick and easy to prepare and lose very little of their nutritional value. Canned peas, on the other hand, lose much more vitamin C and are also generally high in salt. The spring onions and the mint add extra essential oils to boost resistance and energy levels.

**spring onions** 2 large
**frozen peas** 350g (12oz)
**mint** 1 large sprig
**vegetable stock** 850ml (1½ pints) – *see* page 396 or use a good stock cube or bouillon powder

**1** Put all the ingredients into a saucepan and cook gently until the peas are tender.

**2** Reserving 2 tablespoons of the peas, whizz the stock mixture in a food processor or blender – or use a hand blender – until smooth, adding a little boiling water, if necessary.

**3** Serve with the reserved peas floating on top.

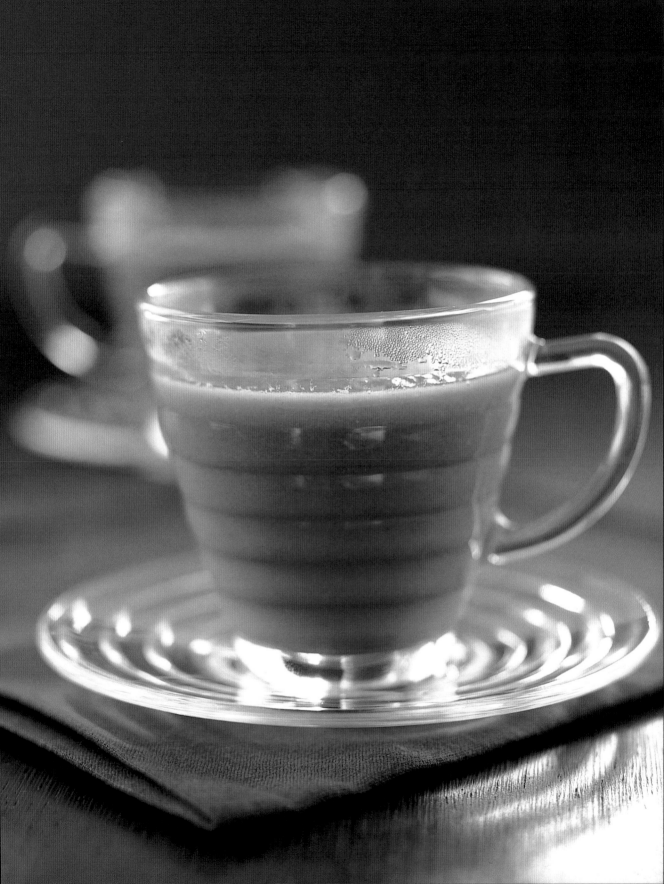

The perfect soup for a boost of slow-release energy. Butter beans are rich in protein, fibre, slow-release energy, B vitamins and natural plant hormones that are a valuable aid to women. Parsley is gently diuretic.

# butter bean, parsley and garlic soup

Butter beans are much loved in middle and southern Europe, as well as the southern United States. This soup is especially good when made with chicken stock, because this adds more healing enzymes. The vegetable option is almost as effective, though, and it will provide more skin-restoring betacarotene.

**extra-virgin olive oil** 4 tbsp

**onion** 1 large, finely chopped

**garlic** 2 cloves, finely chopped

**chicken or vegetable stock** 1.4 litres (2½ pints) – see page 396 or use a good stock cube or bouillon powder

**butter beans** 2 x 400g cans, rinsed

**parsley** 2 large handfuls, very coarsely chopped

**herb croûtons** to serve (see page 95)

1 Heat the oil in a large saucepan over a low heat and sweat the onion and garlic gently until softened.

2 Add the rest of the ingredients.

3 Simmer until the beans are slightly tender – about 15 minutes.

4 Serve with herb croûtons.

This soup will soothe both mind and body. Kidney beans are a source of protein, restorative energy and natural plant hormones, and sage contains essential oils that ease digestion and help regulate moods.

# mushroom and bean broth

When your body or mind – or, worse still, both – have been through the mill, there's no food quite so physically and emotionally restorative as this interesting broth. The subtle flavour and immunity-boosting benefits of mushrooms mix perfectly with the more robust kidney beans to help kick-start the body's regulatory mechanisms.

**dried porcini mushrooms** 25g (1oz)
**freshly boiled water** 1.4 litres (2½ pints)
**celery** 2 sticks, roughly chopped
**leeks** 2 large, chopped
**sage** 1 large sprig
**bay leaves** 3
**kidney beans** 400g can, rinsed
**natural live bio-yogurt** 150ml (¼ pint)

**1** Soak the mushrooms in the water for 15 minutes.

**2** Strain the mushrooms, reserving the liquid, and chop them coarsely.

**3** Pour the liquid into a large saucepan and bring to a simmer.

**4** Add the celery, leeks, sage and bay leaves and simmer for 15 minutes.

**5** Strain again and reserve the liquid.

**6** Add the kidney beans and chopped mushrooms and heat for 10 minutes.

**7** Stir in the yogurt and serve.

Brussels sprouts are rich in cancer-fighting phytochemicals, and garlic and onions supply heart-protective and infection-fighting sulphur compounds. Olive oil provides healing vitamin E. This is the perfect soup to revitalize the system after illness.

# brussels sprouts and stilton soup

What a cornucopia of revitalizing, re-energizing and restorative nutrients! In addition to the benefits of the sprouts, onions and garlic, this soup contains a gentle cleansing action from the parsley, and lots of bone- and body-building calcium from the Stilton. By the way, it tastes absolutely fabulous, too.

**extra-virgin olive oil** 4 tbsp

**red onion** 1 large, finely chopped

**garlic** 2 cloves, finely chopped

**celery** 2 sticks, finely chopped

**vegetable stock** 1.3 litres (2¼ pints) – see page 396 or use a good stock cube or bouillon powder

**brussels sprouts** 500g (1lb 2oz)

**stilton cheese** 300g (10½oz), rind removed and cubed

**parsley** 1 handful, chopped, to serve

**1** Heat the oil in a large saucepan and sweat the onion, garlic and celery gently for 5 minutes.

**2** Add the stock and Brussels sprouts and simmer until the vegetables are tender – about 15 minutes.

**3** Whizz in a food processor or blender – or use a hand blender – until smooth.

**4** Add the cheese, return to a simmer and cook until the cheese has melted.

**5** Serve immediately, with the parsley scattered on top.

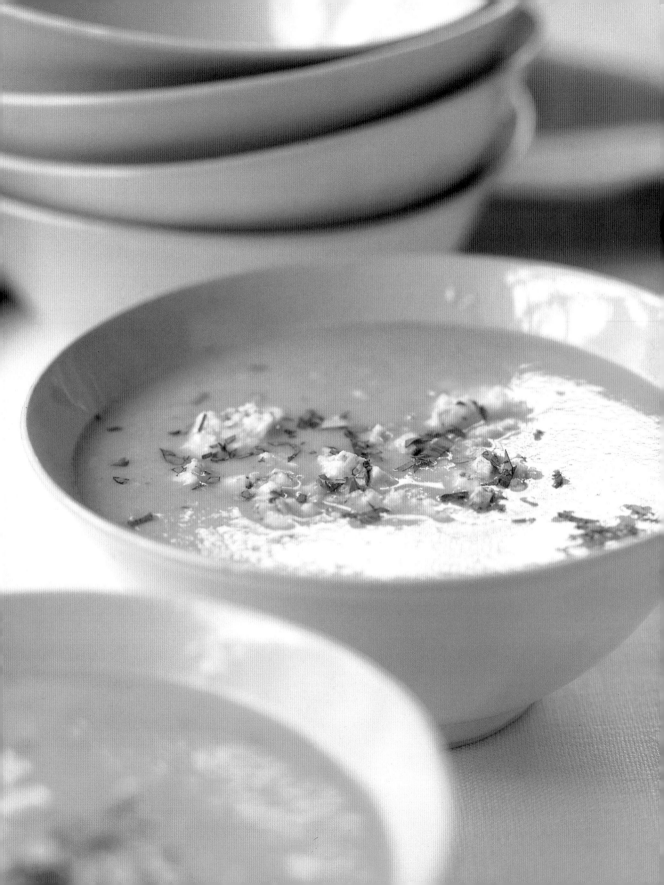

This soup will warm and fortify the constitution. Beef stock is rich in B vitamins; leeks, garlic and onions supply protective phytochemicals; and carrots and mango juice provide vital betacarotene.

# luscious mulligatawny

Like many dishes inherited from the days of the Raj, this soup is not only hot, spicy and warming, but nutritionally valuable as well.

**extra-virgin olive oil** 4 tbsp

**mixed carrots, leeks, celery and parsnips** 500g (1lb 2oz), very finely diced

**spring onions** 4 plump

**garlic** 2 large cloves, finely chopped

**green curry paste** 4 tsp

**beef stock** 1.2 litres (2 pints) – *see* page 397 or use a good stock cube or bouillon powder

**mango** juice of 1 or 100ml (3½fl oz) mango juice

**herb croûtons** to serve (*see* page 95), made with fresh coriander

1 Heat the oil in a large saucepan, add all the vegetables and stir well to coat them in the oil. Cover the pan and sweat gently for 10 minutes.

2 Add the curry paste and continue cooking for another 10 minutes, stirring occasionally.

3 Pour in the stock and simmer until the vegetables are tender.

4 Add the mango juice and heat through.

5 Serve with herb croûtons.

# peas with fish

Fish of all sorts has long been a traditional food in sick-room cooking. For anyone convalescing, the easily digested protein, the absence of artery-clogging saturated fat and the rich spread of vitamins and minerals in the fish in this soup mean several steps up the ladder to recovery. The delicate flavour of smoked haddock gently tempts the taste buds, and the addition of split peas gives an extra energy and fibre boost.

**rapeseed oil** 2 tbsp

**onion** 1, finely chopped

**split peas** 250g (9oz), generously covered with cold water and soaked overnight

**bouquet garni** 3 sprigs each parsley, thyme, and rosemary, tied together with string, or a good commercial bouquet garni bag

**fish or vegetable stock** 1.2 litres (2 pints) – *see* page 396 or use a good stock cube or bouillon powder

**smoked haddock** 400g (14oz), skinless and boneless

**1** Heat the oil in a large saucepan and sauté the onion gently until golden.

**2** Drain the split peas and add to the pan with the bouquet garni and stock.

**3** Bring to the boil, then turn the heat down and simmer until the peas are soft – about 30 minutes.

**4** Remove the bouquet garni.

**5** Whizz in a food processor or blender – or use a hand blender – until smooth, and return to the pan.

**6** Cut the fish into small cubes, add them to the soup and simmer gently until cooked through – about 5 minutes.

Chicken soup is the first choice to speed recovery. Chicken provides healing enzymes, B vitamins and minerals, while eggs are rich in restorative vitamin E.

# chicken soup with matzo dumplings

There cannot be a more renowned natural 'kitchen medicine' than this traditional Jewish chicken soup. Used as the key to recovery by generations of mothers and grandmothers, it is surprisingly easy to make, and its soothing flavour makes it ideal as a first choice for any recovery programme.

**unsalted butter** 100g (3½oz)

**free-range eggs** 2, beaten

**parsley and mint** 4 tsp mixed and chopped

**matzo meal** 90g (3¼oz)

**warm water** 4 tbsp

**chicken stock** 2 litres (3½ pints) – *see* page 396 (no stock cubes allowed here)

1 Mix all the ingredients except the stock together thoroughly in a bowl.

2 Cover and leave in the refrigerator for about 2 hours.

3 Bring the stock to a gentle simmer.

4 Roll the matzo mixture into 8 balls – and don't worry if they're very moist.

5 Drop them into the stock.

6 Bring back to a simmer.

7 Leave to simmer for about 15 minutes.

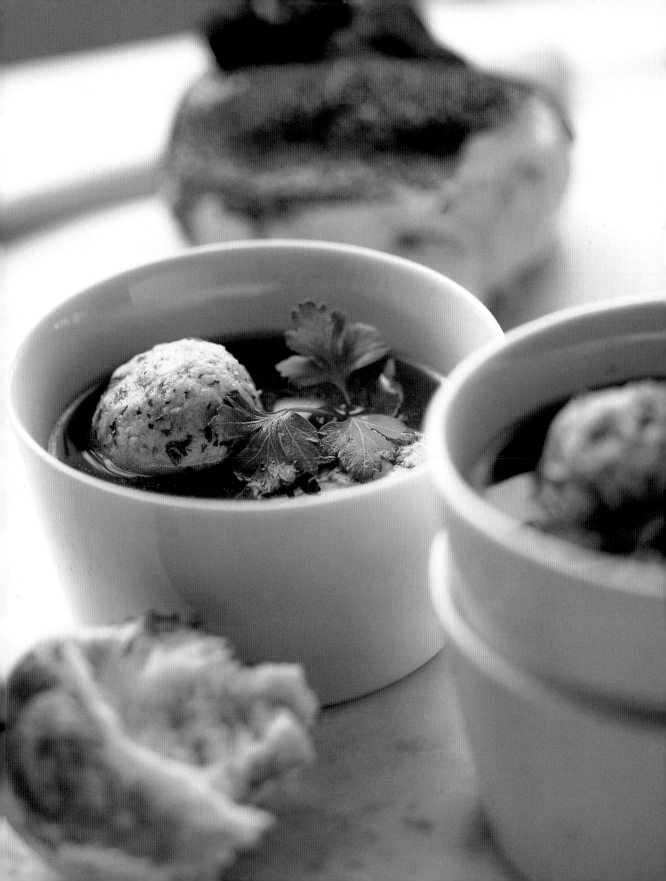

## vital statistics

Parsley is a natural diuretic that helps the body eliminate waste products. The red colouring in beetroot is produced by a natural ingredient that improves the oxygen-carrying capacity of the blood, while the peppers and carrots are a huge source of restorative carotenoids and vitamin C. Watercress is one of nature's most powerful cancer fighters, with a very specific effect on lung tissue.

# pep yourself up

All red, yellow and orange vegetables contain the chemicals your body needs for the replacement of damaged cells. In any illness or at times of excessive stress, overwork and difficult life situations, your body suffers. This really savoury and delicious juice could make all the difference.

**red pepper** 1 small, cored and deseeded
**carrots** 3, trimmed and peeled unless organic
**raw beetroot** 1 small, unpeeled, preferably with leaves, halved
**flat-leaf parsley** 1 handful, with stalks
**watercress leaves** 1 handful

**1** Put all the vegetables, parsley and watercress through a juicer, reserving a few watercress leaves.

**2** Mix thoroughly and serve with a few watercress leaves on top.

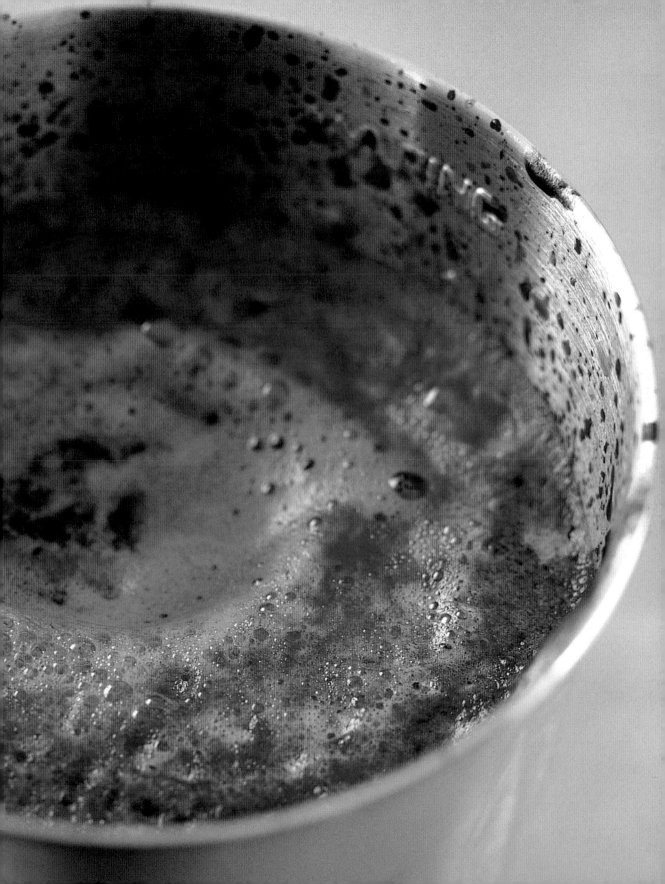

Pineapples are an exceptional source of the enzyme bromelain, which is extremely healing and repairing. Add the phytochemicals in coriander and the soluble fibre in cloudy apple juice, and this makes a potent drink indeed.

# pineapple and coriander cup

This is another delicious, refreshing and restorative summer drink, but it's also great as a digestive aid after any large meal, such as those we tend to have on Christmas Day, Boxing Day or Thanksgiving. As long as your pineapple is ripe, the flavour will be deliciously sweet but offset by the sharp taste of the coriander. Both coriander and pineapple are renowned repairers, and pineapple has the added benefit of healing bruises and improving digestion. This is also a great drink for anyone with a sore throat.

**fresh coriander** 2 sprigs
**pineapple** 1 small, peeled, cored and very finely chopped
**brown caster sugar** 75g (2³/₄oz)
**apple juice** 500ml (18fl oz)

1 Tear the leaves off the sprigs of coriander and chop them very finely.

2 Put the pineapple and coriander into a jug and stir in the sugar.

3 Cover and refrigerate for at least 2 hours.

4 Pour on the apple juice and dilute with water to achieve the required consistency.

## vital statistics

A glass of this juice will give you four times your daily requirement of vitamin C. Its betacarotene and other carotenoids will protect your skin, vision and immunity. Strawberries contain anti-arthritic substances, and kiwi fruit are rich providers of potassium and bioflavonoids, which protect the heart and blood vessels. The grapes not only provide antioxidants, but are also a great source of natural fruit sugars for instant energy.

# a passion for fruit

Not only does this juice taste wonderful, it's a real morning eye opener too. It contains enough nutrients to fuel your body's boiler and provide nutritional protection for hours. Vitamins, minerals and a vast array of plant chemical protectors are things you won't even think about as you enjoy this drink, but they're all there, beavering away to build your defences, nourish your tissues and protect every cell from potential damage. This should be a regular passion for anyone with arthritis, high blood pressure, poor immunity, skin problems, lethargy or chronic fatigue.

**strawberries** 6, hulled

**kiwi fruit** 2, unpeeled

**passion fruit** 2, flesh scooped out

**peaches** 2, unpeeled and stoned

**pomegranate** 1, seeds and flesh scooped out

**seedless grapes** 175g (6oz)

**1** Put all the ingredients through a juicer.

This vitamin C-rich crush has an exceptionally high ORAC score. ORAC stands for oxygen radical absorbence capacity, a measure of food's ability to neutralize free radicals and protect the body from ageing, heart disease, cancer and other degenerative conditions.

# blueberry and raspberry crush

One serving of this will give you more protection from the ravages of free radicals than most people get in three days from the average American, northern European or UK diet. Free radicals attack the body's individual cells, and it's this dangerous chemical activity that's frequently the trigger for heart disease, joint problems, diminishing eyesight and cancer. Although you will certainly lose some of the vitamin C content from both fruits if they're frozen, the protective antioxidants aren't damaged, so you can enjoy this crush all year round.

**blueberries** 200g (7oz)
**raspberries** 200g (7oz)
**crushed ice**

**1** Put the berries into a blender or food processor – or use a hand blender – and whizz until smooth.

**2** Serve in long glasses over the crushed ice.

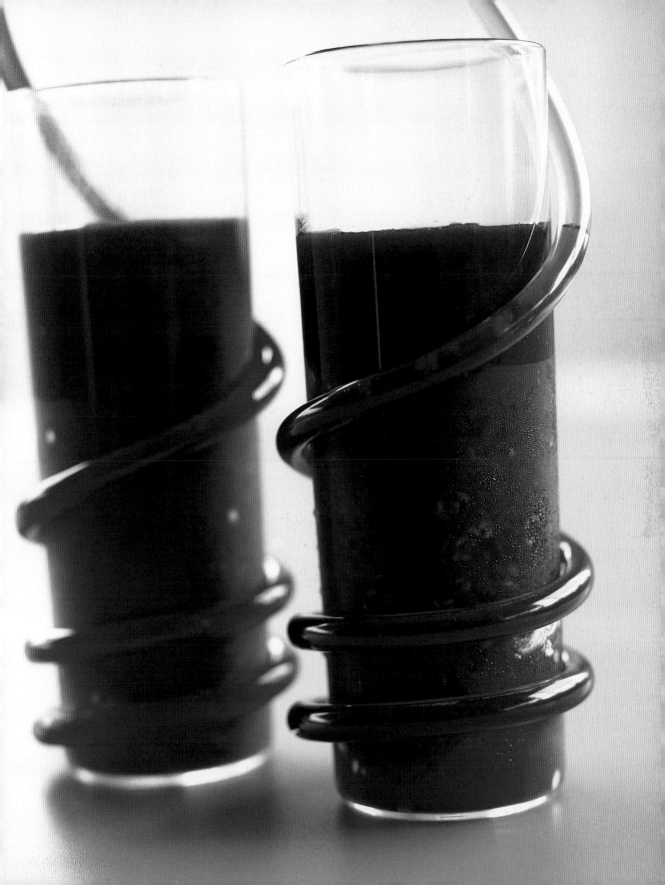

## vital statistics

Having an extremely high ORAC antioxidant score
(*see* page 104), blueberries are one of the most
protective and restorative of all foods. With lots of
calcium to rebuild the bones of anyone who's had a few
weeks in bed and the well-absorbed nutrients and low-
fat content of the semi-skimmed milk, this is a healthy
and ideal treat for men, women and children of all ages.

# blueberry fool

Whoever heard of cheesecake in a health book? Yet this is basically cheesecake without
the cake. The wonderful protection that every cell in your body gets from blueberries,
the rebuilding calcium and protein from the milk, vitamins A and D, some of the Bs and
even more calcium from the ricotta turn this extremely pleasant and simple recipe into
a potent healing potion.

**blueberries** 280g (10oz)
**ricotta cheese** 115g (4oz)
**semi-skimmed milk** about 125ml (4fl oz)

**1** Put the blueberries and ricotta into a blender or
food processor – or use a hand blender – and whizz
until smooth.

**2** Thin with the milk to the desired consistency.

## vital statistics

Almonds provide well-absorbed quantities of protein, B vitamins, zinc and healing essential fatty acids. The milk contains easily used calories for restorative energy, while the raspberries are rich in vitamin C and protective phytochemicals.

# almond and raspberry milk

This is a wonderful sick-room remedy. Like all nuts and seeds, almonds are a considerable source of body-building nutrients. Milk is easily digestible and, to most people, palatable, so it's a simple way of rebuilding run-down bodies. Add all the protective antioxidants and the high ORAC score (*see* page 104) of raspberries for a powerhouse restorative beverage.

**ground almonds** 25g (1oz)
**semi-skimmed milk** 400ml (14fl oz)
**raspberries** 10

1 Wash the ground almonds in a sieve.

2 Drain thoroughly.

3 Put into a jug and mix thoroughly with the milk.

4 Serve with the raspberries on top.

## vital statistics

The combination of crème fraîche and milk provides lots of calcium, protein, potassium and B vitamins and some vitamin A, while the strawberries add plenty of vitamin C and some fibre and folic acid, making this an excellent nutritional package. This drink is a good immunity booster and particularly important for all children and women, because it helps protect and build strong bones.

# strawberry sundae

This is a wonderful milk shake and, without the vodka, an extremely healthy drink for children. It provides lots of nutrients and is a great way of getting good food and vital calories into anyone unable to eat due to mouth or throat problems, or recovering from surgery or major illness. It's important to blend the ingredients together long enough to remove all lumps so that it can be drunk through a straw. It's also best to use ingredients straight from the refrigerator rather than chilling the shake afterwards, because the milk and crème fraîche may separate a bit.

**strawberries** 400g (14oz)
**vodka** ½ standard wine glass (optional)
**crème fraîche** 125ml (4fl oz)
**milk** 75ml (2½fl oz)

**1** Keeping 2 of the strawberries to decorate, if desired, hull the rest and put them into a blender or food processor with the vodka, if using, crème fraîche and milk. Whizz until smooth, thinning with more milk if necessary.

**2** Serve with the reserved strawberries, almost halved and sitting over the rim of the glasses, if desired.

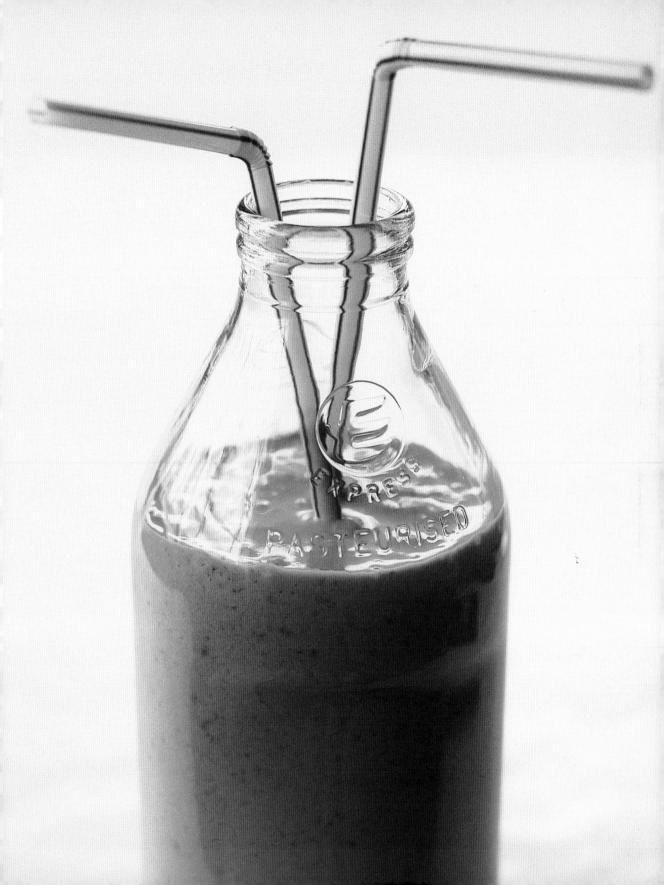

## vital statistics

The natural carbohydrates in the barley and the sugars in the honey combine to make this an effective stimulant that encourages the brain to release soothing tryptophan. There are more than 40 naturally occurring phytochemicals in lavender, including large quantities of healing and relaxing volatile essential oils. As well as being a relaxing drink, this is also useful for toothache, headache, migraine, indigestion and insomnia.

# lavender barley water

Lavender is one of the all-time great herbal relaxants. Although you may be more accustomed to using it as an externally applied oil for aches and pains, or a luxurious and relaxing addition to the bath, this herb is delicious in food and drink. Here, it is combined with the soothing properties of honey and the relaxing effects of barley, creating the ultimate relaxing drink. Because the preparation time is so long, it is wise to double or triple the quantities to keep in the refrigerator and warm as required.

**pot barley** 20g (³/₄oz)
**lavender leaves** 2 heaped tbsp, finely chopped
**freshly boiled water** 425ml (³/₄ pint)
**lavender honey** 2 tbsp

1 Put the barley and lavender into a saucepan.

2 Add the water and simmer for 1¹/₂ hours.

3 Strain through kitchen muslin or a very fine sieve.

4 Reheat if necessary.

5 Stir in the honey before serving.

## vital statistics

Throughout the Mediterranean, mothers know how quickly camomile can calm the most irritable, agitated and fractious child. But it works just as well for adults, especially when combined with the soothing benefits of honey and the calming fragrance of orange blossom.

# orange and camomile cup

One of the most striking characteristics of camomile is its wonderful fragrance. Just inhaling the essential oils has a direct and calming effect on the brain. This explains the wide use of camomile lawns in Elizabethan times, because the long skirts brushed the flowers and released the oils. If you ever visit Kew Gardens on the outskirts of London (and you must), go to Queen Elizabeth I's herb garden, where you'll find a stone bench covered in camomile. Ten minutes in the sun sitting on this seat will be one of the most relaxing times you've ever spent.

**camomile** 1 tsp dried or 1 camomile tea bag
**boiling water** 125ml (4fl oz)
**oranges** 1 large or 2 small
**orange-blossom honey** 1 tbsp

**1** Put the herb or tea bag into a saucepan.

**2** Pour over the water, cover and leave to infuse for 5 minutes.

**3** Meanwhile, juice the orange(s).

**4** Strain out the herb, reserving the liquid, or remove the tea bag.

**5** Pour in the orange juice and warm through.

**6** Pour into a mug or heatproof glass and stir in the honey to serve.

## vital statistics

Nutritionally speaking, juicing your own peaches as you use them provides by far the best results. Peaches are not hugely nutritious to start with, but the fresher the juice, the more vitamin C and betacarotene you'll get. The essential oils from the star anise help to disperse wind in the stomach and colon, and so reduce distension and pain. Star anise is also good for the relief of dry, painful coughs and bronchial congestion.

# starry, starry peach

Peach juice is extremely good to drink, but watch out for cartons or bottles labelled 'peach nectar', because these will have large amounts of added sugar. Although peaches are an excellent source of health-giving carotenoids, they don't possess pain-relieving properties. In this recipe, it's the star anise that will help you overcome the discomfort of abdominal distension and flatulence.

**star anise** 4
**peach juice** 500ml (18fl oz)

**1** Put the star anise into a small heatproof bowl, cover with boiling water and leave for 5 minutes.

**2** Gently heat the peach juice.

**3** Add the star anise and its liquid and simmer gently for 5 more minutes.

**4** Pour into 2 heatproof glasses, leaving the star anise on top as a decoration.

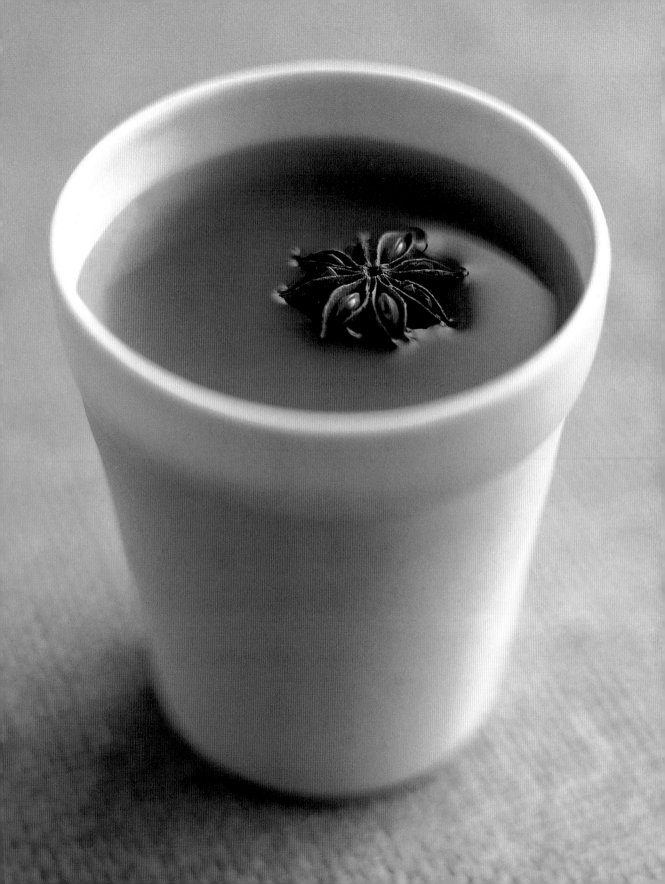

## vital statistics

The essential chemicals in liquorice root are antibacterial, expectorant and healing to the mucous membranes of the mouth and throat. In the stomach, liquorice creates a protective gel that prevents acid damage and relaxes the digestive muscles.

# liquorice and cinnamon booster

This wonderful healing drink combines some of the most ancient remedies known to man: soothing honey, the virtues of which were extolled in the Old Testament; lemons, a traditional cure for scurvy; cinnamon, a stimulant used in Indian Ayurvedic medicine; and the amazing properties of liquorice. For fatigue, coughs, colds, flu, sore throats and even acid indigestion and heartburn, this is the first choice in the sick room.

**liquorice** 1cm (½in) piece
**lemon** juice of ½
**cinnamon stick** 1cm (½in) piece
**honey** 1 generous tsp

1 Put the liquorice into a large mug.

2 Cover with boiling water and leave until dissolved.

3 Add the lemon juice and cinnamon stick.

4 Stir in the honey.

5 Drink while still warm.

## vital statistics

The vitamin C and antiseptic properties of lemon and the soothing, healing value of honey are well known. More surprising, perhaps, are the medicinal benefits of carrageen. Rich in healing chlorophyll and betacarotene and with an abundance of trace minerals from the fertile Irish soil, this moss is a wonderful restorative during or after any illness.

# the luck of the irish

Carrageen, the wonderful Irish moss, has an ancient history of both culinary and medicinal use. It is excellent as a vegetarian substitute for gelatine, and helps to set junkets, jellies and blancmange. You'll find it in most health-food stores. This surprisingly pleasant and satisfying drink is ideal for all stomach and bowel problems, and it is also an excellent remedy for heartburn and acid indigestion.

**carrageen moss** 2 heaped tbsp
**boiling water** 500ml (18fl oz)
**runny honey** 2 tbsp
**unwaxed lemon** ½

1 Preheat the oven to its lowest setting (110°C/225°F/gas mark ¼).

2 Rinse the moss well and put it into a heatproof bowl.

3 Cover with cold water and leave for 10 minutes.

4 Pour over the boiling water.

5 Put into the oven for about 2 hours, topping up with boiling water if necessary.

6 Strain and stir in the honey.

7 Juice the lemon, cut the rind into thin strips and stir the juice and rind into the moss mixture.

8 Serve in mugs or heatproof glasses.

## vital statistics

Barley is a very good source of calcium, potassium and B vitamins. This most ancient of all cultivated cereals, it also has valuable amounts of fibre and, like all starches, helps trigger the release of the natural sleep-inducing chemical tryptophan in the brain. Honey is widely used in folk medicine as a sleep promoter, and it combines perfectly with the other ingredients to make this a most pleasant drink.

# barley broth

Nothing like the apology for barley water you can buy as a cordial, this is the real McCoy. A longtime sick-room favourite for urinary infections such as cystitis, it's also a great aid to a good night's sleep – and doubly valuable because, as well as helping you gently into the land of Nod, it prevents the frequent night-time trips to the bathroom if you have cystitis.

**cold water** 850ml (1½ pints)
**pot barley** 55g (2oz)
**unwaxed lemon** 1 large
**honey** 1 generous tbsp

1 Put the water and barley into a saucepan.

2 Cut the lemon into thin slices and add to the pot.

3 Simmer for 1½ hours.

4 Strain, stir in the honey and pour into cups to serve.

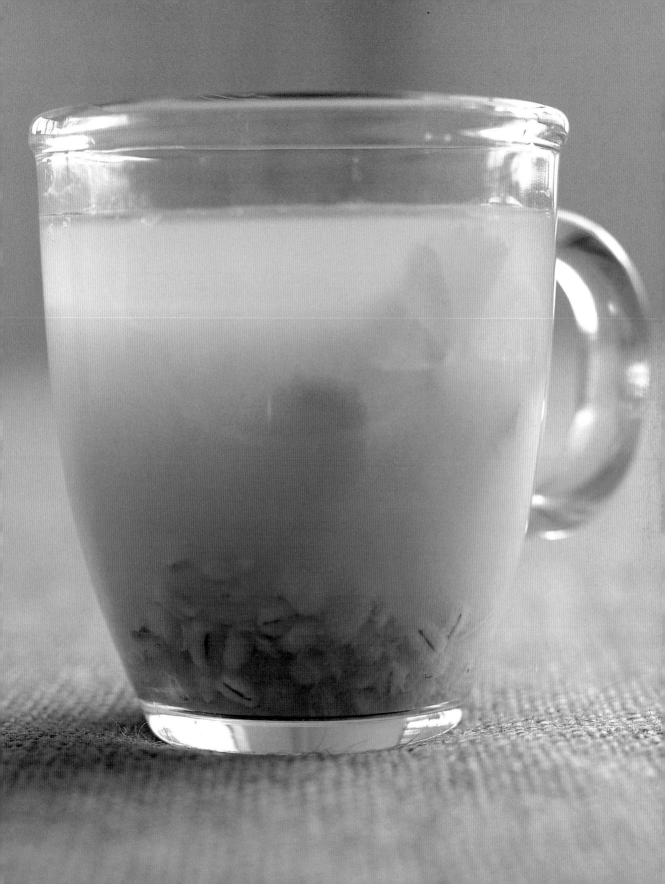

## vital statistics

This drink isn't an analgesic in the pharmaceutical sense, but it is a major bringer of the feel-good factor. It is this sensation, which overrides the pain impulse, that makes you feel positive and relaxed. The theobromine in the chocolate and the gently hallucinogenic properties of the myristicin in the nutmeg generate these feelings – but the rest is pure enjoyment.

# austrian chocolate

Even if it had no pain-relieving properties, this heavenly drink – a variation on the favourite hot chocolate of Viennese coffee shops – would distract you from your discomfort and imbue you with sensations of peace, calm and happiness. What could be more self-indulgent than wonderful chocolate, whipped cream and spices? All this, and it's a pain reliever, too!

**satsuma** 1 organic

**milk chocolate** 85g (3oz) good-quality organic

**ground cinnamon** ½ tsp

**milk** 425ml (¾ pint)

**whipping cream** 125ml (4fl oz)

**nutmeg** 2 pinches freshly ground

**cinnamon sticks** 2

**1** Finely grate the rind of the satsuma (eat the flesh while you're making the drink).

**2** Break the chocolate into small pieces.

**3** Put both ingredients into a saucepan, along with the ground cinnamon and 2 tablespoons of the milk, and heat very gently, stirring continuously, until the chocolate melts.

**4** Add the rest of the milk, continue heating gently until just boiling and pour into mugs.

**5** Whip the cream until stiff and add a heaped tablespoon to each mug.

**6** Serve immediately, sprinkled with nutmeg and with the cinnamon sticks stuck into the cream.

## vital statistics

Chillies contain capsaicin, which is a very powerful circulatory stimulant and an effective analgesic. It can bring great relief to arthritic joints and injured muscles. It's also one of the few treatments that help relieve the pain of chilblains and Raynaud's disease.

# rum-rum, chilli-chilli, rum-rum

I suppose you could say that a generous tot of white rum has some anaesthetic effect, but that's not what provides the real benefits in this delicious, tropical-tasting hot drink. Surprisingly, the chilli is the key ingredient, even though it's the coconut that provides the smell of the Spice Islands.

**red chilli** 1 small
**coconut milk** 300ml (½ pint)
**white rum** 4 tbsp

**1** Bruise the chilli gently.

**2** Put into a saucepan with the coconut milk.

**3** Bring slowly to the boil.

**4** Strain into 2 heatproof glasses to remove any chilli seeds, add the rum and serve.

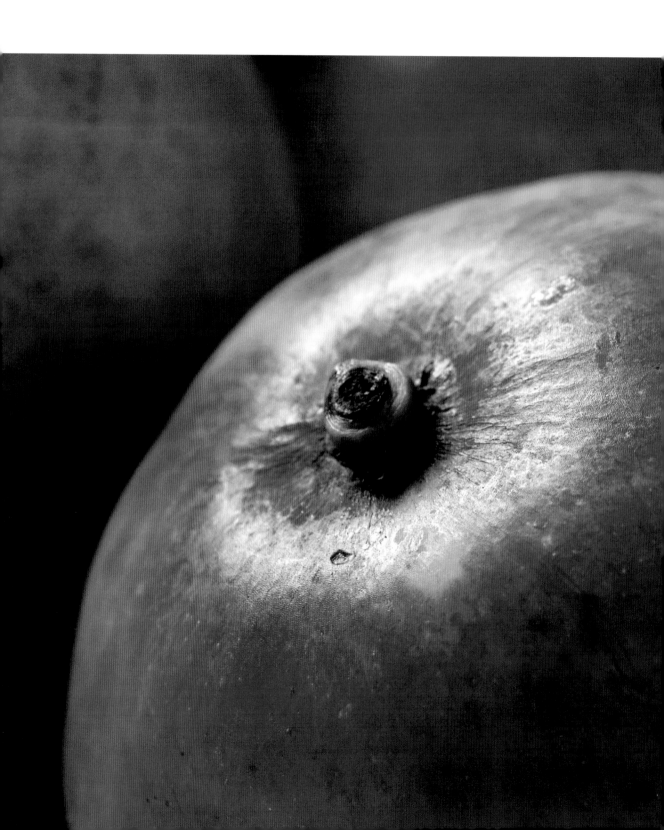

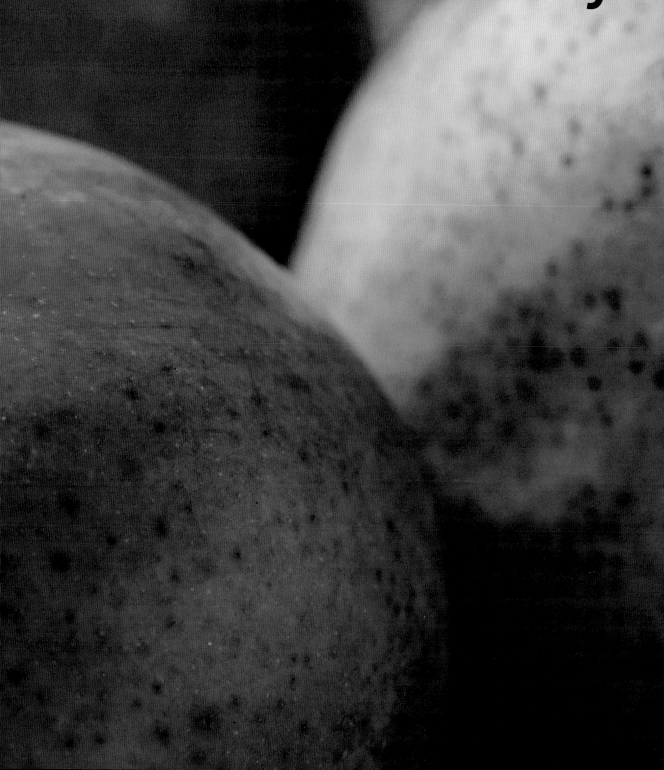

# sensuality

**L**iving in the 21st century poses a string of problems associated with desire, sex and conception. Male impotence, loss of libido in both sexes, fertility problems and the decline of sperm counts by around 50 per cent in the past 30 years are all problems faced by many otherwise happy and compatible couples.

Until recently, the general consensus of medical opinion was that most sexual problems were psychosomatic. While this is true in some cases, many couples experiencing sexual difficulties do so because of a physical problem in either one or both. High blood pressure, raised cholesterol levels, diabetes, narrowed arteries and heart disease, circulatory difficulties, neurological disorders and even diseases of wear and tear, such as osteoarthritis, can all interfere with the ability to perform or enjoy sexual relationships. To make matters worse, the medication prescribed for some of these conditions can also have a devastating effect on libido and erectile function.

Poor diets characterized by the excessive consumption of saturated animal fats, caffeine, alcohol and refined carbohydrates add to the problem. The other side of the coin is a decline in the consumption of fresh fruit and vegetables and foods that provide vitamin E, zinc, selenium, iron, magnesium and the other major nutrients that are essential for sex, fertility, conception and a healthy pregnancy.

This rise in sexual problems has gone hand in hand with a decreasing nutritional content in food caused by intensive farming, and with pollution by insecticides, pesticides and hormone-disrupting chemicals. Even if you try to eat more fresh produce, the vitamin and mineral content of most has fallen dramatically due to these factors. Declining nutritional standards compromise the quality and fertility of eggs and the quantity and quality of sperm.

It's worth noting that over 50 per cent of women attending fertility clinics have been on some form of drastic weight-loss diet in the 12 months prior to their visit. If you want to be sexy and fertile, it's important to eat enough, and even more important to eat the right nutrients.

Strictly speaking, the only aphrodisiacs that work are either illegal or dangerous, but there's no doubt at all that some foods do lend a helping hand by igniting that flickering flame of desire that is all-important in a fulfilling relationship. Folklore is full of magic foods said to awaken that slumbering Greek goddess of love and beauty, Aphrodite. But is there any truth in this? Surprisingly, many of the traditional aphrodisiac foods are indeed rich in nutrients that are vital to sexual performance and fertility. Oysters, for example, are the great traditional aphrodisiac food for men.

These aphrodisiac recipes, soups and juices combine traditional and new ideas and will really help set the scene. Their ingredients have a centuries-old aphrodisiac reputation and harbour no unwanted side effects. Although the recipes are not based on hard scientific evidence, all are good sources of the essential nutrients you need for sexual health. So, whether you're trying to conceive or just want to rekindle old flames, any of these recipes makes a perfect prelude to a night of consuming passion.

# sensuality checklist

- Avoid excessive consumption of artery-clogging, weight-gain-promoting and heart-disease-causing foods such as saturated animal fats, refined carbohydrates, coffee, alcohol and caffeinated drinks.
- Eat plenty of the foods that provide vitamins A, B and E, zinc, selenium, iron and magnesium – major nutrients that are essential for sex, fertility, conception and a healthy pregnancy. Try asparagus for vitamins A and E; oysters and prawns for zinc; nuts and seeds for zinc and selenium; and wheat germ, bananas and avocados for vitamins B and E. Root vegetables such as carrots, celeriac and beetroot are great for essential minerals; rice and potatoes will provide necessary energy; and eggs should be eaten for iron, vitamin E and protein.
- Avoid unwanted synthetic hormones from intensively reared animals and intensively produced dairy produce by buying organic wherever possible.
- Eat some chocolate! It contains amazing substances that generate feelings of euphoria – similar to the feelings experienced while being in love.
- Try herbs and flowers such as bergamot, coriander, nasturtium, rose petals, scented geraniums, rosemary and myrtle, which are all believed to have aphrodisiac qualities.
- Avoid crash diets and extreme weight-loss regimes – these can lead to a lack of essential nutrients and have catastrophic effects on the body's ability to reproduce. They can be equally disastrous when it comes to enjoying a regular, active sex life.

## vital statistics

This vegetarian treat offers plenty of aphrodisiac qualities, since it contains masses of betacarotene, lots of vitamin E, plenty of good, energy-giving calories and the traditional stimulus of pepper.

# vegetable timbale

I first ate these delicious and very professional-looking towers of vegetables in a tiny café overlooking Lake Zürich, in the German-speaking part of Switzerland, which is a wonderful place to eat healthy salads and vegetables. Surprisingly, this nutritious vegetarian treat is also excellent sex food.

**carrots** 2 large, peeled and grated

**celeriac** ½, peeled and grated

**raw beetroot** 2, peeled and grated

**basmati rice** 400g (14oz), cooked and cooled

**flat-leaf parsley** 2 tbsp finely chopped, plus extra to garnish (optional)

**chives** 1 tbsp finely snipped, plus a few whole to garnish (optional)

**black pepper** freshly ground, to taste

**extra-virgin olive oil** 2 tbsp

**1** Thoroughly mix the grated vegetables with the cooked rice.

**2** Add all the chopped parsley and snipped chives, black pepper to taste and oil and mix again.

**3** Firmly press the mixture into 4 timbale pots. Refrigerate for at least 1 hour before serving.

**4** Turn out on to serving plates and garnish with the whole chives, or more parsley if preferred.

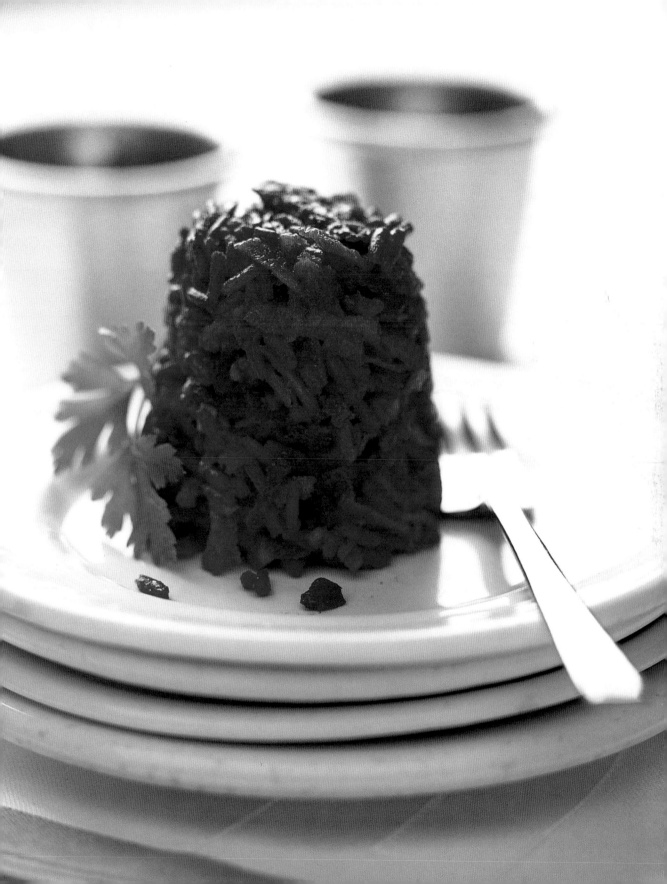

## vital statistics

Avocado is rich in vitamin E (the love vitamin for both sexes), is great for the skin and helps the body get rid of cholesterol. The mustard oils in watercress are a sexual stimulant, and the pine nuts provide even more vitamin E and essential minerals.

# lover's treat

This is a salad that will bring a glint to the eye of any man or woman, because it's a true bringer of jollity and love. The avocado is a much-maligned food, but contrary to received wisdom and dire warnings of ill-informed slimming gurus, it's not fattening.

**avocados** 2 ripe
**watercress** 1 bunch
**pine nuts** 2 tbsp
**salad dressing** 3 tbsp (*see* page 182)

**1** Halve, stone and peel the avocados. Cut each half into thin slices.

**2** Discard any very tough stalks of watercress. Pile the watercress into the centre of a serving plate.

**3** Lay the slices of avocado around the watercress. Sprinkle all over with the pine nuts and drizzle with the salad dressing.

## vital statistics

As well as protein in surprising quantities for a vegetable, asparagus contains the strongly diuretic asparagine and asparagosides – a form of plant hormone – which may explain its reputation as an aphrodisiac. Purslane is one of the few plants that are rich in omega-3 fatty acids, making it a perfect romantic food for women.

# cupid's spears

Asparagus has been used as a medicine for around 3000 years and is known to have been cultivated as a food plant in Egypt since 4000BC. Wherever it's grown, it has a reputation as an aphrodisiac. Eaten here with eggs (the ultimate symbol of fertility), vitamin E-rich walnut oil and the unusual flavour of purslane, it makes a dish Casanova would have been proud to taste.

**asparagus spears** 24, steamed and cooled

**free-range eggs** 2, hard-boiled, cooled and chopped

**purslane** 100g (3½oz), roughly chopped

**herb vinaigrette** 6 tbsp (see page 72), made with walnut oil in place of extra-virgin olive oil

**black pepper** freshly ground, to taste

1 Arrange the asparagus spears on 4 plates.

2 Sprinkle the tips with the hard-boiled eggs.

3 Add a spoonful of purslane to each plate.

4 Drizzle the herb vinaigrette over the asparagus and the purslane.

5 Finish with a dash of black pepper – and draw the curtains.

## vital statistics

Loads of energy-giving calories from the pasta combine with vitamin D and calcium from the goats' cheese and betacarotene from the chard. The essential oils in garlic specifically improve circulation, a benefit that is enhanced by similar properties in the onion, while the oregano helps calm any jangling nerves.

# a touch of venus

This unusual mixture of pasta, greens and goats' cheese is light, full of energy and rich in potassium and calcium – essential for the prevention of cramp! Nervous tension can be a real 'downer' for men; when the vital moment comes, the calming effects of oregano should stave off disaster. Another love herb of the ancient world, oregano was said to be grown by Venus in her own garden of love.

**extra-virgin olive oil** 3 tbsp

**chard** 200g (7oz), stalks removed and cut into strips, green parts roughly torn, or spinach leaves

**red onion** 1, sliced into thin rings

**garlic** 2 cloves, finely chopped

**oregano leaves** a generous sprinkling

**goats' cheese** 100g (3½oz)

**double cream** 4 tbsp

**black pepper** freshly ground, to taste

**spaghettini** 400g (14oz)

**1** Heat the oil in a saucepan and sweat the chard stalks, onion, garlic and half the oregano gently until the onion is soft.

**2** Add the chard (or spinach) leaves with a little water, stirring thoroughly. Cover and cook until wilted.

**3** Beat the goats' cheese, cream, remaining oregano and black pepper to taste together.

**4** Drain the chard (or spinach) and add the goats' cheese mixture to it. Stir thoroughly and keep warm until the pasta is cooked.

**5** Cook the pasta according to the packet instructions until al dente.

**6** Pour the sauce over the pasta and serve.

## vital statistics

This powerful aphrodisiac recipe contains huge amounts of iron and vitamin B12 from the liver, vitamin E from the almonds, crocin from the saffron and the spirit-raising rosmaricine in rosemary.

# lover's liver

Several great 'love foods' are present here. In primitive societies, the liver was considered a guarantee of strength and virility. Almonds were renowned Middle Eastern aphrodisiacs, while rosemary was considered the herb of fidelity. In medieval times, saffron was believed to foster a happy heart. Amaretto, which adds its own heady aroma, completes this romantic dish.

**stale wholemeal breadcrumbs** 100g (3½oz)

**ground almonds** 100g (3½oz)

**garlic** 1 clove, crushed

**rosemary leaves** 1 tbsp, very finely chopped

**saffron threads** 2 generous pinches

**black pepper** freshly ground

**extra-virgin olive oil** 3 tbsp

**butter** 55g (2oz)

**calves' liver** 750g (1lb 10oz) organic, in 4 slices

**amaretto** 2 tbsp

1 Mix the breadcrumbs, almonds, garlic, rosemary, saffron and lots of black pepper together with 1 tablespoon of the oil.

2 Melt the butter with the remaining oil in a large frying pan and sauté the liver slices for 1–2 minutes.

3 Turn and cook for a further 1–2 minutes.

4 Remove the liver with a slotted spoon, set aside and keep warm.

5 Put the breadcrumb mixture into the pan and mix well with the pan juices. Simmer briskly for 1 minute, stirring continously.

6 Add the amaretto, simmer for 1 minute and spoon over the liver to serve.

## vital statistics

This is a sensual salad with a symbolic twist. Eggs are the ultimate symbol of fertility, and when put together with the sexually stimulating mustard oils in the cress, this is not a dish I'd recommend for breakfast – unless you have the morning off!

# quail's nest

I'd never eaten quails' eggs until 1969, when I spent Easter weekend in a beautiful hotel near Hilversum, in Holland. It had been a royal palace and was set in stunning grounds. As I sat in the elegant dining room for breakfast on Easter morning, they served this traditional Dutch Easter breakfast. I think it was meant more as a religious symbol than an aphrodisiac, but it serves both purposes.

**quails' eggs** 1 dozen
**growing cress** 3 packs
**celery** 2 sticks, preferably with leaves
**radishes** 10
**salad dressing** 2 tbsp (see page 182)
**celery salt** to serve

**1** Hard-boil the quails' eggs – don't cook than longer than 5 minutes.

**2** Shell the eggs.

**3** Snip the cress from the packs.

**4** Cut the celery into 2.5cm (1in) chunks, then slice into batons. Chop any leaves.

**5** Slice the radishes thinly.

**6** Make a nest of cress on each plate. Surround it with the celery batons and radishes.

**7** Put 3 eggs into the centre of each nest and drizzle a little dressing over the salad.

**8** Put a pile of celery salt on the edge of each plate – it's the traditional accompaniment to quails' eggs.

**9** Sprinkle with the chopped celery leaves.

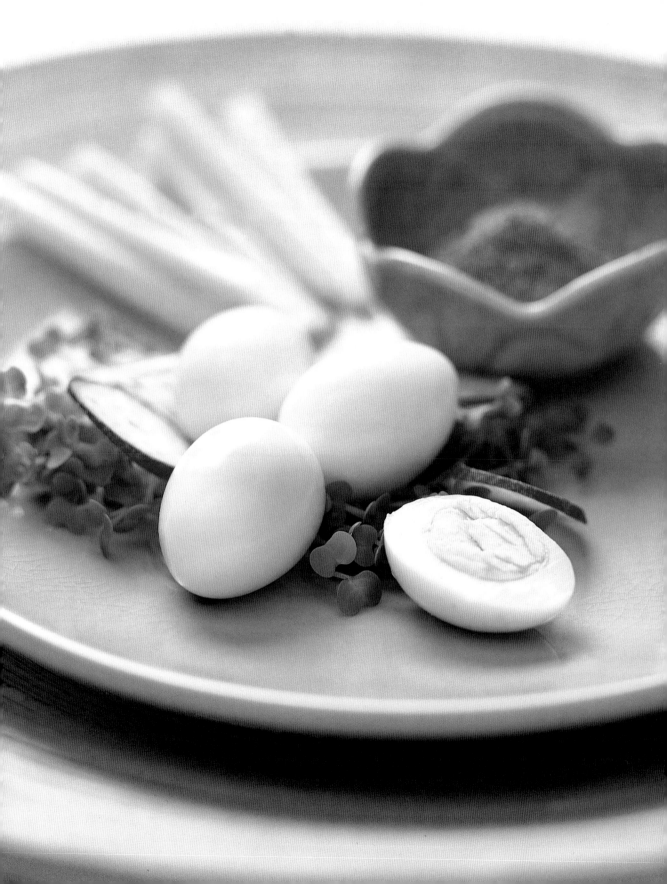

## vital statistics

Shellfish are aphrodisiacs because they're rich in zinc, which is essential for male sexual performance, and essential fatty acids, which are good for both sexes.

# casanova's salad

Casanova was reputed to eat 70 oysters a day – usually while sharing a bath with his latest paramour. If you had to open 70 oysters, you'd have no need of any aphrodisiacs since, unless you're one of those amazing men behind the shellfish counters of Paris, you'd have no time for anything else. Vongole are wonderful baby clams, widely used in the Mediterranean. Nothing could be simpler, healthier or more delicious than this salad, dedicated to the greatest lover of all time.

**vongole (baby clams)** 1kg (2lb 4oz)

**new potatoes** 500g (1lb 2oz)

**unsalted butter** 2 knobs

**onion** 1 small, finely chopped

**dry white wine** 1 glass

**flat-leaf parsley** 1 bunch, chopped

**black pepper** freshly ground, to taste

**1** Wash the vongole, discarding any open ones.

**2** Scrub but don't peel the potatoes and put them on to cook.

**3** Put the vongole into a saucepan with 1cm (½in) depth of water in the bottom.

**4** Cover tightly and boil briskly for 5 minutes.

**5** Line a sieve with a double layer of kitchen muslin. Strain the vongole, returning the liquid to the saucepan.

**6** Add a knob of butter to the pan with the onion.

**7** Bring to the boil, add the wine and boil until reduced by half.

**8** When the potatoes are cooked, strain and toss in the remaining butter as well as the chopped parsley.

**9** Add the vongole to the potatoes, season to taste with black pepper and pour the wine sauce over the top. Serve warm.

## vital statistics

Prawns are rich in zinc, iodine and protein, and avocado is a good source of monounsaturated fatty acids and vitamin E, essential for sexual function and fertility.

# prawn avodisia

If you're old enough to remember the prawn cocktail of the 1960s, you probably need help with your love life. This is it. Use the best prawns, a perfectly ripe avocado and, if you can't be bothered to make your own, a good commercial mayonnaise. This a real his n hers aphrodisiac: plenty of zinc for him, vitamin E for her and the side effects you'll both derive from fresh coriander, which contains the volatile oil coriandrol and angelicin, and has been regarded as an aphrodisiac in Europe since the Middle Ages.

**avocados** 2 ripe
**dublin bay prawns** 12, cooked
**fresh coriander** 3 tbsp chopped
**mayonnaise** 8 large tbsp

**1** Halve, stone and peel the avocados, then slice each half lengthways into 6 slivers.

**2** Arrange the avocado slices on 4 plates along with the prawns.

**3** Mix the coriander with the mayonnaise and put 2 tablespoons on each plate.

## vital statistics

The easily digested protein and high mineral content of cod make this a perfect romantic supper. The complex flavour of coriander comes from volatile oils, flavonoids and phenolic acids, which produce the aphrodisiac effect. Saffron contains volatile oil and bitter glycosides, especially crocin. It also has carotenoids and vitamins B1 and B2, helps menstrual problems and indigestion and is reputed to be an aphrodisiac.

# passionate poisson

Extremely healthy, with classic visual, aroma and taste appeal, this dish is easily digestible and spiked with the aphrodisiactic properties of fresh coriander and saffron. Widely used in Mediterranean countries, saffron has a delicate flavour that is of much greater value than the cheery yellow colour it gives to food.

**extra-virgin olive oil** 3 tbsp

**cod fillets** 4

**stale wholemeal breadcrumbs** 100g (3½oz)

**parsley** 1 tbsp chopped

**fresh coriander** 1 tbsp chopped

**garlic** 1 clove, finely chopped

**saffron threads** ½ tsp

**lemon** juice of 1

**1** Preheat the oven to 190°C/375°F/gas mark 5.

**2** Line an ovenproof dish with enough foil to make a lid as well.

**3** Brush the foil with a little of the oil.

**4** Lay the fish fillets on the foil.

**5** Mix the breadcrumbs, 2 tablespoons of the remaining oil, parsley, coriander, garlic and saffron into a paste, adding the rest of the oil if necessary.

**6** Spread over the fish and drizzle with the lemon juice.

**7** Fold over the foil and bake for 20 minutes. Meanwhile, preheat the grill to high.

**8** Remove the foil and sear under the grill for 1 minute or until brown.

# exotic herbal chicken

The smells coming from the kitchen are enough to set the mood for a night of romance. The pungency of cider and thyme, the exotic aromas of cloves and nutmeg and the perfumed hint of bergamot... These should put anybody in a loving frame of mind.

**extra-virgin olive oil** 3 tbsp

**onion** 1 large, chopped

**garlic** 2 cloves, chopped

**nutmeg** 1 generous pinch freshly grated

**cloves** 4

**bergamot leaves** 2, chopped

**chicken pieces** 1.5kg (3lb 5oz)

**very dry cider** 300ml (½ pint)

**cider vinegar** 2 tbsp

**thyme** 2 good-sized sprigs

**peppers** 1 red, 1 green, cored, deseeded and diced

**vegetables** a good selection, to serve

**1** Heat the oil in a large saucepan and sauté the onion gently for 3 minutes. Add the garlic, nutmeg, cloves and bergamot and cook for 2 minutes.

**2** Add the chicken and cook gently, turning until browned all over.

**3** Pour in the cider and vinegar and add the thyme. Simmer, covered, for 20 minutes.

**4** Add the peppers and simmer for another 20 minutes, until the chicken is cooked and tender.

**5** Remove the thyme. Serve surrounded by vegetables and covered in the cooking juices.

## vital statistics

Theobromine, which induces feelings of love and romance, as well as protein, iron and magnesium are all found in the chocolate. Plus, you'll get some circulatory stimulus from the rum.

# tango with mango

Here's an exotic soup to conjure up the romance of the tropics. With the traditional aphrodisiac properties of mango, the passion of passion fruit and chocolate, the original food of love, how could this one fail? It was originally reserved for the Aztec royal family, and it's no accident that the botanical genus name for the cocoa tree is *Theobroma*, meaning 'food of the Gods'.

**cold water** 850ml (1½ pints)

**cane sugar** about 150g (5½oz)

**mangoes** 3 large ripe, peeled, stoned and cut into very small dice (reserve any juices that try to escape)

**white rum** 4 tbsp

**passion fruit** 2

**dark chocolate** 8 squares good-quality minimum 70 per cent cocoa solids, grated

**1** Put the water into a large saucepan. Add the sugar, stir well and heat very gently for 10 minutes until it has dissolved.

**2** Tip in the mango and any reserved juices and continue cooking for 5 more minutes. Leave to cool.

**3** Pour in the rum and mix well. Cover and leave in the refrigerator for at least 8 hours.

**4** Scoop the flesh out of the passion fruit, mix with the mango and put into serving bowls.

**5** Serve with the grated chocolate scattered on top.

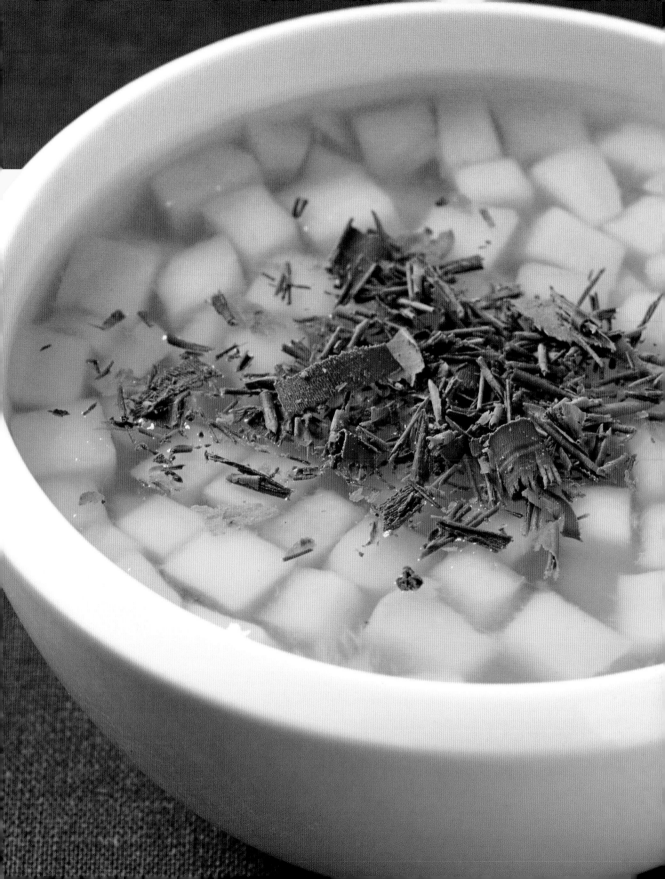

## vital statistics

Plums are a rich source of betacarotene, vitamins C and E and malic acid, which promote a healthy heart and good circulation. Geranium leaves contain calming volatile oils used in aromatherapy for reducing stress.

# scented plums

The luscious English Victoria plum is one of the world's great fruit treats. It's not just the flavour that makes it a national treasure but its all-round health benefits. With a scant dab of butter and hardly any sugar divided between four generous portions, this dessert will leave you guilt-free and licking your lips with delight and desire.

**butter** 30g (1oz)

**honey** 3 tbsp

**red plums** 8 just ripe

**scented geranium leaves** 4 torn, 4 whole to decorate

**sweet white wine** 300ml (½ pint)

**caster sugar** 1 tbsp

1 Preheat the oven to 180°C/350°F/gas mark 4.

2 Put the butter into a flameproof dish large enough to hold the halved plums in a single layer. Heat gently until melted.

3 Stir in the honey and heat until runny.

4 Halve the plums, remove the stones and set, cut side down, on the butter mixture.

5 Add the torn geranium leaves to the wine and pour over the plums. Sprinkle with the sugar.

6 Cook, uncovered, in the oven for 25 minutes or until the plums are soft.

7 Serve decorated with the whole geranium leaves.

# angel's kiss

From India to the Middle East, ancient Greece to the modern Mediterranean, fresh figs have been a traditional symbol of love and sexual prowess. Angelica is often confined to the crystallized green bits used in cakes, but the real treat lies in its leaves: they have a delicate, sweet aromatic flavour that, combined with the figs, makes this a heavenly dish indeed.

**ready-made puff pastry** 1 sheet, completely defrosted if frozen

**fresh figs** 8 ripe, quartered

**natural live bio-yogurt** 300ml (½ pint)

**brandy** 1 tbsp

**caster sugar** 60g (2¼oz)

**free-range eggs** 2 large

**angelica leaves** 2 tbsp chopped

**1** Preheat the oven to 200°C/400°F/gas mark 6.

**2** Use the pastry to line a greased 20 x 28cm (8 x 11in) loose-bottomed tart tin.

**3** Arrange the quartered figs on the pastry.

**4** Beat the yogurt, brandy and all but 2 tablespoons of the sugar together in a bowl.

**5** Beat the eggs and add to the yogurt mixture. Stir in the angelica leaves.

**6** Pour the yogurt mixture over the figs and sprinkle over the remaining sugar.

**7** Bake for 30–40 minutes until risen, firm and dark golden brown. Don't worry if it falls after cooling; the flavour stays great!

## vital statistics

The essential oils in bergamot – especially thymol – are a stimulant and also help control menstrual irregularities. Mint is a natural digestive, preventing any embarrassment during the romantic sequel.

# myrtle magic

Certain romance writers maintain that only men who eat plenty of red meat make good lovers; certainly there has been a link between meat and virility since men were hunters. The natural high from the instant energy contained in grapes makes this the perfect dessert for the end of a romantic meal. Ginger, rosemary and sesame seeds are regarded as aphrodisiacs all over the world, and myrtle – once dedicated to Aphrodite, goddess of love – adds the final touch. All, of course, impart superb flavour, too.

**white wine** 450ml (16fl oz)

**caster sugar** 175g (6oz)

**earl grey tea** 3 bags

**white seedless grapes** 500g (1lb 2oz), sliced

**mint leaves** 15, finely chopped

**1** Put the wine, sugar and tea bags into a large saucepan and boil until the liquid thickens.

**2** Add the grapes to the wine mixture and simmer gently for 5 minutes.

**3** Remove the tea bags.

**4** Serve sprinkled with the mint.

## vital statistics

Vitamin C is a major constituent of grapefruit and lemons, but grapefruit has the added benefit of naringin, which prevents clotting and lowers cholesterol levels, thus improving circulation. Rose petals supply important natural chemicals that improve blood flow.

# pink passion

You may think the use of rose petals and rosewater in this dish is just for visual effect. They certainly make this sorbet look beautifully romantic and give it a wonderfully refreshing taste. Yet inhabitants of the Middle East have gathered rose flowers at the end of the summer for more than 3000 years for their medicinal benefits – which have been highly regarded ever since.

**caster sugar** 200g (7oz)

**rosewater** 250ml (9fl oz)

**pink grapefruit juice** 350ml (12fl oz)

**lemon juice** 3 tbsp

**pink grapefruit** 1, peeled and white pith and pips removed, cut into segments

**rose petals** 1 handful

**1** Put the sugar and rosewater into a saucepan and boil for 4–5 minutes. Leave to cool.

**2** Mix the grapefruit juice and lemon juice together.

**3** Combine the juices with the sugared rosewater, then pour into a freezerproof dish, cover and freeze until almost firm.

**4** Break into chunks and reduce to a slush in a food processor, or put into a bowl and use a mouli.

**5** Return to the freezer, cover and freeze until firm.

**6** Serve several mounds on each plate, with the grapefruit segments arranged around the side and rose petals scattered over the top.

This broth is great for a boost of sensual nutrients. Eggs supply protein, iron and vitamin E, all of which are vital to healthy sexual performance.

# vegetable broth with poached egg

Eggs are the ultimate symbol of fertility. Poached gently in this nutrient-rich stock, they provide much-needed essential ingredients for a night of consuming passion.

**vegetable stock** 1.4 litres (2½ pints) – *see* page 396 (no stock cubes allowed here)

**carrots** 2 large, trimmed and peeled unless organic, finely diced

**small turnip** 1, peeled and finely diced

**mixed herbs** such as sage, thyme, rosemary and bay leaves, 1 large handful

**free-range eggs** 4

**flat-leaf parsley** chopped, to garnish

**1** Bring the stock to simmering point in a large saucepan. Add the vegetables and herbs and boil briskly until reduced by about a quarter – usually 15 minutes.

**2** Strain out the vegetables and herbs, then pour the broth back into the pan.

**3** Place the eggs – still in their shells – in the simmering stock for about 20 seconds (this holds the egg whites together).

**4** Crack the eggs and poach carefully in the stock until just set – about 4 minutes.

**5** Serve the soup with the eggs floating on top and garnished with the parsley.

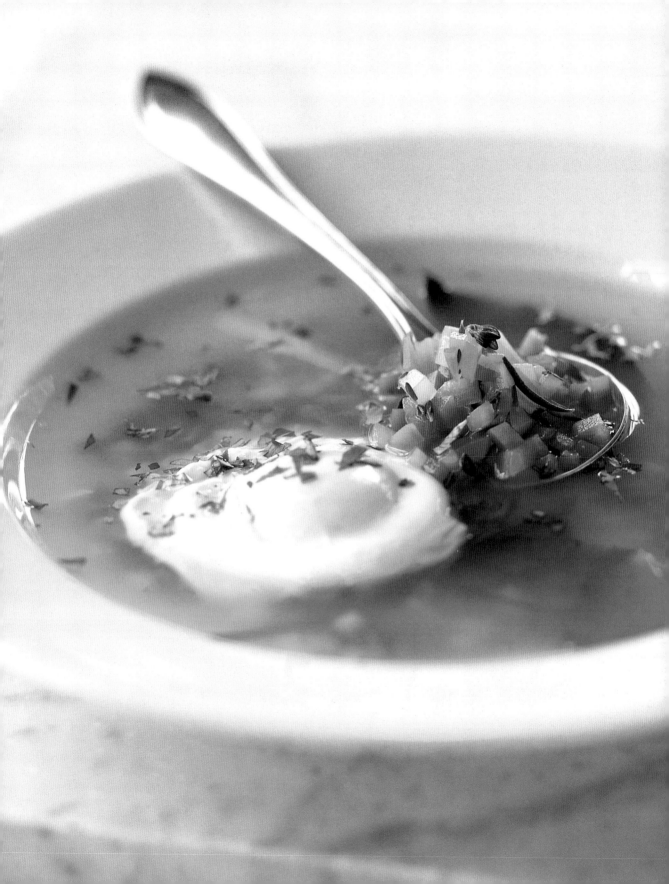

# chilled yogurt and cucumber soup

Throughout Greece and the Middle East, tzatziki is renowned as a potent aphrodisiac. This soup combines the traditional ingredients of yogurt, mint and garlic with a lavish helping of tomato juice.

**cucumbers** 1 large or 2 small, peeled and deseeded

**salt**

**natural live bio-yogurt** 500ml (18fl oz)

**tomato juice** 300ml (½ pint)

**garlic** 1 large clove, finely chopped

**chilled vegetable stock** 1 litre (1¾ pints) – *see* page 396 or use a good stock cube or bouillon powder

**mint** 1 large bunch, woody stalks removed, finely chopped

**worcestershire sauce** 1 tsp

**1** Slice the cucumber finely and put it in layers into a colander, covering each layer with a sprinkling of salt. Leave to stand for 1 hour to allow the excess moisture to run out.

**2** Meanwhile, mix the yogurt, tomato juice, garlic, stock and most of the mint together.

**3** Tip the cucumber on to a clean tea towel and squeeze out the rest of the moisture. If necessary, chop gently again.

**4** Stir the cucumber into the yogurt mixture.

**5** Serve with a dash of Worcestershire sauce in each bowl and scatter with the rest of the mint.

## vital statistics

Asparagus contains plant hormones called asparagosides, which balance hormones and are mildly diuretic. Oysters are rich in zinc, which is vital for sexual function. This is the perfect soup for an aphrodisiac boost.

# asparagus soup

Of all vegetables, asparagus is regarded as the most potent aphrodisiac, with celery following a close second. Asparagus is one of the oldest cultivated vegetables and has been grown as food for more than 6000 years. Adding oysters, the most potent of all the aphrodisiac foods, guarantees that this will be the sexiest soup you've ever tasted.

**unsalted butter** 50g (1¾oz)

**spring onions** 4 large, thinly sliced

**celery** 2 sticks, very thinly sliced

**plain flour** 3 tbsp

**vegetable stock** 1.2 litres (2 pints) – *see* page 396 or use a good stock cube or bouillon powder

**asparagus spears** 500g (1lb 2oz) (trimmed weight); use canned only if you must

**natural live bio-yogurt** 200ml (⅓ pint)

**tarragon** ½ a handful of sprigs

**oysters** 4, the flat, native variety if possible

**1** Melt the butter in a large saucepan and sweat the spring onions and celery gently for about 5 minutes.

**2** Mix in the flour and stir to coat the vegetables.

**3** Pour in the stock and add the asparagus.

**4** Bring to the boil, then turn the heat down and simmer until the asparagus is tender – about 8 minutes if fresh, or just to boiling point if using canned.

**5** Remove 8 asparagus pieces and set aside.

**6** Whizz the soup in a food processor or blender – or use a hand blender – until smooth. Return to the rinsed-out saucepan.

**7** Add the yogurt and whisk thoroughly.

**8** Tip in the reserved asparagus pieces and sprigs of tarragon and heat to a simmer.

**9** Serve with the oysters floating on top.

## vital statistics

The phytochemicals in pumpkin are known for their aphrodisiac effect. Vitamin E from wheat germ and the circulatory benefits of garlic improve blood flow, and oregano is valued for its role as a stimulant.

# cinderella soup

Halloween is a dreadful waste of pumpkins; such a nourishing vegetable deserves a better fate. This soup not only contains some vital ingredients for sexual function and fertility, it also has romantic eye appeal. The peppery nasturtium contrasts deliciously with the oregano and curry plant, making an ideal start to a long, loving evening. Nasturtium flowers contain glucocyanates, which are the substances responsible for Peruvian tribesmen's belief in its aphrodisiac powers.

**extra-virgin olive oil** 2 tbsp

**onion** 1 large, sliced

**garlic** 1 clove, chopped

**pumpkin** 750g (1lb 10oz), peeled, deseeded and cubed

**vegetable stock** 1 litre (1¾ pints) – *see* page 396 or use a good stock cube or bouillon powder

**curry-plant leaves** 2 tsp chopped

**dried oregano** 1 tsp

**crème fraîche** 250ml (9fl oz)

**wheat germ** 1 tbsp

**nasturtium flowers** 8, to garnish

**1** Heat the oil in a large saucepan and sweat the onion until softened. Add the garlic and cook, stirring, for 2 minutes.

**2** Add the pumpkin and cook gently for 2 minutes, stirring to coat thoroughly in the oil.

**3** Add the stock, curry-plant leaves and oregano. Bring to the boil, then turn the heat down and simmer for 35 minutes.

**4** Whizz the soup in a food processor or blender – or use a hand blender – and reheat.

**5** Stir in the crème fraîche and wheat germ thoroughly.

**6** Serve with the nasturtium flowers floating on top.

## vital statistics

This delicious soup supplies fortifying essential nutrients. Game birds provide B vitamins, natural enzymes and minerals, which all promote sexual function and a healthy heart.

# game soup

This is just the soup to get you in the mood for the game of love. Although it might sound rich and heavy, it's actually a very delicate and nourishing broth that is extremely low in fat, very rich in vital sexual nutrients and enhanced by the sensual aromatic oils in rosemary, sage and thyme. All game birds, such as wild duck, pheasant, partridge and grouse, are delicious in roasts or in casseroles and stews. With this recipe, you can enjoy eating them one day and having the soup the next.

**cooked game carcasses** 1 duck or pheasant, 2 pigeons or other smaller birds or a combination

**cold water** 2 litres (3½ pints)

**onion** 1 large, finely chopped

**leek** 1 large, coarsely chopped

**celery** 2 large sticks, chopped

**rosemary** 1 large sprig

**parsley** ½ large bunch

**sage** 1 large sprig

**thyme** 2 large sprigs

**bay leaves** 3

**root vegetables** about 200g (7oz) of any kind, cut into julienne strips

**port** ½ wine glass

**1** Put the carcass or carcasses into a large saucepan and cover with the water.

**2** Bring to the boil, then turn the heat down and simmer for about 1 hour.

**3** Add the onion, leek, celery and herbs.

**4** Bring back to the boil, then simmer for 40 minutes.

**5** Strain through kitchen muslin or a fine sieve.

**6** Leave to cool until the fat rises to the top, then skim off any fat.

**7** Add the julienned root vegetables and simmer until just tender.

**8** Tip in the port and serve.

## vital statistics

Stimulating gingeroles in the ginger improve the vitally important blood flow. Potassium from the vegetable stock prevents cramp. Volatile oils in the turmeric and curry powder provide a stimulating effect.

# turmeric, ginger and acorn squash

The great 18th-century British wit (and clergyman) Dr Sydney Smith wrote a great deal about food. One of my favourite quotes is: 'Soup and fish explain half the emotions of human life.' When it comes to the emotions of sex, this soup is a winner. The stimulus of ginger, the spice of turmeric and the heat of curry, all combined with the exotic and romantic flavours of coconut, are almost guaranteed to make this dish an enjoyable aphrodisiac.

**vegetable stock** 1 litre (1¾ pints) – *see* page 396 or use a good stock cube or bouillon powder

**onion** 1, finely sliced

**garlic** 2 large cloves, flattened with the blade of a large knife and finely chopped

**fresh root ginger** 2.5cm (1in) piece, peeled and grated

**turmeric** 1 tsp

**curry powder** 1 tsp

**squash or pumpkin flesh** about 700g (1lb 9oz), cubed

**coconut milk** about 250ml (9fl oz)

**1** Put 1 tablespoon of the stock into a large saucepan.

**2** Add the onion, bring to a simmer and cook for 5 minutes, stirring occasionally.

**3** Add the garlic and ginger and cook for 2 more minutes.

**4** Add the turmeric and curry powder and mix well.

**5** Pour in the rest of the stock and add the squash or pumpkin flesh.

**6** Bring to a simmer and cook until the vegetables are tender – about 10 minutes.

**7** Stir in the coconut milk.

**8** Whizz in a food processor or blender – or use a hand blender – until smooth.

## vital statistics

Fish stock offers plenty of minerals and B vitamins, while prawns provide protein, zinc and selenium. The spices in curry powder stimulate circulation. Coconut milk adds the sensuous perfume of the tropics.

# curried coconut

There's nothing quite so romantic as images of tropical islands, coconut palms and blue seas. It only takes a hint of coconut aroma to transport us to sun-drenched tropical shores. For years, coconut and coconut oil have been thought of as unhealthy, whereas the opposite is actually true. There is saturated fat in coconut, but 60 per cent is the healthiest type, easily digested and quickly converted into energy. These fats protect the circulation because they don't end up as fatty deposits in the arteries. Add the natural aphrodisiacs in the prawns and the exotic hint of curry – what more could you desire?

**olive oil** 2 tbsp

**shallots** 2 large or 3 small

**garlic** 2 cloves, finely chopped

**curry powder** 1 tbsp

**coconut milk** 300ml (½ pint)

**fish stock** 700ml (1½ pints) – *see* page 396 or use a good stock cube or bouillon powder

**crème fraîche** 100ml (3½fl oz)

**lemon liqueur** 4 tbsp (optional)

**prawns** 12, cooked and peeled

**1** Heat the oil in a large saucepan. Add the shallots and garlic, sprinkle on the curry powder and mix well. Sauté gently until the shallots are soft.

**2** Add the coconut milk and stock and bring to the boil, then turn the heat down and simmer for 5 minutes.

**3** Add the crème fraîche.

**4** Whizz in a food processor or blender – or use a hand blender – until smooth.

**5** Leave to cool, then chill well in the refrigerator.

**6** Before serving, stir in the lemon liqueur, if using.

**7** Serve with the prawns scattered on top.

# simple bouillabaisse

Bouillabaisse is a miracle, and one that you can produce easily in your own kitchen. Fish is always a good choice as a prelude to romance: it's light and easily digested. Fish, and especially shellfish, contain nutrients essential for sexual performance. There is energy for physical activity, protection for the circulation and nutrients to enhance sensuality.

**olive oil** 3 tbsp

**onion** 1, finely chopped

**fennel** 1 bulb, very finely chopped

**garlic** 2 cloves, finely chopped

**new potatoes** 3, cubed

**fish stock** 1.4 litres (2½ pints) – *see* page 396 or use a good stock cube or bouillon powder

**unwaxed lemon** grated rind of 1

**tomato purée** 2 tbsp

**bouquet garni** 3 sprigs each parsley, thyme and rosemary, tied together with string or a good commercial bouquet garni bag

**mixed white fish** such as halibut, turbot etc., skinless and boneless, cut into 2.5cm (1in) cubes

**prawns** 12, uncooked and peeled

**1** Heat the oil in a large, wide saucepan and sweat the onion, fennel and garlic until softened.

**2** Add the potatoes and stir until they are coated with the oil.

**3** Pour in the stock, add the lemon rind, tomato purée and bouquet garni and simmer for 20 minutes.

**4** Add the fish and prawns and continue cooking for another 10 minutes.

## vital statistics

Use this soup to promote good sexual function. Prawns are rich in zinc, which is vital for the formation of sperm, and contain essential fatty acids that help maintain fertility.

# thai sweet-and-sour soup

This deliciously light soup is a delight for all the senses. By combining prawns with the tang of fresh coriander (which has a long tradition in Asia as an aphrodisiac) and the heady, aromatic oils in lemon grass, you've got a sure-fire winner for a night of passion.

**fish stock** 1 litre (1¾ pints) – *see* page 396 or use a good stock cube or bouillon powder

**limes** juice of 2

**runny honey** 2 tbsp

**lemon grass** 5cm (2in) stalk, crushed

**fresh coriander leaves** 1 handful, chopped, plus extra leaves to garnish

**prawns** 500g (1lb 2oz), uncooked and peeled

1 Warm the stock in a large saucepan over a low heat.

2 Mix the lime juice with the honey and lemon grass and heat gently with half the stock for 5 minutes.

3 Remove the lemon grass and pour the honey mixture into the rest of the stock with the chopped coriander.

4 Simmer for 2 minutes, stirring continuously.

5 Add the prawns and poach gently for 5 minutes.

6 Serve sprinkled with coriander leaves.

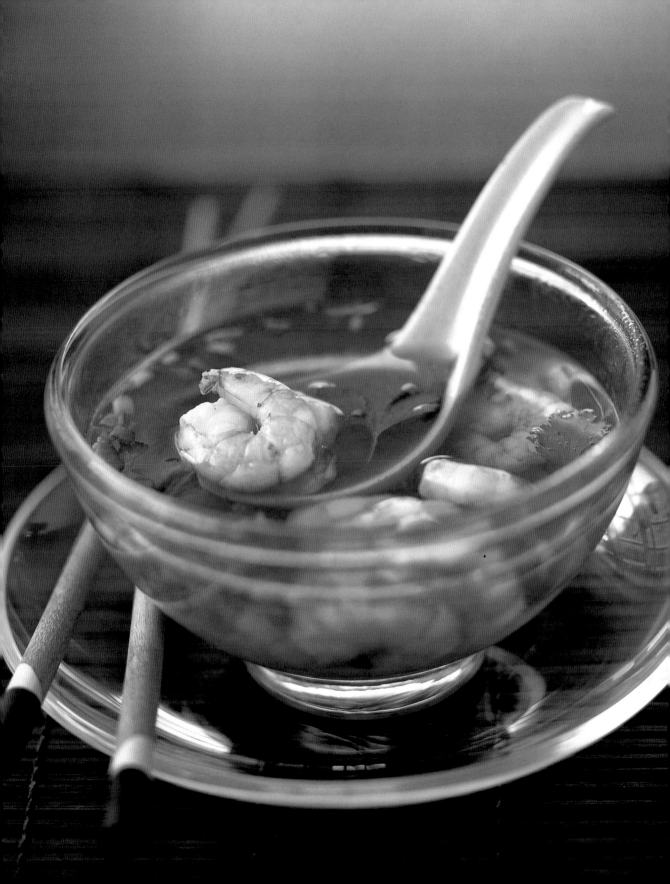

## vital statistics

Sweet potatoes are a great source of complex carbohydrates – and therefore of energy. They provide a huge quantity of different carotenoids, and it's these and the other phytochemicals that make them an exceptional cancer-fighting food, especially if you're a smoker. It's the trace minerals in all the root vegetables that make them so useful as potential aphrodisiacs.

# raunchy roots

This is another strange-sounding mixture that most people would not associate with all-consuming passion (it really tastes much, much nicer than it sounds). Thanks to the root vegetables, it's a cornucopia of nutrients needed for sex, and if you love root vegetables, then this is just the one for you.

**turnip** 1 small, with top
**raw beetroot** 2 small, with leaves
**parsnip** 1
**sweet potato** 1 small
**carrots** 2, trimmed and peeled unless organic

**1** Put all the ingredients through a juicer.

## vital statistics

The plant chemical asparagine gives asparagus its diuretic effect and the unmistakable smell in your urine after eating it. It's great if you've got rheumatism or arthritis, but avoid it if you have gout. Pumpkin seeds add zinc, often lacking and essential not only for the health of the prostate gland but also for male sexuality. Chard and pak choi provide iron, which helps guard against anaemia, another cause of impotence.

# love in a glass

Asparagus is one of the traditional aphrodisiac foods. It has been used for medical purposes for at least 500 years and cultivated as a vegetable for more than 2000. This is a vegetable that really does need to be eaten in season if you're going to enjoy its maximum flavour and benefits. In this juice you can't detract from its health benefits by smothering it in butter, mayonnaise, hollandaise sauce or piles of grated cheese.

**asparagus spears** 4
**carrots** 3, trimmed and peeled unless organic
**chard leaves** 1 handful
**pak choi** 2 heads
**pumpkin seeds** 2 tsp

**1** Put all the ingredients except the pumpkin seeds through a juicer.

**2** Sprinkle the pumpkin seeds on top of the juice.

## vital statistics

This dish is rich in vitamins A and C and contains some B vitamins, folic acid and potassium. The plant chemicals in pumpkin have a gentle aphrodisiac effect, but it's the capsaicin in the chilli pepper that is a remarkable circulatory stimulant. It has a dramatic effect on blood flow and male potency. A glass at bedtime should almost guarantee a hot and juicy night.

# hot and juicy

In the traditional Ayurvedic medicine of India – home of the fabled *Kama Sutra* – the pumpkin is believed to preserve and increase male virility. In Hot and Juicy, its cool, health-giving juice is combined deliciously with the distinctive flavour of apple and the unusual, slightly nutty taste of lamb's lettuce. The sting in the tail comes from the red chilli – so be prepared for fireworks!

**apple** 1, unpeeled, uncored and quartered
**pumpkin** 350g (12oz), peeled
**red chilli** ½ small, deseeded
**lamb's lettuce** 1 handful

**1** Put all the ingredients through a juicer.

Super-rich in vitamins A, C and carotenoids and also rich in vitamin E, B vitamins and zinc, Passionate Pumpkin makes a potent remedy for both sexes, which also encourages the production of healthy sperm. What's more, it makes a perfect drink at any time of the day. The volatile constituents from saffron also help soothe menstrual cramps and pain.

# passionate pumpkin

It's the tiny pinch of saffron that adds the vibrant colour tones to this already bright-yellow juice. Certainly the most expensive spice in the world – it takes more than 20,000 hand-picked stigmas and styles from the saffron crocus to make 115g (4oz) – saffron is also highly prized for its aphrodisiac properties. Used in ancient India, Greece and Rome, it was also reputed by medieval herbalists to quicken the spirit and heart.

**apricots** 2, stoned
**mango** 1, peeled and stoned
**pumpkin** 1 slice, peeled
**wheat germ** 1 dessertspoon
**sesame seeds** 1 tsp
**saffron threads** 1 tiny pinch
**ice cubes** 1 handful

**1** Put the apricots, mango and pumpkin through a juicer.

**2** Put the juices into a blender or food processor –or use a hand blender – with the remaining ingredients and whizz until blended.

## vital statistics

Much prized by the Roman physicians and equally popular with 18th-century European herbalists, celery is a gentle but effective diuretic and a treatment for kidney and urinary infections. The essential oils have a strong calming effect and help overcome nervousness and anxiety – just what you need in intimate situations.

# celery special

From a strictly nutritional standpoint, celery is a pretty poor source of vitamins and minerals, although it does contain some folic acid and potassium. If you have the unblanched, green celery and you also eat the leaves, you'll get a modest amount of betacarotene, too. And yes, it's probably true that you use more calories chewing it than you consume by eating it – that's why it's every slimmer's friend. It's the other substances in both the seeds and the rest of the plant that give it its reputation as a gentle aphrodisiac.

**celery** 2 large heads, with leafy tops
**celery seeds** 1 tsp, crushed
**cold water** 600ml (1 pint)

**1** Cut the celery tops off, reserving 2 sprigs and the outer stalks. (Keep the hearts to use in salads or as a braised vegetable.)

**2** Slice the tops and outer stalks, and put them with the seeds into a medium saucepan.

**3** Cover with the water.

**4** Bring to the boil, then turn the heat down and simmer for 1 hour.

**5** Strain into heatproof glasses and serve with the reserved sprigs floating on top.

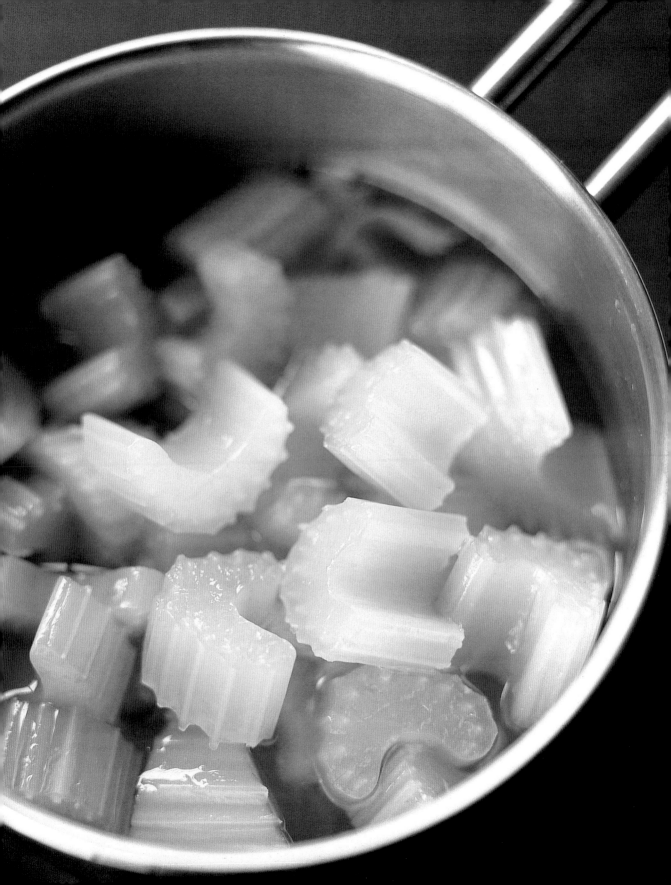

## vital statistics

Rich in vitamins A, C and E. Contains chlorophyll, magnesium, potassium and silicon. As a bonus, the French Kicker is a really good hair tonic – but you're not thinking about that now! Just enjoy the calming natural opiates in the lettuce, the stimulating sulphur compounds in the garlic and the bioflavonoids in the lime that strengthen the circulatory system. It's enough to make anyone say ooh la la!

# french kicker

Garlic as an aphrodisiac? Mais, oui! After all, 50 million Frenchmen can't be wrong! Combining it with a selection of colourful salad leaves (make sure that you add plenty of the darker-coloured and red ones), this juice is a sexual stimulant and has a calming effect on the mind. Hence, it takes away all those anxieties that so commonly lead to poor performance.

**carrots** 2, trimmed and peeled unless organic

**garlic** 1 clove, peeled

**lime** 1, unpeeled

**mixed salad leaves** 350g (12oz)

**1** Put all the ingredients through a juicer.

## vital statistics

Rich in vitamins A and C. Contains some calcium and B vitamins. Femme Fatale gets a hefty shot of phyto-oestrogens from the radishes, sensuous volatile oils from the apples and calming B vitamins from the alfalfa sprouts. Add the essential fatty acids and bladder-calming substances derived from the purslane, and this is just the juice to trigger a fatal attraction.

# femme fatale

Unless you have North African or Arabic friends, or you have travelled to these parts of the world, you may never have heard of, let alone tasted, purslane. But it has been used as a medicinal plant since Roman times and eaten as a vegetable long before that. It's one of the few plant sources of omega-3 fatty acids – and these are the ingredients that make it a mood-enhancing food for women. You should be able to find it in ethnic shops that stock African or Moroccan foods.

**dessert apples** 4 sweet, unpeeled, uncored and quartered

**radishes** 4

**purslane** 225g (8oz)

**alfalfa sprouts** 1 handful

**1** Put all the ingredients through a juicer.

## vital statistics

The red colouring in beetroot improves the oxygen-carrying capacity of blood, which in turn helps boost the circulation – a prime requirement for male potency. Another essential nutrient is vitamin E, supplied by the avocado. The mango contains betacarotene, some of which the body converts into vitamin A – essential for the health and protection of mucous membranes.

# mangavo

Whether it's a lack of libido in either partner or male impotence that's causing a problem, there are foods that might help. Over the centuries, many things have acquired a reputation as aphrodisiacs, and just knowing that can be enough to heighten sexual arousal. Avocados and mangoes both fall into this category. Used here with the mood-enhancing effects of coriander, they're certain to help put you in the mood.

**mango** 1 large, peeled, stoned and cut into chunks
**raw beetroot** 2
**fresh coriander leaves** 2 tbsp
**hass avocado** 1 large, peeled, stoned and cut into chunks
**goats' milk** 200ml (⅓ pint)

**1** Put the mango, beetroot and coriander through a juicer.

**2** Put into a blender or food processor – or use a hand blender – with the avocado and goats' milk and whizz until smooth.

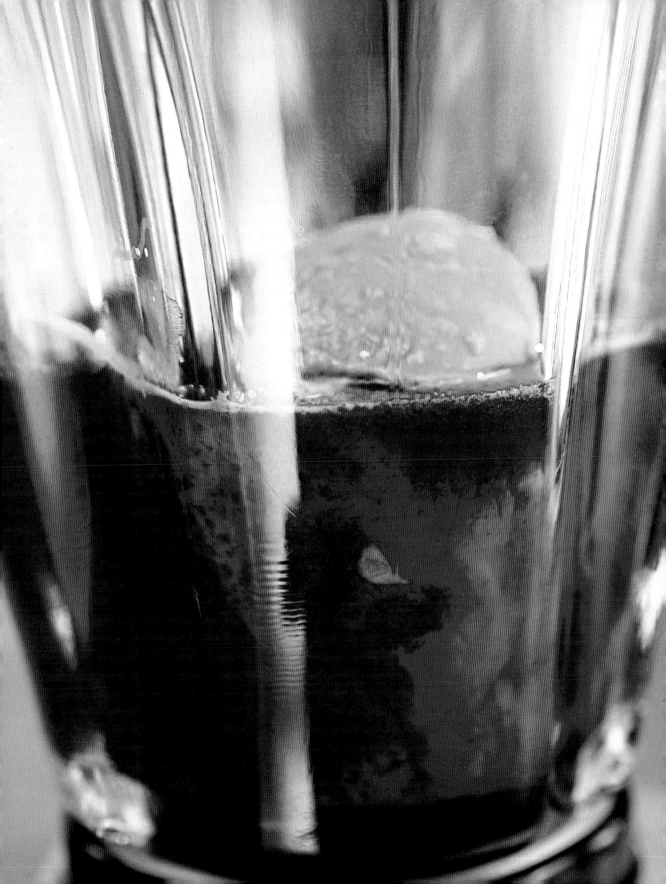

## vital statistics

Super-rich in vitamin C, rich in potassium and full of healing and stimulating enzymes, Oriental Magic gets its punch from the volatile oils of ginger and the flavonoids, coumarins and other plant chemicals found in coriander.

# oriental magic

The aphrodisiac properties of ginger are reinforced in this recipe by coriander, one of the most ancient culinary and medicinal plants. Over the past 3500 years, its use has spread from ancient Egypt and China, through Asia, North Africa and into Europe, where it has been used as an aphrodisiac since the Middle Ages. A candlelit supper, a smouldering incense stick, a glass of Oriental Magic and a rug in front of the fire... Well, need I say more. The contrasting flavours of pineapple and ginger, together with the powerful phytochemicals present in coriander, give this juice a surprising but nonetheless delicious flavour.

**pineapple** ½, with skin, cut to fit juicer
**fresh root ginger** 15g (½ oz)
**fresh coriander** 1 small bunch

**1** Put all the ingredients through a juicer.

## vital statistics

This juice is super-rich in vitamins A and C. All three ingredients are bursting with volatile oils and hormone-stimulating properties. The high quantity of fruit sugars provide instant energy, while the digestion-improving enzymes from the papaya make it the ideal accompaniment to a meal when your planned dessert is, shall we say, more interesting than ice cream.

# eastern promise

This most potent of aphrodisiac juices has a history shrouded in the mists of time. The sacred fig tree of India has been worshipped for 5000 years, and the Spartan athletes of ancient Greece were fed a diet rich in figs to improve their performance – and not just in the arena. Add the noblest of fruits (the grape), which is cooling and aphrodisiac in itself, plus the Oriental aroma of papaya, and you truly have a juice that is filled with Eastern promise.

**fresh figs** 2 large
**papaya** 1, deseeded and flesh scooped out
**black seedless grapes** 225g (8oz)

**1** Put all the ingredients through a juicer.

As well as having renowned properties for the relief of headaches, lavender is a mood-enhancing and calming plant, too. The elderflowers contain rutin, which helps protect and strengthen the tiniest capillary blood vessels that play such a vital role in the art of love.

# elderflower and lavender kiss

Elder trees were known and used by the ancient Greeks and the Anglo-Saxons, and they are still popular today. In ancient times, growing elder outside your house was supposed to keep the witches away, but in this drink, it will certainly help attract the romantic intentions of the person you're sharing it with – witch or not. This is a very simple but delicious and effective drink with which to ply your partner.

**elderflower cordial** 300ml (½ pint), diluted according to the bottle instructions

**lavender** 2 long stalks, preferably with young flowers

1 Pour the diluted cordial into a saucepan.

2 Cut the flowers from the lavender stalks and reserve.

3 Add the lavender stalks and leaves to the cordial.

4 Bring slowly to the boil.

5 Strain out the lavender.

6 Serve in heatproof glasses with the flowers floating on top.

Almonds are an extremely rich source of protein, minerals and vitamins, but they also contain the heart- and circulatory-protective monounsaturated fatty acids. These help ensure efficient circulation and are aided and abetted by substantial amounts of vitamin E. The added bonus of protective antioxidants in the green tea makes this a wonderfully sexy drink.

# amaretto cup

Almonds are an ancient and traditional aphrodisiac. Wherever they grow naturally, they're associated with sex, love and romance. In ancient cultures they were treasured by chieftains, medicine men and religious leaders. As Christianity spread through the Middle and Near East and southern Europe, so these wonderful nuts became linked with wedding ceremonies. To this day, almonds are part of the traditional food given to the guests at wedding feasts in many cultures.

**green tea** 300ml (½ pint), made according to the packet instructions from leaf tea or tea bags

**amaretto** 2 tbsp

**crushed almonds** 15g (½oz)

**double cream** 100ml (3½fl oz)

1 Strain the tea or remove the tea bags.

2 Pour into 2 heatproof glasses.

3 Add the amaretto, but don't stir.

4 Add the crushed almonds to the cream and whip until it forms peaks.

5 Serve with the whipped almond cream on top of the tea.

# raw ingredients a–z

| ingredient | source of |
|---|---|
| **Alfalfa sprouts** | Calcium, silicon, vitamins A, B complex, C, E and K |
| **Apples** | Carotenes, ellagic acid, pectin, potassium, vitamin C |
| **Apricots** | Betacarotene, iron, potassium, soluble fibre |
| **Artichokes, Jerusalem** | Inulin, iron, phosphorus |
| **Asparagus** | Asparagine, folic acid, phosphorus, potassium, riboflavin, vitamin C |
| **Bananas** | Energy, fibre, folic acid, magnesium, potassium, vitamin A |
| **Basil** | Volatile oils: estragole, limonene, linalol |
| **Beetroot** | Betacarotene, calcium, folic acid, iron, potassium, vitamins B6 and C |
| **Blackcurrants** | Anti-inflammatory and cancer-fighting phytochemicals, carotenoids, vitamin C |
| **Blueberries** | Antibacterial and cancer-fighting phytochemicals, carotenoids, vitamin C |
| **Brazil nuts** | Protein, selenium, vitamins B and E |
| **Brewer's yeast** | B vitamins, biotin, folic acid, iron, magnesium, zinc |
| **Broccoli** | Cancer-fighting phytochemicals, folic acid, iron, potassium, riboflavin, vitamins A and C |
| **Cabbage family** | Cancer-fighting phytochemicals, folic acid, potassium, vitamins A, C and E |
| **Carrots** | Carotenoids, folic acid, magnesium, potassium, vitamin A |
| **Celery** | Coumarins, potassium, vitamin C |
| **Chard (Swiss)** | Calcium, cancer-fighting phytochemicals, carotenes, iron, phosphorus, vitamins A and C |
| **Cherries** | Cancer-fighting phytochemicals, flavonoids, magnesium, potassium, vitamin C |
| **Chicory** | Bitter, liver-stimulating terpenoids, folic acid, iron, potassium, vitamin A (if unblanched) |
| **Chives** | Betacarotene, cancer-fighting phytochemicals, vitamin C |
| **Cinnamon** | Coumarins, tannins and volatile oils with mild sedative/analgesic blood-pressure-lowering effects |
| **Cloves** | Volatile oil (especially eugenol) with anti-nausea, antiseptic, antibacterial and analgesic properties |
| **Coconut milk** | Calcium, magnesium, potassium, small quantities of B vitamins |

| ingredient | source of |
| --- | --- |
| **Coriander** | Coumarins, flavonoids, linalol |
| **Cottage cheese** | Calcium, folic acid, magnesium, protein, vitamins A and B |
| **Cranberries** | Cancer-fighting phytochemicals, specific urinary antibacterials, vitamin C |
| **Cucumber** | Folic acid, potassium, silica, small amounts of betacarotene in the skin |
| **Cumin seeds** | Flavonoids that relieve intestinal wind and spasm, volatile oils |
| **Dandelion** | Betacarotene, diuretic and liver-stimulating phytochemicals, iron, other carotenoids |
| **Dates** | Fibre, folic acid, fruit sugar, iron, potassium |
| **Fennel** | Volatile oils: fenchone, anethole and anisic acid – all liver and digestive stimulants |
| **Figs** | Betacarotene, cancer-fighting phytochemicals, fibre, ficin (a digestive aid), iron, potassium |
| **Garlic** | Antibacterial and antifungal sulphur compounds, cancer- and heart-disease-fighting phytochemicals |
| **Ginger** | Circulation-stimulating zingiberene and gingerols |
| **Grapefruit** | Betacarotene, bioflavonoids  (especially naringin, which thins the blood and lowers cholesterol), vitamin C |
| **Grapes** | Natural sugars, powerful antioxidant flavonoids, vitamin C |
| **Horseradish** | Natural antibiotics, protective phytochemicals, vitamin C |
| **Jalapeño pepper** | Capsaicin (a circulatory stimulant), carotenoids, flavonoids |
| **Kale** | Betacarotene, calcium, cancer-fighting phytochemicals, folic acid, iron, phosphorus, sulphur, vitamin C |
| **Kiwi fruit** | Betacarotene, bioflavonoids, fibre, potassium, vitamin C |
| **Kohlrabi** | Cancer-fighting phytochemicals, folic acid, potassium, vitamin C |
| **Lamb's lettuce** | Folic acid; iron; potassium; vitamins A, C and B6; zinc. Also contains calming phytochemicals |
| **Lecithin** | Phospholipids extracted from soya beans – heart protective and beneficial to nerves |
| **Leeks** | Anti-arthritic, anti-inflammatory substances, cancer-fighting phytochemicals, diuretic substances, folic acid, potassium, vitamins A and C |
| **Lemon** | Bioflavonoids, limonene, potassium, vitamin C |
| **Lettuce** | Calcium, folic acid, phosphorus, potassium, sleep-inducing phytochemicals, vitamins A and C |
| **Lime** | Bioflavonoids, limonene, potassium, vitamin C |

| ingredient | source of |
| --- | --- |
| Mango | Betacarotene, flavonoids, potassium, other antioxidants, vitamin C |
| Mangosteen | Digestion-friendly mucilage, potassium, vitamin C |
| Melon | Folic acid, potassium, vitamins A and C, small amounts of B vitamins, |
| Milk | Calcium, protein, riboflavin, zinc |
| Mint | Antispasmodic volatile oils, flavonoids, menthol |
| Mixed salad leaves | Calcium, folic acid, phosphorus, potassium, sleep-inducing phytochemicals (the darkest leaves contain the most nutrients), vitamins A and C |
| Molasses | Calcium, iron, magnesium, phosphorus |
| Mooli | Iron, magnesium, phytochemicals that stimulate the gall bladder and heal mucous membranes, potassium, vitamin C |
| Nutmeg | Myristicin (mood enhancing and hallucinogenic in excess), phytochemicals that aid sleep and digestion |
| Oranges and citrus fruits (including mandarins, satsumas and tangerines) | Bioflavonoids, calcium, folic acid, iron, limonene, potassium, thiamine, vitamin B6 and C |
| Pak choi | Betacarotene, cancer-fighting phytochemicals, folic acid, vitamins B and C |
| Papaya | Betacarotene, flavonoids, magnesium, papain (a digestive enzyme), vitamin C |
| Parsley | Calcium, iron, potassium, vitamins A and C |
| Parsnip | Folic acid, inulin, potassium, vitamins B and E |
| Passion fruit | Betacarotene; phytochemicals that are antiseptic, sedative and mildly laxative; vitamin C |
| Peaches | Betacarotene, flavonoids, potassium, vitamin C |
| Peanuts | B vitamins, folic acid, iron, protein, zinc |
| Pears | Soluble fibre, vitamin C |
| Peppers | Betacarotene, folic acid, phytochemicals that prevent blood clots, strokes and heart disease, potassium, vitamin C |
| Pineapple | Enzymes (especially bromelain, helpful for angina, arthritis and physical injury), vitamin C |
| Plums | Betacarotene, malic acid (an effective aid to digestion), vitamins C and E |
| Pomegranate | Betacarotene, enzymes with antidiarrhoeal properties, heart-protective phytochemicals, vitamin E |
| Prunes | Betacarotene, fibre, iron, niacin, potassium, vitamin B6 |
| Pumpkin | Folic acid, potassium, vitamins A and C, small amounts of B vitamins |
| Purslane | Essential fatty acids and cleansing bitter alkaloids, folic acid, vitamins C and E |

| ingredient | source of |
|---|---|
| **Radishes** | Iron, magnesium, phytochemicals that stimulate the gall bladder and heal mucous membranes, potassium, vitamin C |
| **Rosemary** | Flavonoids, volatile oils: borneol, camphor, limonene |
| **Sage** | Phenolic acids, phyto-oestrogens, thujone (an antiseptic) |
| **Sauerkraut** | Calcium, cancer-fighting phytochemicals, gut-protective lactic acid, potassium, vitamin C |
| **Seaweed** | Betacarotene, calcium, iodine, iron, magnesium, potassium, protein, soluble fibre, vitamin B12, zinc |
| **Sesame seeds** | Calcium, folic acid, magnesium, niacin, protein, vitamins B and E |
| **Sorrel** | Carotenoids, iron, protective phytochemicals, vitamin C |
| **Soya milk** | Calcium, phyto-oestrogens (especially genistein, a powerful breast- ovarian- and prostate-cancer fighter), protein. If fortied, also vitamin D |
| **Spinach** | Betacarotene, cancer-fighting phytochemicals, chlorophyll, folic acid, iron, lutein, xeaxanthine |
| **Spring greens** | Betacarotene, cancer-fighting phytochemicals, carotenoids, iron, vitamin C |
| **Spring onions** | Anti-arthritic and anti-inflammatory substances, cancer-fighting phytochemicals, diuretic, folic acid, potassium, vitamins A and C |
| **Stinging nettle** | Betacarotene, calcium, iron, vitamin C |
| **Strawberries** | Anti-arthritic phytochemicals, betacarotene, vitamins C and E |
| **Sweet potato** | Betacarotene and other carotenoids, cancer-fighting phytochemicals, protein, vitamins C and E |
| **Tahini** | Calcium, folic acid, magnesium, niacin, protein, vitamins B and E |
| **Thyme** | Flavonoids, volatile oils: antiseptic thymol and carvol |
| **Tomatoes** | Betacarotene, lycopene, potassium, vitamins C and E |
| **Watercress** | Antibacterial mustard oils, betacarotene, iron, phenethyl isothiocyanate (specific lung- cancer-fighter for smokers), vitamins C and E |
| **Watermelon** | Folic acid, potassium, vitamins A and C, small amounts of B vitamins |
| **Wheat germ** | Folic acid, iron, magnesium, potassium, vitamins B and E |
| **Yogurt: milk** | Beneficial bacteria, calcium, protein, riboflavin, zinc |
| **Yogurt: soya** | Calcium, phyto-oestrogens, especially genistein (a powerful breast-, ovarian- and prostate-cancer fighter). If fortified, also contains vitamin D |

# vitamins and minerals a–z

| vitamins | essential for | best food sources |
|---|---|---|
| A | Growth, skin, colour and night vision, immunity | Butter, cheese, chicken livers, cod-liver oil, eggs, herring, lambs' liver, mackerel, salmon |
| B1 (Thiamine) | Conversion of starchy foods into energy | Brewer's yeast (dried), peanut butter, peanuts, pork and pork products, sunflower seeds, veggie burger mixes, wheat germ, yeast extract |
| B2 (Riboflavin) | Converting fats and proteins into energy; also for mucous membranes and skin | Brewer's yeast, cheese, eggs, green leafy vegetables, liver, meat, soya products, wheat germ, yeast extracts, yogurt |
| B3 (Niacin) | Brain and nerve function, healthy skin, tongue and digestive organs | Brewer's yeast (dried), cheese, dried fruits, eggs, nuts, oily fish, pigs' liver, poultry, wholegrain cereals, yeast extracts |
| B6 (Pyridoxine) | Protein conversion, protection against heart disease, regulation of menstrual cycle, growth, nervous and immune systems | Bananas, beef, brewer's yeast, cod, herring, lentils, poultry, salmon, walnuts, wheat germ |
| B12 | Metabolism, nervous system, prevention of pernicious anaemia, proper formation of blood cells. With B6, controls levels of homocysteine, which may cause heart disease | Beef, cheese, eggs, lamb, liver, oily fish, pork, seaweed |
| Betacarotene | Essential in its own right for protection against heart disease, cancer and as an immune booster. Not a vitamin in its own right, but listed here because it is converted by the body into vitamin A (see above) | Apricots, chard, dark green and red leaf lettuce, dark leafy greens, mangoes, old carrots, pumpkin, red and yellow peppers, spinach, squashes, sweet potatoes, tomatoes, watercress, yellow melon |
| C | Natural immunity, wound healing, iron absorption; extremely powerful antioxidant that protects against heart disease, circulatory problems and cancers | All citrus fruits, all green vegetables, berries, currants, lettuces, peppers, potatoes, tomatoes, tropical fruits such as guavas, kiwi fruit, mangoes and pineapple |

| vitamins | essential for | best food sources |
|---|---|---|
| Calcium | Bone formation and prevention of osteoporosis, proper functioning of heart muscles and nerves | Brazil nuts, canned sardines, cheese, chickpeas, dried seaweed, figs, greens, milk, shellfish, tofu, whitebait, yogurt |
| D | Bone formation, protection from osteoporosis and rickets | Canned sardines, cod-liver oil, eggs, fresh tuna, herring, kipper, mackerel, salmon, trout |
| E | Antioxidant protection of the heart and blood vessels, skin, immune-boosting and cancer-fighting | Avocado, broccoli, nuts and seeds, peanut butter, safflower/sunflower/olive and other seed oils, spinach, sweet potatoes, watercress, wheat germ |
| Folic acid | Blood cells, prevention of birth defects; protects against anaemia | Brewer's yeast (dried), citrus fruit, eggs, dried fruit, fresh nuts, green leafy vegetables, liver, oats, pulses, soya flour, wheat germ |
| Iodine | Normal functioning of the thyroid gland | Cockles, cod, haddock (fresh or smoked), milk, mussels, seaweed, smoked mackerel, whelks |
| Iron | Red blood cells | Beef and other meats, dark green leafy vegetables, dates, dried apricots, kidney, legumes, lentils, liver, nuts, prunes, pumpkin and sesame seeds, raisins, spinach, wholemeal bread |
| Magnesium | Energy-producing processes, the functions of vitamins B1 and B6, growth and repair | Almonds, Brazil nuts, brown rice, cashew nuts, peas, pine nuts, sesame and sunflower seeds, soya-based protein, soya beans |
| Potassium | Normal cell function, nerves, control of blood pressure | Bananas, cheese, dried fruit, eggs, fresh fruit, fruit juices, molasses, nuts, raw vegetables, tea, wholemeal bread |
| Selenium | Powerful antioxidant – protects against heart disease, prostate cancer and lung cancer | Brazil nuts, dried mushrooms, lambs' kidneys and liver, lentils, sardines, sunflower seeds, tuna, walnuts, white fish, wholemeal bread |
| Zinc | Growth, hormone function, male fertility, liver function, immunity, taste | Cheese, dried seaweed, eggs, liver, oysters, pumpkin/sesame/sunflower seeds, pine nuts, shellfish, wholemeal bread |

# health boosters a–z

| ailment | booster | effect |
|---|---|---|
| Acne | Artichoke, Dandelion | Artichoke improves liver function and fat digestion. Dandelion is both cleansing and diuretic. |
| Anxiety | Passionflower, Valerian | Both are calming and mild tranquillizers. |
| Arthritis | Devil's claw, Glucosamine, Pycnogenols | Devil's claw and pycnogenols are both anti-inflammatories, while glucosamine sulphate helps repair damaged cartilage. |
| Back pain | Chilli, Devil's claw | Chilli stimulates the circulation and promotes healing of damaged tissues. Devil's claw is a natural anti-inflammatory. |
| Boils | Garlic, Tea tree | Both are powerful antibacterials (eat one clove of garlic a day or take as tablets; apply tea-tree oil directly to the boil). |
| Bruising | Horse chestnut, Pycnogenols | Horse chestnut improves capillary blood flow. Pycnogenols are natural anti-inflammatories. |
| Chilblains | Chilli, Ginger, Vitamin E | All stimulate and improve circulation to the extremities. |
| Cholesterol | Evening primrose oil, Folic acid, Garlic | Evening primrose oil is anti-inflammatory and protects the arteries. Folic acid controls levels of heart-damaging homocysteine. Garlic helps reduce blood cholesterol. |
| Chronic fatigue | Bio-Strath Elixir, Coenzyme Q10, Ginseng, St John's wort | Bio-Strath is an immunity-booster, protects against infection and improves nutrient uptake. Coenzyme Q10 improves energy release from food. Ginseng boosts energy. St John's wort helps with depression that accompanies chronic fatigue. |
| Circulation problems | Ginger, Ginkgo biloba, Vitamin E | Ginger stimulates circulation and improves blood flow. Ginkgo biloba helps dilate the tiny capillaries at the end of the circulatory system. Vitamin E strengthens blood-vessel walls. |
| Colds | Devil's claw, Echinacea, Lapacho | Devil's claw lessens aches and pains. Echinacea and lapacho are both immune boosters. |
| Cough | Garlic, Liquorice, Valerian | Garlic is antibacterial. Liquorice is an effective expectorant. Valerian improves sleep that is interrupted by coughing. |

| ailment | booster | effect |
| --- | --- | --- |
| Cramps | Chilli, Ginger, Vitamin E | All stimulate and improve circulation. |
| Cystitis | Cranberry, Dandelion | Cranberry protects against urinary bacteria. Dandelion is diuretic. |
| Depression | Kava kava, Lemon balm, St John's wort | Kava kava eases stress and anxiety. Lemon balm relieves physical tension. St John's wort helps moderate depression. |
| Fever | Camomile, Feverfew, Tea tree | Camomile helps ease fevers, especially for children. Feverfew helps lower body temperature. Tea tree is antibacterial. |
| Flatulence | Fennel, Peppermint | Both relieve symptoms. |
| Fluid retention | Dandelion | Dandelion leaves are powerfully diuretic. |
| Gallstones | Artichoke, Fenugreek | Artichoke stimulates the gall bladder and improves liver function. Fenugreek protects and stimulates the liver. |
| Gastritis | Camomile, Fennel, Peppermint | Camomile relieves stomach pain. Fennel seeds relieve gastric discomfort. Peppermint reduces stomach acidity. |
| Gout | Dandelion, Devil's claw, Lemon balm, Pycnogenols | Dandelion's diuretic action helps remove uric acid, which causes the pain of gout. Devil's claw and pycnogenols are anti-inflammatories. Lemon balm relieves muscle spasms. |
| Hair problems | Camomile, Bio-Strath Elixir, Red clover | Camomile helps strengthen weak hair (drink as tea or use tea as a rinse after washing). Bio-Strath improves nutrient absorption to aid hair health. Red clover provides plant hormones that may help reduce hair loss. |
| Headache | Artichoke, Dong quai, Feverfew | Artichoke cleanses the liver (good for hangover headaches). Dong quai relieves vascular spasm, so may help headaches associated with blood flow. Feverfew eases headaches. |
| Heart disease | Folic acid, Garlic, Lycopene, Selenium, Vitamin E | Folic acid controls homocysteine levels, a predictor of heart disease. Garlic lowers blood pressure and cholesterol, as well as reducing the   stickiness of blood. Lycopene is a protective antioxidant. Selenium is an essential mineral. Vitamin E protects both heart and arteries against oxidative damage. |
| Hepatitis | Artichoke, Milk thistle | Artichoke stimulates the liver and gall bladder and improves fat digestion. Milk thistle is useful for all liver problems. |

| ailment | booster | effect |
|---|---|---|
| **Herpes** | Garlic, Lemon balm | Both are specifically antiviral. Dab the cut end of a garlic clove on to affected areas, eat garlic in food or take as tablets. Take lemon balm as tea; use cold tea as a lotion on any areas affected by the herpes virus. |
| **Hypertension** | Coenzyme Q10, Flaxseeds, Garlic | Coenzyme Q10 may lead to significant reduction in blood pressure. Flaxseed oil aids cholesterol and blood-pressure reduction. Garlic lowers blood pressure and cholesterol. |
| **Impotence** | Catuaba, Muira puama, Pfaffia | Catuaba stimulates the central nervous system. Muira puama helps improve sexual function. Pfaffia helps combat stress. |
| **Indigestion** | Camomile, Fennel seeds, Peppermint | Camomile relieves stomach pain. Fennel seeds relieve flatulence. Peppermint reduces stomach acidity. |
| **Influenza** | Cat's claw, Echinacea, Turmeric | Cat's claw is a great immune booster. Echinacea protects against viruses. Turmeric is antibacterial and antiviral. |
| **Insomnia** | Passionflower, St John's wort, Valerian | Passionflower is calmative. St John's wort is an anti-depressant; insomnia can be a symptom of depression. Valerian encourages deeper sleep and prevents waking in the small hours. |
| **Memory loss** | Ginkgo biloba, Phosphatidylserine | Ginkgo biloba stimulates blood flow to the smallest blood vessels of the brain, specifically improving short-term memory loss. Phosphatidylserine is a vital regulator of brain function and helps improve general memory. |
| **Menstrual problems** | Black cohosh, Camomile, Dandelion | Black cohosh helps regulate general physical and emotional disruptions of the menstrual cycle. Camomile eases painful breasts before and during periods. Dandelion helps correct fluid retention that causes menstrual discomfort. |
| **Mouth ulcers** | Garlic, Lemon balm, Probiotics | Garlic oil is excellent for healing mouth ulcers (rub the ulcers with the cut, squeezed end of a clove). Lemon balm is antiviral and prevents secondary infections (use lemon balm tea as an antiviral mouthwash). Probiotics replace the friendly bacteria in the mouth and digestive tract that protect against infections. |
| **Prostate problems** | Zinc, Oyster extract | Zinc is essential for proper functioning of the prostate – oysters are one of the richest of all sources. |
| **Raynaud's syndrome** | Chilli, Ginger, Ginkgo biloba, Vitamin E | All stimulate and improve circulation to the extremities. |

| ailment | booster | effect |
|---|---|---|
| **Seasonal affective disorder (SAD)** | Ginseng, Lemon balm, St John's wort | While none of these is a true treatment for the condition (light therapy is most effective), together they can produce a remarkable improvement. Ginseng provides an energy boost, which at least enables sufferers to be more active. Lemon balm relaxes physical tension and aids wellbeing. St John's wort helps overcome the inevitable depression of SAD. |
| **Tired-all-the-time syndrome** | Bio-Strath Elixir, Guarana, Kelp, Schisandra | Bio-Strath promotes wellbeing. Guarana provides a gentle, slow-release energy boost. Kelp stimulates the thyroid, which is commonly, though subclinically, underactive. Schisandra restores the zest for life and improves mental state. |
| **Varicose veins** | Chilli, Garlic, Ginger, Horse chestnut, Vitamin E | All stimulate and improve circulation to the extremities. Vitamin E in particular helps strengthen vein walls. |

# stocks

## chicken stock

**chicken carcass** 1

**cold water** 2 litres (3½ pints)

**spring onions** 6, green tips left on

**leek** 1 large, coarsely chopped

**celery** 2 large sticks, chopped

**rosemary, sage and thyme**
1 generous bunch, tied together (or 2 bouquets garnis)

**parsley** ½ large bunch

**bay leaves** 3

**white peppercorns** 10

**salt** ½ tsp

**1** Put the chicken carcass into a large saucepan. Cover with the water and bring to the boil, then simmer, uncovered, for about 30 minutes.

**2** Add the rest of the ingredients, return to the boil, then simmer for another 40 minutes.

**3** Strain through kitchen muslin or a fine sieve.

## ham stock

**ham bones** about 900g (2lb)

**red onions** 2 large, coarsely chopped

**carrots** 2 large, trimmed and peeled unless organic

**leek** 1 large, coarsely chopped

**celery** 2 large sticks, chopped

**cloves** 6

**ground allspice** 1 tsp

**bay leaves** 5

**peppercorns** 10

**cold water** 2 litres (3½ pints)

**salt** about ⅓ tsp

**1** Put all the ingredients into a large saucepan.

**2** Bring to the boil, then simmer slowly, uncovered, for about 4 hours, skimming regularly with a slotted spoon to remove the fat.

**3** Strain through kitchen muslin or a fine sieve.

**4** Leave, covered, until completely cold.

**5** Skim off any solidified fat.

## fish stock

**fish trimmings and bones** 100g (3½oz), washed and dried

**carrots** 3, trimmed and peeled unless organic, cubed

**white spanish onions** 2, chopped

**leek** 1 large, coarsely chopped

**flat-leaf parsley** 1 generous bunch

**rosemary, mint and tarragon**
1 generous bunch tied together (or 2 bouquets garnis)

**cold water** 1.4 litres (2½ pints), or 1 litre (1¾ pints) water and 500ml (18fl oz) dry white wine

**white peppercorns** 8

**salt** ½ tsp

**1** Put all the ingredients into a large saucepan and bring to the boil, then simmer gently, uncovered, for 30 minutes, skimming the surface regularly.

**2** Strain through kitchen muslin or a fine sieve.

# vegetable stock

**onions** 2 large, unpeeled and halved

**celery sticks** 3, with leaves, chopped

**carrots** 5 large, trimmed and peeled unless organic, chopped

**turnips** 3, chopped

**leeks** 3 large, chopped (including green part)

**garlic** 1 head, unpeeled and halved horizontally

**plum tomatoes** 3 ripe, quartered

**flat-leaf parsley** 1 generous bunch

**thyme, rosemary and bay leaves** 1 generous bunch, tied together (or 2 bouquets garnis)

**peppercorns** 5

**cold water** 4 litres (7 pints)

**1** Put the ingredients into a large saucepan and bring to the boil, then simmer gently, uncovered, for 2 hours.

**2** If using a large basket to hold the vegetables, lift it out and use a wooden spoon to press the vegetables in order to extract the maximum flavour and nutrients. If you haven't got a basket, pour through the biggest sieve you have, again using a wooden spoon to squeeze the vegetables. The stock will keep in the refrigerator for several days or for up to 3 months in the freezer.

# beef, lamb or pork stock

**meat bones** about 900g (2lb), chopped into 4cm (1½in) pieces by your butcher

**red onions** 2 large, coarsely chopped

**carrots** 2 large, trimmed and peeled unless organic

**leek** 1 large, coarsely chopped

**celery** 2 large sticks, chopped

**sage** 1 large bunch

**rosemary sprig** 1

**bay leaves** 5

**peppercorns** 10

**cold water** 2 litres (3½ pints)

**salt** about ½ tsp

**1** Preheat the oven to 220°C/ 425°F/gas mark 7. Roast the meat bones for about 30 minutes.

**2** Put the bones and any scrapings into a large saucepan.

**3** Add the rest of the ingredients.

**4** Bring to the boil, then simmer slowly, uncovered, for about 4 hours, skimming regularly with a slotted spoon to remove the fat. Top up the water if it seems to be drying up.

**5** Strain through kitchen muslin or a fine sieve.

**6** Leave, covered, until completely cold.

**7** Skim off any solidified fat.

# index